Fundamentals of

Anatomy and Physiology Workbook

A Study Guide for Nursing and Healthcare Students

Ian Peate, OBE
Professor of Nursing
Head of School
School of Health Studies
Gibraltar
Visiting Professor
St George's, University of London
Kingston University, London

WILEY Blackwell

This edition first published 2017 © 2017 by John Wiley & Sons Ltd.

Registered Office
John Wiley & Sons Ltd., The Atrium, Southern Gate, Chichester, West Sussex, PO19 8SQ, UK

Editorial Offices
9600 Garsington Road, Oxford, OX4 2DQ, UK
111 River Street, Hoboken, NJ 07030-5774, USA

For details of our global editorial offices, for customer services and for information about how to apply for permission to reuse the copyright material in this book please see our website at www.wiley.com/wiley-blackwell.

The right of the author to be identified as the author of this work has been asserted in accordance with the UK Copyright, Designs and Patents Act 1988.

Library of Congress Cataloging-in-Publication Data

Names: Peate, Ian.
Title: Fundamentals of anatomy and physiology workbook : a study guide for nursing and
    healthcare students / Ian Peate.
Other titles: Complemented by (expression): Fundamentals of anatomy and physiology for
    nursing and healthcare students. 2nd ed.
Description: Oxford : John Wiley & Sons Ltd., 2017. | Includes index. |
    Companion to Fundamentals of anatomy and physiology for nursing and healthcare students /
    edited by Ian Peate, Muralitharan Nair. 2nd ed. 2017.
Identifiers: LCCN 2016022483 | ISBN 9781119130093 (paperback)
Subjects: | MESH: Anatomy | Physiological Phenomena | Examination Questions
Classification: LCC QP34.5 | NLM QS 18.2 | DDC 612–dc23
LC record available at https://lccn.loc.gov/2016022483

A catalogue record for this book is available from the British Library.

Wiley also publishes its books in a variety of electronic formats. Some content that appears in print may not be available in electronic books.

Cover images: Main image: Gettyimages/SCIEPRO. Image of pencils: Gettyimages/comzeal.

Set in 10/12pt Myriad Pro by SPi Global, Pondicherry, India.

1 2017

Contents

Preface

Learning and naming the various parts and systems that make up the human body is interesting; it is also an essential prerequisite for the provision of care that is safe and effective. At the same time this can also be a daunting task for many healthcare students. This text, an accompaniment to the very popular Fundamentals of Anatomy and Physiology for Nursing and Healthcare Students, can help to make learning much easier. With a number of anatomically accurate line drawings portraying the many body parts, readers are encouraged to identify the component parts of the figures and colour them in using various colours. A systems approach is used to order the chapters.

Using such an approach to learning aims to help readers memorise and recall important anatomical features. This is a simple yet effective activity that is intended to help make later visualisation and recall much easier, helping the reader to revise and remember important elements. The text should be seen as a revision aid to be used with core reading such as Fundamentals of Anatomy and Physiology for Nursing and Healthcare Students.

Other highlights of the book include a range of self-tests that challenge the reader to relate the anatomy and physiology to people that they may care for. They include:

- A scramble exercise where the reader unscrambles a jumbled word to form another one related to the subject matter in the chapter
- Match the pairs: the reader has to choose from a selection of partially completed sentences associated with the system being discussed in order to form a correct sentence

Each chapter concludes with:

- A clinically related snap shot focusing on the topic in the chapter
- A crossword
- Fill in the blanks to complete the paragraphs
- Word search
- Ten multiple choice questions

Most chapters ask you to complete tables. This requires the reader to think about what they might want to write in the table; they may wish to seek other resources (human and material) to help complete the tables.

The reader is provided with a list of normal values as well as a comprehensive list of prefixes, suffixes and roots.

I hope that you enjoy using this book and that it stimulates you and encourages you to learn more about the human body that is just as beautiful on the inside as it is on the outside.

Ian Peate, OBE
Gibraltar

Acknowledgements

I would like to thank Mrs Frances Cohen for her help and support, and Jussi Lahtinen for his encouragement. The team from Wiley have been absolutely outstanding in helping me arrive at this point.

Prefixes, suffixes

Prefix: a prefix is positioned at the beginning of a word to modify or change its meaning. 'Pre' means 'before'. Prefixes may also indicate a location, number or time.

Suffix: the ending part of a word that changes the meaning of the word.

Prefix or suffix	Meaning	Example(s)
a-, an-	not, without	analgesic, apathy
ab-	from; away from	abduction
abdomin(o)-	of or relating to the abdomen	abdomen
acous(io)-	of or relating to hearing	acoumeter, acoustician
acr(o)-	extremity, topmost	acrocrany, acromegaly, acro-osteolysis, acroposthia
ad-	at, increase, on, toward	adduction
aden(o)-, aden(i)-	of or relating to a gland	adenocarcinoma, adenology, adenotome, adenotyphus
adip(o)-	of or relating to fat or fatty tissue	adipocyte
adren(o)-	of or relating to adrenal glands	adrenal artery
-aemia	blood condition	anaemia
aer(o)-	air, gas	aerosinusitis
-aesthesio-	sensation	anaesthesia
alb-	denoting a white or pale colour	albino
-alge(si)-	pain	analgesic
-algia, alg(i)o-	pain	myalgia
all(o-)	denoting something as different, or as an addition	alloantigen, allopathy
ambi-	denoting something as positioned on both sides; describing both of two	ambidextrous
amni-	pertaining to the membranous fetal sac (amnion)	amniocentesis
an-	not, without	analgesia
ana-	back, again, up	anaplasia
andr(o)-	pertaining to a man	android, andrology
angi(o)-	blood vessel	angiogram

Prefix or suffix	Meaning	Example(s)
ankyl(o)-, ancyl(o)-	denoting something as crooked or bent	ankylosis
ante-	describing something as positioned in front of another thing	antepartum
anti-	describing something as 'against' or 'opposed to' another	antibody, antipsychotic
arteri(o)-	of or pertaining to an artery	arteriole, artery
arthr(o)-	of or pertaining to the joints, limbs	arthritis
articul(o)-	joint	articulation
-ase	enzyme	lactase
-asthenia	weakness	myasthenia gravis
ather(o)-	fatty deposit, soft gruel-like deposit	atherosclerosis
atri(o)-	an atrium (especially heart atrium)	atrioventricular
aur(i)-	of or pertaining to the ear	aural
aut(o)-	self	autoimmune
axill-	of or pertaining to the armpit (uncommon as a prefix)	axilla
bi-	twice, double	binary
bio-	life	biology
blephar(o)-	of or pertaining to the eyelid	blepharoplast
brachi(o)-	of or relating to the arm	brachium of inferior colliculus
brady-	'slow'	bradycardia
bronch(i)-	bronchus	bronchiolitis obliterans
bucc(o)-	of or pertaining to the cheek	buccolabial
burs(o)-	bursa (fluid sac between the bones)	bursitis
carcin(o)-	cancer	carcinoma
cardi(o)-	of or pertaining to the heart	cardiology
carp(o)-	of or pertaining to the wrist	carpopedal
-cele	pouching, hernia	hydrocele, varicocele
-centesis	surgical puncture for aspiration	amniocentesis
cephal(o)-	of or pertaining to the head (as a whole)	cephalalgy
cerebell(o)-	of or pertaining to the cerebellum	cerebellum
cerebr(o)-	of or pertaining to the brain	cerebrology
chem(o)-	chemistry, drug	chemotherapy

Prefix or suffix	Meaning	Example(s)
chol(e)-	of or pertaining to bile	cholecystitis
cholecyst(o)-	of or pertaining to the gall bladder	cholecystectomy
chondr(i)o-	cartilage, gristle, granule, granular	chondrocalcinosis
-chrom(ato)-	colour	haemochromatosis
-cidal, -cide	killing, destroying	bacteriocidal
cili-	of or pertaining to the cilia, the eyelashes; eyelids	ciliary
circum-	denoting something as 'around' another	circumcision
col-, colo-, colono-	colon	colonoscopy
colp(o)-	of or pertaining to the vagina	colposcopy
contra-	against	contraindicate
coron(o)-	crown	coronary
cost(o)-	of or pertaining to the ribs	costochondral
crani(o)-	belonging or relating to the cranium	craniology
-crine, -crin(o)-	to secrete	endocrine
cry(o)-	cold	cryoablation
-cutane-	skin	subcutaneous
cyan(o)-	denotes a blue color	cyanopsia
cycl-	circle, cycle	cyclical
cyst(o)-, cyst(i)-	of or pertaining to the urinary bladder	cystotomy
cyt(o)-	cell	cytokine
-cyte	cell	leucocyte
-dactyl(o)-	of or pertaining to a finger, toe	dactylology, polydactyly
dent-	of or pertaining to teeth	dentist
dermat(o)-, derm(o)-	of or pertaining to the skin	dermatology
-desis	binding	arthrodesis
dextr(o)-	right, on the right side	dextrocardia
di-	two	diplopia
dia-	through, during, across	dialysis
digit-	of or pertaining to the finger [rare as a root]	digit
-dipsia	suffix meaning '(condition of) thirst'	polydipsia, hydroadipsia, oligodipsia
dors(o)-, dors(i)-	of or pertaining to the back	dorsal, dorsocephalad

Prefix or suffix	Meaning	Example(s)
duodeno-	duodenum	duodenal atresia
dynam(o)-	force, energy, power	hand strength dynamometer
-dynia	pain	vulvodynia
dys-	bad, difficult, defective, abnormal	dysphagia, dysphasia
ec-	out, away	ectopia, ectopic pregnancy
ect(o)-	outer, outside	ectoblast, ectoderm
-ectasia, -ectasis	expansion, dilation	bronchiectasis, telangiectasia
-ectomy	denotes a surgical operation or removal of a body part; resection, excision	mastectomy
-emesis	vomiting condition	haematemesis
encephal(o)-	of or pertaining to the brain; also see **cerebr(o)-**	encephalogram
endo-	denotes something as 'inside' or 'within'	endocrinology, endospore
eosin(o)-	red	eosinophil granulocyte
enter(o)-	of or pertaining to the intestine	gastroenterology
epi-	on, upon	epicardium, epidermis, epidural, episclera, epistaxis
erythr(o)-	denotes a red colour	erythrocyte
-oesophageal, -oesophago-	gullet	oesophagus
ex-	out of, away from	excision, exophthalmos
exo-	denotes something as 'outside' another	exoskeleton
extra-	outside	extradural haematoma
faci(o)-	of or pertaining to the face	facioplegic
fibr(o)	fibre	fibroblast
fossa	a hollow or depressed area; trench or channel	fossa ovalis
front-	of or pertaining to the forehead	frontonasal
galact(o)-	milk	galactorrhoea
gastr(o)-	of or pertaining to the stomach	gastric bypass
-genic	formative, pertaining to producing	cardiogenic shock
gingiv-	of or pertaining to the gums	gingivitis
glauc(o)-	denoting a grey or bluish-grey colour	glaucoma
gloss(o)-, glott(o)-	of or pertaining to the tongue	glossology
gluco-	sweet	glucocorticoid

Prefix or suffix	Meaning	Example(s)
glyc(o)-	sugar	glycolysis
-gnosis	knowledge	diagnosis, prognosis
gon(o)-	seed, semen; also, reproductive	gonorrhoea
-gram, -gramme	record or picture	angiogram
-graph	instrument used to record data or picture	electrocardiograph
-graphy	process of recording	angiography
gyn(aec)o-	woman	gynaecomastia
halluc-	to wander in mind	hallucinosis
haemat-, haemato- (haem-,)	of or pertaining to blood	haematology
haemangi-, haemangio-	blood vessels	haemangioma
hemi-	one-half	cerebral hemisphere
hepat- (hepatic-)	of or pertaining to the liver	hepatology
heter(o)-	denotes something as 'the other' (of two), as an addition, or different	heterogeneous
hist(o)-, histio-	tissue	histology
home(o)-	similar	homeopathy
hom(o)-	denotes something as 'the same' as another or common	homosexuality
hydr(o)-	water	hydrophobe
hyper-	denotes something as 'extreme' or 'beyond normal'	hypertension
hyp(o)-	denotes something as 'below normal'	hypovolaemia
hyster(o)-	of or pertaining to the womb, the uterus	hysterectomy, hysteria
iatr(o)-	of or pertaining to medicine, or a physician	iatrogenic
-iatry	denotes a field in medicine of a certain body component	podiatry, psychiatry
-ics	organised knowledge, treatment	obstetrics
ileo-	ileum	ileocaecal valve
infra-	below	infrahyoid muscles
inter-	between, among	interarticular ligament
intra-	within	intramural
ipsi-	same	ipsilateral hemiparesis
ischio-	of or pertaining to the ischium, the hip-joint	ischioanal fossa
-ism	condition, disease	dwarfism

Prefix or suffix	Meaning	Example(s)
-ismus	spasm, contraction	hemiballismus
iso-	denoting something as being 'equal'	isotonic
-ist	one who specialises in	pathologist
-itis	inflammation	tonsillitis
-ium	structure, tissue	pericardium
juxta- (iuxta-)	near to, alongside or next to	juxtaglomerular apparatus
karyo-	nucleus	eukaryote
kerat(o)-	cornea (eye or skin)	keratoscope
kin(e)-, kin(o)-, kinesi(o)-	movement	kinesthaesia
kyph(o)-	humped	kyphoscoliosis
labi(o)-	of or pertaining to the lip	labiodental
lacrim(o)-	tear	lacrimal canaliculi
lact(i)-, lact(o)-	milk	lactation
lapar(o)-	of or pertaining to the abdomen wall, flank	laparotomy
laryng(o)-	of or pertaining to the larynx, the lower throat cavity where the voice box is	larynx
latero-	lateral	lateral pectoral nerve
-lepsis, -lepsy	attack, seizure	epilepsy, narcolepsy
lept(o)-	light, slender	leptomeningeal
leuc(o)-, leuk(o)-	denoting a white colour	leucocyte
lingu(a)-, lingu(o)-	of or pertaining to the tongue	linguistics
lip(o)-	fat	liposuction
lith(o)-	stone, calculus	lithotripsy
-logist	denotes someone who studies a certain field	oncologist, pathologist
-logy	denotes the academic study or practice of a certain field	haematology, urology
lymph(o)-	lymph	lymphoedema
lys(o)-, -lytic	dissolution	lysosome
-lysis	destruction, separation	paralysis
macr(o)-	large, long	macrophage
-malacia	softening	osteomalacia
mamm(o)-	of or pertaining to the breast	mammogram

Prefix or suffix	Meaning	Example(s)
mammill(o)-	of or pertaining to the nipple	mammilloplasty, mammillitis
manu-	of or pertaining to the hand	manufacture
mast(o)-	of or pertaining to the breast	mastectomy
meg(a)-, megal(o)-, -megaly	enlargement, million	splenomegaly, megameter
melan(o)-	black colour	melanin
mening(o)-	membrane	meningitis
meta-	after, behind	metacarpus
-meter	instrument used to measure or count	sphygmomanometer
-metry	process of measuring	optometry
metr(o)-	pertaining to conditions or instruments of the uterus	metrorrhagia
micro-	denoting something as small, or relating to smallness, millionth	microscope
milli-	thousandth	millilitre
mon(o)-	single	infectious mononucleosis
morph(o)-	form, shape	morphology
muscul(o)-	muscle	musculoskeletal system
my(o)-	of or relating to muscle	myoblast
-myc(o)-	fungus	onychomycosis
myel(o)-	of or relating to bone marrow or spinal cord	myeloblast
myri-	ten thousand	myriad
myring(o)-	eardrum	myringotomy
narc(o)-	numb, sleep	narcolepsy
nas(o)-	of or pertaining to the nose	nasal
necr(o)-	death	necrosis, necrotising fasciitis
neo-	new	neoplasm
nephr(o)-	of or pertaining to the kidney	nephrology
neur(i)-, neur(o)-	of or pertaining to nerves and the nervous system	neurofibromatosis
normo-	normal	normocapnia
ocul(o)-	of or pertaining to the eye	oculist
-odont(o)-	of or pertaining to teeth	orthodontist
odyn(o)-	pain	stomatodynia

Prefix or suffix	Meaning	Example(s)
-oesophageal, oesophago-	gullet	gastro-oesophageal reflux
-oid	resemblance to	sarcoidosis
-ole	small or little	arteriole
olig(o)-	denoting something as 'having little, having few'	oliguria
-oma (singular), **-omata** (plural)	tumour, mass, collection	sarcoma, teratoma
onco-	tumour, bulk, volume	oncology
onych(o)-	of or pertaining to the nail (of a finger or toe)	onychophagy
oo-	of or pertaining to the an egg, a woman's egg, the ovum	oogenesis
oophor(o)-	of or pertaining to the woman's ovary	oophorectomy
ophthalm(o)-	of or pertaining to the eye	ophthalmology
optic(o)-	of or relating to chemical properties of the eye	opticochemical
orchi(o)-, orchid(o)-, orch(o)-	testis	orchiectomy, orchidectomy
-osis	a condition, disease or increase	harlequin type ichthyosis, psychosis, osteoperosis
osseo-	bony	osseous
ossi-	bone	peripheral ossifying fibroma
ost(e)-, oste(o)-	bone	osteoporosis
ot(o)-	of or pertaining to the ear	otology
ovo-, ovi-, ov-	of or pertaining to the eggs, the ovum	ovogenesis
pachy-	thick	pachyderma
paed-, paedo-	of or pertaining to the child	paediatrics. paedophilia
palpebr-	of or pertaining to the eyelid [uncommon as a root]	palpebra
pan-, pant(o)-	denoting something as 'complete' or containing 'everything'	panophobia, panopticon
papill-	of or pertaining to the nipple (of the chest/breast)	papillitis
papul(o)-	indicates papulosity, a small elevation or swelling in the skin, a pimple, swelling	papulation
para-	alongside of, abnormal	paracyesis
-paresis	slight paralysis	hemiparesis
parvo-	small	parvovirus
path(o)-	disease	pathology

Prefix or suffix	Meaning	Example(s)
-pathy	denotes (with a negative sense) a disease, or disorder	sociopathy, neuropathy
pector-	breast	pectoralgia, pectoriloquy, pectorophony
ped-, -ped-, -pes	of or pertaining to the foot; -footed	pedoscope
pelv(i)-, pelv(o)-	hip bone	pelvis
-penia	deficiency	osteopenia
-pepsia	denotes something relating to digestion, or the digestive tract	dyspepsia
peri-	denoting something with a position 'surrounding' or 'around' another	periodontal
-pexy	fixation	nephropexy
phaco-	lens, lens-shaped	phacolysis, phacometer, phacoscotoma
-phage, -phagia	forms terms denoting conditions relating to eating or ingestion	sarcophagia
-phago-	eating, devouring	phagocyte
-phagy	forms nouns that denotes 'feeding on' the first element or part of the word	haematophagy
pharmaco-	drug, medication	pharmacology
pharyng(o)-	of or pertaining to the pharynx, the upper throat cavity	pharyngitis, pharyngoscopy
phleb(o)-	of or pertaining to the (blood) veins, a vein	phlebography, phlebotomy
-phobia	exaggerated fear, sensitivity	arachnophobia
phon(o)-	sound	phonograph, symphony
phot(o)-	of or pertaining to light	photopathy
phren(i)-, phren(o)-, phrenico	the mind	phrenic nerve, schizophrenia
-plasia	formation, development	achondroplasia
-plasty	surgical repair, reconstruction	rhinoplasty
-plegia	paralysis	paraplegia
pleio-	more, excessive, multiple	pleiomorphism
pleur(o)-, pleur(a)	of or pertaining to the ribs	pleurogenous
-plexy	stroke or seizure	cataplexy
pneum(o)-	of or pertaining to the lungs	pneumonocyte, pneumonia
pneumat(o)-	air, lung	pneumatocele

Prefix or suffix	Meaning	Example(s)
-poiesis	production	haematopoiesis
poly-	denotes a 'plurality' of something	polymyositis
post-	denotes something as 'after' or 'behind' another	postoperation, postmortem
pre-	denotes something as 'before' another (in [physical] position or time)	premature birth
presby(o)-	old age	presbyopia
prim-	denotes something as 'first' or 'most important'	primary
proct(o)-	anus, rectum	proctology
prot(o)-	denotes something as 'first' or 'most important'	protoneurone
pseud(o)-	denotes something false or fake	pseudoephedrine
psych(e)-, psych(o)-	of or pertaining to the mind	psychology, psychiatry
psor-	itching	psoriasis
-ptosis	falling, drooping, downward placement, prolapse	apoptosis, nephroptosis
-ptysis	(a spitting), spitting	haemoptysis
pulmon-, pulmo-	of or relating to the lungs	pulmonary
pyel(o)-	pelvis	pyelonephritis
py(o)-	pus	pyometra
pyr(o)-	fever	antipyretic
quadr(i)-	four	quadriceps
radio-	radiation	radiowave
ren(o)-	of or pertaining to the kidney	renal
retro-	backward, behind	retroversion, retroverted
rhin(o)-	of or pertaining to the nose	rhinoplasty
rhod(o)-	denoting a rose-red colour	rhodophyte
-rrhage	burst forth	haemorrhage
-rrhagia	rapid flow of blood	menorrhagia
-rrhaphy	surgical suturing	gastrorrhaphy
-rrhexis	rupture	karyorrhexis
-rrhoea	flowing, discharge	diarrhoea
-rupt	break or burst	erupt, interrupt
salping(o)-	of or pertaining to tubes, e.g. fallopian tubes	salpingectomy, salpingopharyngeus muscle

Prefix or suffix	Meaning	Example(s)
sangui-, sanguine-	of or pertaining to blood	sanguine
sarco-	muscular, fleshlike	sarcoma
scler(o)-	hard	scleroderma
-sclerosis	hardening	atherosclerosis, multiple sclerosis
scoli(o)-	twisted	scoliosis
-scope	instrument for viewing	endoscope
-scopy	use of instrument for viewing	endoscopy
semi-	one-half, partly	semiconscious
sial(o)-	saliva, salivary gland	sialagogue
sigmoid(o)-	sigmoid, s-shaped curvature	sigmoid colon
sinistr(o)-	left, left side	sinistrocardia
sinus-	of or pertaining to the sinus	sinusitis
somat(o)-, somatico-	body, bodily	somatic
-spadias	slit, fissure	hypospadias, epispadias
spasmo-	spasm	spasmodic dysphonia
sperma-, spermo-, spermato-	semen, spermatozoa	spermatogenesis
splen(o)-	spleen	splenectomy
spondyl(o)-	of or pertaining to the spine, the vertebra	spondylitis
squamos(o)-	denoting something as 'full of scales' or 'scaly'	squamous cell
-stalsis	contraction	peristalsis
-stasis	stopping, standing	cytostasis, homeostasis
-staxis	dripping, trickling	epistaxis
-stenosis	abnormal narrowing in a blood vessel or other tubular organ or structure	restenosis, stenosis
stomat(o)-	of or pertaining to the mouth	stomatogastric, stomatognathic system
-stomy	creation of an opening	colostomy
sub-	beneath	subcutaneous tissue
super-	in excess, above, superior	superior vena cava
supra-	above, excessive	supraorbital vein
tachy-	denoting something as fast, irregularly fast	tachycardia

Prefix or suffix	Meaning	Example(s)
-tension, -tensive	pressure	hypertension
tetan-	rigid, tense	tetanus
thec-	case, sheath	intrathecal
therap-	treatment	hydrotherapy, therapeutic
therm(o)-	heat	thermo regulation
thorac(i)-, thorac(o)-, thoracico-	of or pertaining to the upper chest, chest; the area above the breast and under the neck	thorax
thromb(o)-	of or relating to a blood clot, clotting of blood	thrombus, thrombocytopenia
thyr(o)-	thyroid	thyroxine
thym-	emotions	dysthymia
-tome	cutting instrument	osteotome
-tomy	act of cutting; incising, incision	gastrostomy
tono-	tone, tension, pressure	tonometer
-tony	tension	neurotony
top(o)-	place, topical	topical anaesthetic
tort(i)-	twisted	torticollis
tox(i)-, tox(o)-, toxic(o)-	toxin, poison	toxoplasmosis
trache(a)-	trachea	tracheotomy
trachel(o)-	of or pertaining to the neck	tracheloplasty
trans-	denoting something as moving or situated 'across' or 'through'	transfusion
tri-	three	triangle
trich(i)-, trichia, trich(o)-	of or pertaining to hair, hair-like structure	trichocyst
-tripsy	crushing	lithotripsy
-trophy	nourishment, development	pseudohypertrophy
tympan(o)-	eardrum	tympanocentesis
-ula, -ule	small	nodule
ultra-	beyond, excessive	ultraviolet
un(i)-	one	unilateral hearing loss
ur(o)-	of or pertaining to urine, the urinary system; (specifically) pertaining to the physiological chemistry of urine	urology
uter(o)-	of or pertaining to the uterus or womb	uterus

Prefix or suffix	Meaning	Example(s)
vagin-	of or pertaining to the vagina	vagina
varic(o)-	swollen or twisted vein	varicose
vas(o)-	duct, blood vessel	vasoconstriction
vasculo-	blood vessel	vascular
ven-	of or pertaining to the (blood) veins, a vein	vein, venospasm
ventr(o)-	of or pertaining to the belly; the stomach cavities	ventrodorsal
ventricul(o)-	of or pertaining to the ventricles; any hollow region inside an organ	cardiac ventriculography
-version	turning	anteversion, retroversion
vesic(o)-	of or pertaining to the bladder	vesical arteries
viscer(o)-	of or pertaining to the internal organs, the viscera	viscera
xanth(o)-	denoting a yellow colour	xanthopathy
xen(o)-	foreign, different	xenograft
xer(o)-	dry, desert-like	xerostomia
zo(o)-	animal, animal life	zoology
-zym(o)-	fermentation	enzyme, lysozyme

How to use your textbook

It is entirely up to you how you use this book, each of us knows best how we learn. You can dip in and out of the chapters as you wish. The first four chapters set the scene and it may be advisable to consider these chapters first prior to moving into the various systems.

The icons used:

 Colouring. You are asked to colour in the elements of the diagram. The more colours that you have available to you, the more effective and enjoyable your artistic work will be. You should have at least a range of ten colours. Using felt-tipped pens is not recommended as this may cause the colours to 'bleed' through the page. If lighter colours are used they are less likely to cover up detail.

Generally, you should use what ever colours please you. There are universally agreed colours that are used in anatomy texts, for example:

- red for arteries
- blue for veins
- purple for capillaries
- yellow for nerves
- green for lymph vessels and lymph nodes.

 Identifying. Invites you to identify the various components/structures in the diagram; label the diagram.

 Pairing. Here you are required to match the pairs. You are provided with a range of sentences that should be paired up to make meaningful paragraphs

 Scrambled words. Time yourself to unscramble the words.

Wordplay. A number of activities to test your knowledge of terminology and concepts are included, such as **crosswords** and **word searches**.

Chapter 1

Basic scientific principles of physiology

Physiology is the study of how living things function; it differs from anatomy, which studies human form, yet it relies heavily on anatomical and biological concepts. An understanding of the basic principles of physiology is an essential component of any healthcare student's repertoire of understanding. Physiology integrates biology, chemistry, physics and even human behaviour.

The body is a very complex organism and is made up of many components. The smallest of these components is the atom and concludes with the organism itself – organismal level (Figure 1.1).

Fundamentals of Anatomy and Physiology Workbook: A Study Guide for Nursing and Healthcare Students, First Edition. Ian Peate.
© 2017 John Wiley & Sons Ltd. Published 2017 by John Wiley & Sons Ltd.

2

Question 1

(a) In Figure 1.1, identify the levels of organisation of the body tissue from the atomic level to the organismal level.

(b) At system level (level 5), complete the labels for the following:

- pharynx
- oesophagus
- liver
- stomach
- pancreas
- gallbladder
- small intestine
- large intestine.

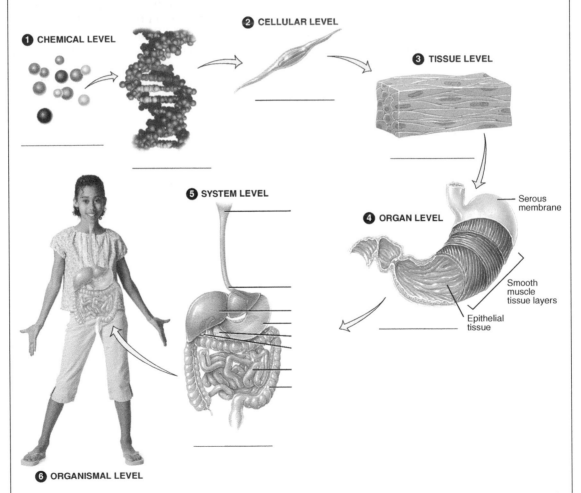

Figure 1.1 Levels of organisation of the body tissue. *Source*: Tortora 2009. Reproduced with permission of John Wiley & Sons.

Question 2   Match the pairs.

The most abundant substance found in the body	Atmospheric and hydrostatic
Supplies the energy for the organism to fulfil all the essential characteristics compatible with life	Water
Forms 20% of air, is used in the release of energy from the assimilated nutrients	Heat
A form of energy that partially controls the rate at which metabolic reactions happen	Oxygen
Two types of pressure that are required by an organism	Food

 Question 3   Time yourself to unscramble these words.

Scrambled	Answer
CHAOSTEMPRI	
SYPHIGOYLO	
SONGMAIR	
ATOMBLICE	
LAMIECHOBCANI	
REMYSCHIT	
AMTONYA	
UHNAM	

4

Question 4
(a) Figure 1.2 shows the components of an atom. Label this diagram with the following labels:

- Proton
- Electron
- Neutron
- Paths of orbit
- Nucleus

(b) Colour in:

- Proton
- Electron
- Neutron
- Nucleus

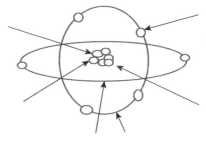

Figure 1.2 Schematic diagram of an atom. *Source*: Peate 2015. Reproduced with permission of John Wiley & Sons.

Question 5 Match the pairs.

Always central	Atoms
The building blocks of life	The nucleus
Carry a positive electrical charge	Electrons
Carry a negative electrical charge	Protons

Question 6   Time yourself to unscramble these words.

Scrambled	Answer
TORPON	
BORTI	
CETRENLO	
VISITOPE	
VENEGIAT	
THAP	
LELSH	
DUBLINGI	

Carbon atom

Carbon is a very important atom for life forms, as we are all carbon-based entities. Carbon is used to demonstrate the make-up of an actual atom.

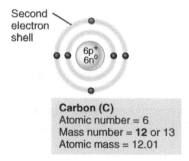

Second electron shell

Carbon (C)
Atomic number = 6
Mass number = **12** or 13
Atomic mass = 12.01

Figure 1.3   Carbon atom. *Source*: Peate 2015. Reproduced with permission of John Wiley & Sons.

Question 7   In Figure 1.4, identify the atomic number for nitrogen.

Nitrogen (N)
Atomic number = ?
Mass number = **14** or 15
Atomic mass = 14.01

Figure 1.4   Nitrogen atom. *Source*: Peate 2015. Reproduced with permission of John Wiley & Sons.

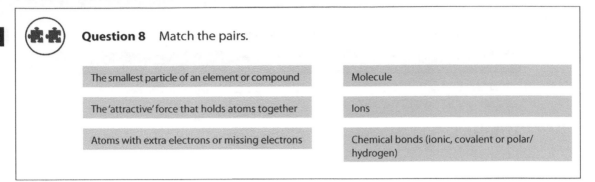

Question 8 Match the pairs.

The smallest particle of an element or compound	Molecule
The 'attractive' force that holds atoms together	Ions
Atoms with extra electrons or missing electrons	Chemical bonds (ionic, covalent or polar/hydrogen)

Elements

A chemical element is a material that cannot be broken down or changed into another substance using chemical means. Elements are the basic chemical building blocks of matter. There are 117 or 118 known elements. Some common examples of elements found in the body include:

- iron
- hydrogen
- carbon
- nitrogen
- oxygen
- calcium
- potassium
- sodium
- chlorine
- sulphur
- phosphorus

Question 9 Time yourself to unscramble these words.

Scrambled	Answer
BARCON	
RAGECH	
BATSIYLIT	
RATTYLENUI	
TROGENIN	
VACOLENT	
CINIO	
DOGYRHEN	

Question 10 Complete Table 1.1. Identify the chemical symbol representing the elements and also identify those that are metals and non-metals.

Table 1.1 Elements.

Element	Chemical symbol	Metal	Non-metal
Iron			
Hydrogen			
Carbon			
Nitrogen			
Oxygen			
Calcium			
Potassium			
Sodium			
Chlorine			
Sulphur			
Phosphorus			

Question 11 In Figure 1.5, colour in the metals, metalloids and non-metals on the periodic table.

1																17	18
1 I H	2												13	14	15	16	1 H	2 He
3 Li	4 Be												5 B	6 C	7 N	8 O	9 F	10 Ne
11 Na	12 Mg	3	4	5	6	7	8	9	10	11	12	13 Al	14 Si	15 P	16 S	17 Cl	18 Ar
19 K	20 Ca	21 Sc	22 Ti	23 V	24 Cr	25 Mn	26 Fe	27 Co	28 Ni	29 Cu	30 Zn	31 Ga	32 Ge	33 As	34 Se	35 Br	36 Kr
37 Rb	38 Sr	39 Y	40 Zr	41 Nb	42 Mo	43 Tc	44 Ru	45 Rh	46 Pd	47 Ag	48 Cd	49 In	50 Sn	51 Sb	52 Te	53 I	54 Xe
55 Cs	56 Ba	71 Lu	72 Hf	73 Ta	74 W	75 Re	76 Os	77 Ir	78 Pt	79 Au	80 Hg	81 Tl	82 Pb	83 Bi	84 Po	85 At	86 Rn

☐ Metals   ☐ Metalloids   ☐ Non-metals

Figure 1.5 The periodic table.

Question 12   Match the pairs.

A pure substance made up of two or more elements chemically bonded together	KCl
They donate electrons (to other atoms to make molecules)	Metalloids
They accept electrons (from donor atoms)	Metals
They are neither metals nor non-metals – they are sometimes referred to as semi-metals	Non-metals
NaHCO$_3$	A compound such as H$_2$O (water), NaCl (salt), CO$_2$ (carbon dioxide)
Potassium chloride	Sodium bicarbonate

SC^{R}A-MBLE   **Question 13**   Time yourself to unscramble these words.

Scrambled	Answer
MOPSITASU	
DELTOILSAM	
DUMPNOOCS	
LAMECHIC	
TEEMLEN	
MYSOBL	
DROIPIEC	
RODNO	

Electrolytes

A development of bonding is the production of electrolytes. These are substances that move to oppositely charged electrodes in fluids. Electrolytes include, for example,

- sodium
- potassium
- calcium
- bicarbonate
- magnesium
- chloride

Electrolytes are particularly important for three things within the body:

1. many are essential minerals
2. control the process of osmosis
3. help to maintain the acid–base balance required for normal cellular activity.

Question 14 Complete Table 1.2 by identifying the difference in conduction of electrical current between strong electrolytes, weak electrolytes and non-electrolytes.

Table 1.2 Types of electrolyte.

Type of electrolyte	Conduction of electrical current
Strong electrolytes	
Weak electrolytes	
Non-electrolytes	

Acid and base (pH)

It is important to understand pH values, along with alkalinity and acidity, as we depend upon the relationship between acidity and alkalinity in order to survive.

- Acids are substances that donate hydrogen ions (H^+) into a solution.
- Alkalis (also known as soluble bases) are substances that donate hydroxyl ions (OH^-) into a solution or accept H^+ ions from a solution.

The pH scale measures how acidic or basic (alkaline) a substance is. The pH scale ranges from 0 to 14. A pH of 7 is neutral. A pH less than 7 is acidic. Pure water is neutral, pH of 7.0. Vinegar and lemon juice, for example, are acidic, whilst laundry detergents and ammonia are basic.

Question 15 Complete Table 1.3, showing whether substances are acidic, alkaline (base) or neutral.

Table 1.3 Acidic, alkaline and neutral substances.

Substance	pH (acidic, alkaline or neutral)
Milk	
Water	
Vinegar	
An orange	
Coconut water	
Salt	
Ammonia	
Tea	
Oven cleaner	
Liquid used in car battery	
Blood	

Question 16
(a) In Figure 1.6, complete the boxes below to indicate neutral, acidic, alkaline, very acidic and very alkaline.

(b) Insert the following substances in the appropriate boxes:

- blood
- salt
- sugar
- vinegar
- ammonia

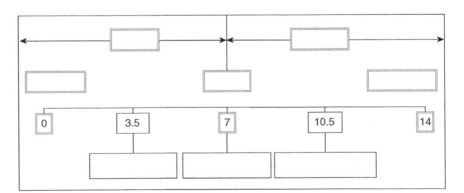

Figure 1.6 Simplified diagram of a pH scale. *Source*: Peate 2011. Reproduced with permission of John Wiley & Sons.

Question 17   Match the pairs.

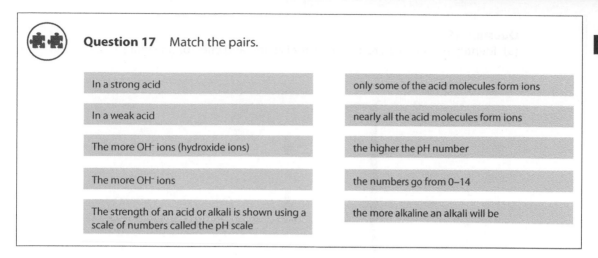

In a strong acid	only some of the acid molecules form ions
In a weak acid	nearly all the acid molecules form ions
The more OH⁻ ions (hydroxide ions)	the higher the pH number
The more OH⁻ ions	the numbers go from 0–14
The strength of an acid or alkali is shown using a scale of numbers called the pH scale	the more alkaline an alkali will be

Question 18   Time yourself to unscramble these words.

Scrambled	Answer
ECLULEMO	
SOSCIDIDATE	
NIMRALES	
BLANCAE	
AILLY TINKA	
UNISTOOL	
DACICI	
TREAVICE	

Homeostasis

Homeostasis refers to the ability of the body or a cell to seek and maintain a condition of equilibrium within its internal environment when dealing with external changes. It is a state of equilibrium for the body allowing the organs of the body to function effectively in a broad range of conditions.

Question 19
(a) Identify the stimulus, receptor, control centre and effector on Figure 1.7.

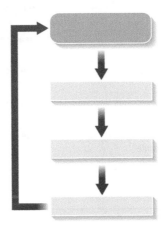

Figure 1.7 Components of a negative feedback system. *Source*: Peate 2015. Reproduced with permission of John Wiley & Sons.

(b) Now use temperature as the stimulus and complete the negative feedback diagram in relation to raised body temperature (Figure 1.8).

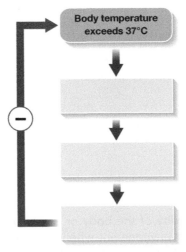

Figure 1.8 Negative feedback of raised temperature. *Source*: Peate 2015. Reproduced with permission of John Wiley & Sons.

(c) In Figure 1.9, place the correct label in each ovals for 1. Stimulus; 2. Receptor; 3. Control centre; 4. Effector; 5. Effector.

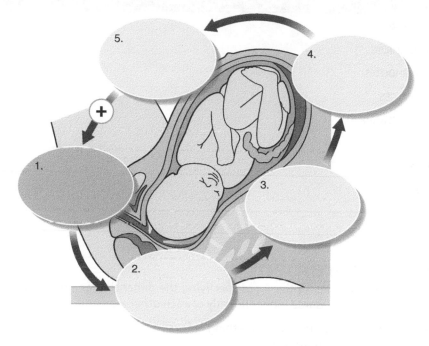

Figure 1.9 Positive feedback of childbirth. *Source*: Peate 2015. Reproduced with permission of John Wiley & Sons.

Question 20 Match the pairs.

Certain nerve endings in the skin sense temperature change	a body system such as the skin, blood vessels or the blood that receives the information from the control centre, producing a response to the condition
The control centre is	something that can elicit or evoke a response in a cell, a tissue, or an organism. A stimulus can be internal or external
An effector is	they detect changes such as a sudden rise or drop in body temperature
Homeostasis is	the brain (the hypothalamus in body temperature regulation)
A stimulus is	a reaction to a specific stimulus
A response is	a state of balance within the body

Question 21   Time yourself to unscramble these words.

Scrambled	Answer
LAXETERN	
MEQUILIRIBU	
MASSIHOOTES	
TROFFECES	
TROVEMENNIN	
KCABDEEF	
LOONTRC	
LIMTUUSS	

Units of measurement

A unit is a standardised, descriptive word specifying the dimension of a number. Properties of matter that have been measured independently of each other are:

- time – measures the duration that something occurs
- length – measures the length of an object
- mass – measures the mass (commonly taken to be the weight) of an object
- current – measures the amount of electric current that passes through an object
- temperature – measures how hot or cold an object is
- amount – measures the amount of a substance that is present
- luminous intensity – measures the brightness of an object.

Question 22   Complete Table 1.4.

Table 1.4   Units of measurement.

Quantity	Name	Symbol
Length	metre	
Mass	kilogram	
Time	second	
Current	ampere	
Temperate	Kelvin	
Amount of substance	mole	
Luminous intensity	candela	

Prefix	Symbol	Meaning	Scientific notation
tera	T		10^{12}
giga	G		10^{9}
mega	M		10^{6}
kilo	k		10^{3}
hecto	h		10^{2}
deca	da		10^{1}
deci	d		10^{-1}
centi	c		10^{2}
milli	m		10^{-3}

1 kilogram = _____ grams
1 gram = _____ milligrams
1 milligram = _____ grams
1 microgram = _____ grams

1 litre = _____ millilitres
100 millilitre = _____ decilitre
1 millilitre = _____ microlitres

Snap shot

Body temperature represents heat production and heat loss. If heat generated equals heat lost, the core body temperature will be stable and there will be a state of homeostasis.

1. What are the various sites and methods used for temperature taking?
2. What are the clinical indications for temperature taking?
3. What are the intrinsic factors that may influence temperature?
4. Define hypothermia.
5. Define fever.
6. Define hyperthermia.

Word search

O	I	S	N	O	R	T	U	E	N	S	J	D	D	O	J	L	E	T	Z
J	E	J	H	W	S	A	L	E	L	E	C	T	R	O	N	F	L	M	R
M	K	Y	Y	L	F	V	W	R	R	E	L	F	S	L	O	I	E	C	W
S	F	R	A	F	J	M	B	Z	D	Q	S	S	G	C	N	S	M	Z	V
S	M	T	O	E	D	D	E	C	T	V	T	R	U	E	V	P	E	T	S
A	E	E	L	J	M	C	I	T	A	T	S	O	R	D	Y	H	N	H	P
M	T	G	F	G	W	V	A	X	A	A	C	I	D	H	J	O	T	S	U
C	A	D	C	B	U	O	E	Y	B	B	D	Q	S	G	E	M	C	N	F
K	L	S	A	I	E	F	K	C	Y	C	O	T	Q	X	L	E	W	O	W
E	L	E	C	T	R	I	C	I	T	Y	E	L	A	H	E	O	P	T	S
N	O	V	T	E	M	Q	I	C	N	U	R	U	I	T	C	S	K	O	U
I	I	E	X	A	Q	O	O	N	T	Y	L	C	I	C	T	T	C	R	M
L	D	H	O	M	E	O	S	T	A	S	I	S	Y	U	R	A	A	P	S
A	S	O	U	O	R	H	C	P	I	G	B	J	E	M	O	S	R	Y	I
K	P	M	O	T	A	V	J	X	H	M	H	W	N	O	L	I	B	L	N
L	T	Q	M	L	G	R	M	F	M	E	T	A	L	S	Y	S	O	S	A
A	Y	K	Y	K	B	Z	T	O	M	S	R	T	L	W	T	Y	N	G	G
Z	P	I	K	N	E	O	C	O	W	Z	I	I	M	Z	E	Y	I	O	R
B	S	G	M	E	F	X	Y	D	N	M	X	Y	C	C	S	U	I	E	O
F	B	C	O	T	B	B	I	R	E	T	A	W	Q	F	E	I	M	G	L

ORGANISM	METALLOIDS	ATMOSPHERIC
HEAT	METALS	HYDROSTATIC
TIME	NON	ELECTRON
MASS	NEUTRON	ATOM
WATER	PROTONS	ELECTRICITY
ACID	ELECTROLYTES	METABOLIC
ALKALINE	ELEMENT	CARBON
FOOD	HOMEOSTASIS	BLOOD

Crossword

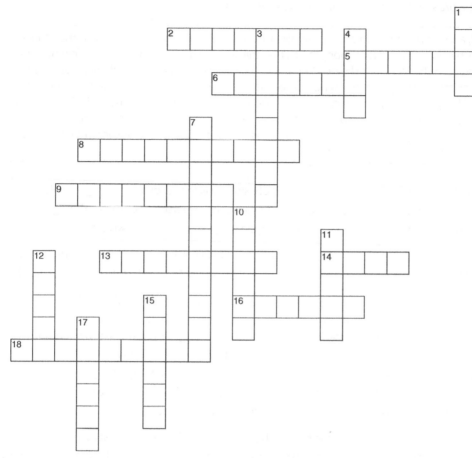

Across

2. The combining power of atoms
5. These solutions have pH values more than 7
6. Ions that carry a positive electrical charge
8. The study of how living things function
9. An element with properties of both metals and non-metals
13. This carries a negative electric charge
14. The smallest component of the human body
16. The eighth element of the period table
18. Elements that are neither metals nor non-metals

Down

1. This chemical turns blue litmus paper pink
3. Chemical element with the symbol N
4. Another name for an alkaline substance
7. Maintainence of a stable internal environment
10. This carries a positive electric charge
11. The most abundant substance found in the body
12. Unit of energy
15. Ions that carry a negative electrical charge
17. A very important element for life forms

Fill in the blanks

Use the words in the box to complete the sentences:

(OH⁻), 7, abundant, acid, acidic, acids, air, alkali, atmospheric, atom, atom, atom, atoms, atoms, balance, bases/alkaline, blood, body, body, breathing, broken, carbon-based, cells, changing, charge, chemical, complex, conduct, dissociated, electrolytes, electrons, electrons, element, element, energy, energy, energy, energy, environment, environment, equal, external, fluids, function, function, growth, H⁺, hydrogen, hydrostatic, hydroxyl, independently, interdependent, ionically, ions, ions, metabolic, metals, molecule, molecule, molecules, neutrons, oppositely, organism, organism, organism, oxygen, pH, pH, poor, positive, protons, protons, pure, rate, raw, semi-metals, soluble, stable, structure, structure, structured

1. Anatomy is the study of _____ and physiology is the study of _____ . However, _____ is always related to function because the structure determines the _____ , which in turn determines how the body/organ is _____ – the two are _____ .

2. The _____ is a very _____ organism which consists of many components, starting with the smallest of them – the _____ – and concluding with the _____ itself.

3. Water is the most _____ substance in the _____ . Food supplies the _____ for the _____ . It also supplies the _____ materials for _____ . _____ forms 20% of _____ and is used in the release of _____ from the assimilated nutrients. Heat is a form of _____ that partly controls the _____ at which _____ reactions occur. There are two types of pressure that are required by an _____ : _____ pressure, which is important in the process of _____ , and _____ pressure, which keeps the _____ flowing through the body.

4. The smallest building block of the body is the _____ . An atom consists of _____ , _____ and _____ . Carbon is a very important _____ for life forms, as we are all _____ entities. A _____ is the smallest particle of an _____ or compound which exists _____ . It contains _____ that have bonded together. The formation of chemical bonds also results in the release of _____ previously contained in the _____ .

5. An ion is an atom or a _____ in which the total number of _____ is not _____ to the total number of _____ – hence the atom or molecule has a net _____ or negative electrical _____ .

6. Electrolytes are substances that move to _____ charged electrodes in _____ . If _____ that are bonded together _____ are dissolved in water within the body _____ , they undergo a process where the _____ separate; they become _____ . These ions are now known as _____ .

7. A chemical _____ is a _____ chemical substance which cannot be _____ down into anything simpler by _____ means. Metals _____ heat and electricity. Non-metals are _____ conductors of heat and electricity. Metalloids are neither _____ nor non-metals – they are sometimes referred to as _____ .

8. An _____ is any substance which donates _____ ions (H^+) into a solution. An _____ (also known as a _____ base) is any substance which donates _____ _____ _____ into a solution or accepts _____ ions from a solution. Solutions with a _____ lower than 7 are _____ , and those with a _____ greater than _____ are _____ / _____ . The further away from a pH of 7 a solution becomes the more _____ or alkaline it is.

9. Homeostasis is the body's attempt to maintain a _____ internal _____ by achieving _____ . The body is normally able to achieve a relatively stable internal _____ even though the _____ environment is constantly _____ .

Multiple choice questions

1. The ionisation of NaCl

   (a) Is a enzymatic reaction
   (b) Has no impact on pH
   (c) Produces a cation (Na^+) and an anion (Cl^-)
   (d) Causes acidosis

2. What is true of iodine and radioactive iodine?

   (a) They both have the same atomic numbers
   (b) None have an atomic mass
   (c) Neither has electrons
   (d) Both create a biohazard

3. Which of the following is not true of sodium?

   (a) It is called the non-potassium ion
   (b) It has more protons than electrons
   (c) It is measured by volume
   (d) It is measured by pH

4. What is true of water?

   (a) It is a molecule
   (b) It is an aqueous solvent
   (c) It is a compound
   (d) All of the above

5. Which of the following best describes ATP?

   (a) It is a buffer, adding K^+ to a solution
   (b) It is an energy transfer molecule
   (c) It is an enzyme
   (d) It is measured by light

6. Out of the following which has donated an electron?

   (a) ATP
   (b) Cl^-
   (c) Na^+
   (d) HCO_3^-

7. The building blocks of life are known as:

   (a) Enzymes
   (b) Proteins
   (c) Atoms
   (d) All of the above

8. Which of the following carries a positive electrical charge?

   (a) Enzymes
   (b) Proteins
   (c) Atoms
   (d) Protons

9. Which of the following carries a negative electrical charge?

   (a) Electrons
   (b) Proteins
   (c) Atoms
   (d) Protons

10. What is the chemical notation for potassium chloride?

   (a) KCl
   (b) Cl
   (c) NaCl
   (d) Ca

References

Peate, I. and Nair, M. (2011) *Fundamentals of Anatomy and Physiology for Student Nurses*. Oxford: John Wiley & Sons, Ltd.

Peate, I. and Nair, M. (2015) *Anatomy and Physiology for Nurses at a Glance*. Oxford: John Wiley & Sons, Ltd.

Tortora, G.J. and Derrickson, B.H. (2009) *Principles of Anatomy and Physiology*, 12th edn. Hoboken, NJ: John Wiley & Sons, Inc.

Chapter 2
Cells

The basic structural, functional and biological unit of all known living organisms is the cell. Humans are multicellular; this is in comparison with some organisms such as bacteria (unicellular). Cells take in nutrients, convert these nutrients into energy, carry out specialised functions and reproduce as necessary.

The cells

Cells are the smallest independent units of life with different parts performing various functions. For cells to survive there are various fundamental chemical activities that occur within the cell, such as cellular growth, metabolism and reproduction.

There are four basic parts within the cell:

1. the cell membrane
2. cytoplasm
3. the nucleus
4. nucleoplasm.

Fundamentals of Anatomy and Physiology Workbook: A Study Guide for Nursing and Healthcare Students, First Edition. Ian Peate.
© 2017 John Wiley & Sons Ltd. Published 2017 by John Wiley & Sons Ltd.

Question 1

(a) In Figure 2.1, there are examples of some cells of the human body. Identify the five cell types.

(b) Identify and draw a circle around the head, body and tail of the sperm cell. On the smooth muscle cell encircle the nucleus of the cell.

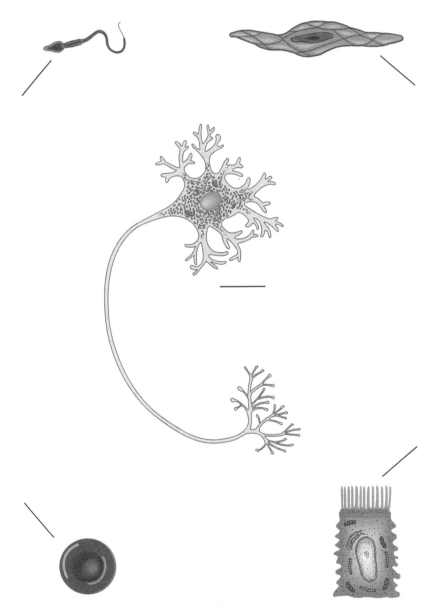

Figure 2.1 Examples of some cells of the human body. *Source*: Tortora and Derrickson, 2009. Reproduced with permission of John Wiley & Sons.

Question 2   Identify the functions of the cell components.

Components	Functions
Centrioles	
Chromatin	
Cilia	
Cytoplasm	
Cytoskeleton	
Endoplasmic reticulum (rough and smooth)	
Glycogen granules	
Golgi complex	
Intermediate filament	
Lysosomes	
Microfilaments	
Microtubules	
Microvilli	
Mitochondria	
Nucleolus	
Nucleus	
Peroxisomes	
Plasma membrane	
Ribosomes	
Secretory vesicles	

Question 3 Match the pairs.

Humans are	unicellular
Some organisms such as bacteria are	multicellular
Fluid and electrolytes are constantly moved between	there are various fundamental chemical activities occurring within the cell, for example, cellular growth, metabolism and reproduction
The basic structural, functional and biological unit of all known living organisms	the cell membrane
For cells to survive	is the cell
One of the four basic aspects associated with the cell is	the intracellular and extracellular compartments

Question 4 Time yourself to unscramble these words.

Scrambled	Answer
MAGICMOSRONIR	
CEARILUNLLU	
BRACEITA	
BREENMAM	
YOKCROPARTI	
BOTEMMLISA	
TEXUALLRACELR	
OBLIOGICAL	

Cell structure

Question 5

(a) From the list below add the labels to Figure 2.2.

- Microfilament
- Mitochondrion
- Golgi complex
- Plasma membrane
- Ribosome
- Lysosome

- Smooth endoplasmic reticulum
- Rough endoplasmic reticulum
- Flagellum
- Nucleus
- Cytoplasm

(b) Colour in the nucleus, mitochondrion and the flagellum.

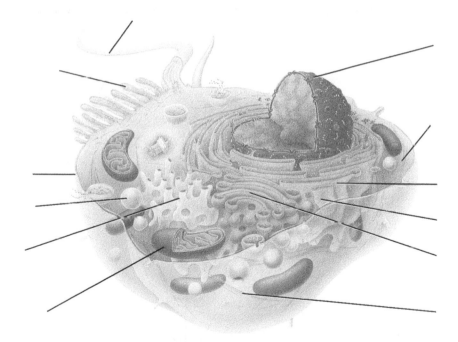

Figure 2.2   Structure of a cell. *Source*: Nair and Peate, 2009. Reproduced with permission of John Wiley & Sons.

Cell membrane

The cell membrane separates and protects a cell from its surrounding environment and is primarily made up of a double layer of proteins and lipids (fat-like molecules). Within this membrane are embedded a variety of other molecules acting as channels and pumps, transporting different molecules into and out of the cell. The cell membrane can vary in thickness from 7.5 nanometres (nm) to 10 nm.

Question 6

(a) In Figure 2.3, identify:

- phospholipids
- glycolipids
- glycoproteins
- lipid bilayer

(b) Colour in the cytosol, the extracellular fluid and the integral proteins and carbohydrates. Now identify and colour in the hydrophobic and hydrophilic phospholipids.

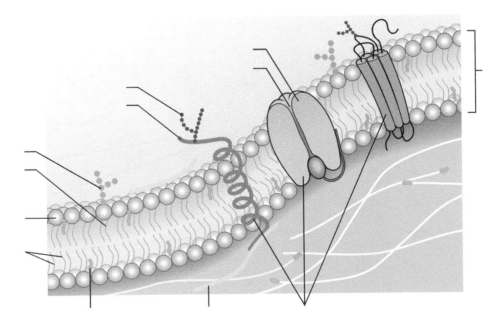

Figure 2.3 Cell membrane. *Source*: Peate and Nair, 2015. Reproduced with permission of John Wiley & Sons.

Question 7 Match the pairs.

Cell membrane	varies from 7.5 nm to 10 nm
Cell membranes are made up mostly from	separates and protects a cell from its surrounding environment
Cell membrane thickness	a double layer of proteins and lipids (fat-like molecules)
Hydrophilic refers to	self-sealing
Hydrophobic refers to	water loving
The bilayer is	water hating

Question 8 Time yourself to unscramble these words.

Scrambled	Answer
CYPRHOHILID	
LAYBIER	
POPPIDHOHSLIS	
POCYGLOTREINS	
SECLUMOLE	
PIDIL	
BLEEPMEMIRA	
DRATYOBHECARS	

The mitochondria

The cell's power producers are called the mitochondria. They convert energy into a form that is usable by the cell, and they also produce cholesterol. The mitochondria are located in the cytoplasm; they are the sites of cellular respiration which eventually generate the fuel that is required for the cell's various activities. Mitochondria are also concerned with cell division and growth, and cell death.

Question 9

(a) Identify the various parts of the mitochondrion in Figure 2.4.

(b) Use different colours to differentiate between the various components of the mitochondrion.

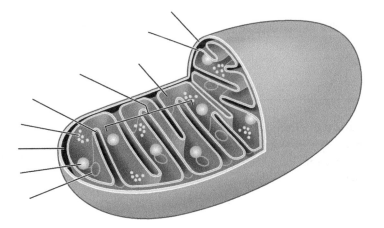

Figure 2.4   The mitochondrion. *Source*: Peate and Nair, 2015. Reproduced with permission of John Wiley & Sons.

Question 10   Match the pairs.

The cell's power producers	in the mitochondrion
The mitochondria are located in	adenosine triphosphate
Cellular respiration occurs	the cytoplasm
The mitochondria are also involved in	are the mitochondria
The mitochondria	cell division, growth and death
The energy made by the mitochondria is in the form of a chemical called	generate fuel for cell activity

Question 11   Time yourself to unscramble these words.

Scrambled	Answer
RENGEY	
ROWEP	
CHOMDRIAINOT	
DENISEAON	
PHATSOTHERIOP	
CIHOOTMINDRON	
RATIONSPIRE	
SCHOOLLETER	

Endoplasmic reticulum

The endoplasmic reticulum is an organelle of cells and is an interconnected network of membrane vesicles. The endoplasmic reticulum is classified into two types, rough endoplasmic reticulum and smooth endoplasmic reticulum.

Question 12

(a) On Figure 2.5 identify the smooth endoplasmic reticulum and the rough endoplasmic reticulum (remember rough endoplasmic reticulum has a rough sandpaper-like appearance). Locate the nuclear envelope and the ribosomes.

(b) Colour in the smooth endoplasmic reticulum and the rough endoplasmic reticulum.

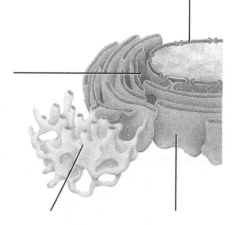

Figure 2.5   The endoplasmic reticulum. *Source*: Jenkins and Tortora, 2013. Reproduced with permission of John Wiley & Sons.

Question 13 Match the pairs.

The endoplasmic reticulum	in abundance in mammalian liver and gonad cells
The endoplasmic reticulum	works closely with the Golgi apparatus
Cells with large amount of endoplasmic reticulum	is an organelle of the cell
Rough endoplasmic reticulum	are found in the pancreas and liver
Smooth endoplasmic reticulum	has ribosomes attached to its surface
The smooth endoplasmic reticulum is found	is a smooth network without any ribosomes

Question 14 Time yourself to unscramble these words.

Scrambled	Answer
RANGELELO	
TRICULUME	
COFIXTATIONIDE	
CLASPENDOMI	
BROOMEISS	
GROUH	
DANGO	
GIGOL	

The nucleus

The cell nucleus contains the genetic information of the cell packaged in the form of chromatin; it is a double-membrane-bound organelle. The nucleus is a characteristic feature of most eukaryotic cells. The nucleus is said to be one of the most important structures of eukaryotic cells. It serves the functions of information storage, and retrieval and duplication of genetic information; it is the control centre of the cell, the brain of the cell.

The key functions of the cell nucleus include deoxyribonucleic acid (DNA) replication and control of gene expression during the cell cycle. The nucleus provides functional compartmentalisation inside the cell allowing higher levels of gene regulation.

Within the cell nucleus is the nucleolus, a round body. There is no membrane surrounding it; it sits in the nucleus.

Question 15

(a) On Figure 2.6 identify the components of the nucleus.

(b) Colour in the chromatin, the nuclear pores, the nuclear envelope and the nucleolus. Note that the nucleolus has no envelope.

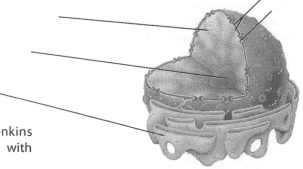

Figure 2.6 The nucleus. *Source*: Jenkins and Tortora, 2013. Reproduced with permission of John Wiley & Sons.

Question 16   Match the pairs.

The genetic information of cell is packaged in the form of	is deoxyribonucleic acid (DNA) replication
The nucleus is a characteristic feature of	it sits in the nucleus
One of the key functions of the cell nucleus	ribosomal subunits from proteins and ribosomal RNA (rRNA)
Within the cell nucleus is the	most eukaryotic cells
There is no membrane surrounding the nucleolus	nucleolus
The nucleolus makes	chromatin

Question 17   Time yourself to unscramble these words.

Scrambled	Answer
GEENCIT	
SLUCNUE	
MOMOCHORES	
TAPECLIRION	
LYCEC	
CLOUNLUSE	
TINPORES	
ROACHMTIN	

Cytoplasm, lipid bilayer and membrane proteins

Cytoplasm (sometimes referred to as cytosol) is the substance that fills the cell. It is a jelly-like material composed of 80% water and is usually clear in colour. It resembles more a viscous (thick) gel as opposed to a watery substance; when shaken or stirred it liquefies.

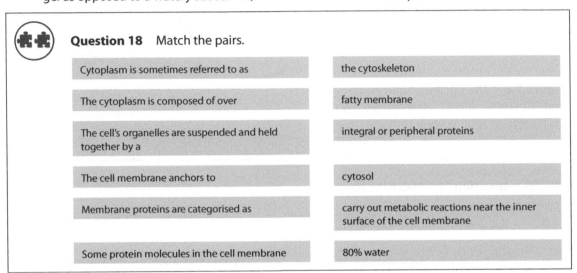

Question 18   Match the pairs.

Cytoplasm is sometimes referred to as	the cytoskeleton
The cytoplasm is composed of over	fatty membrane
The cell's organelles are suspended and held together by a	integral or peripheral proteins
The cell membrane anchors to	cytosol
Membrane proteins are categorised as	carry out metabolic reactions near the inner surface of the cell membrane
Some protein molecules in the cell membrane	80% water

Question 19   Time yourself to unscramble these words.

Scrambled	Answer
SYCTOOL	
PYSCOLMATIC	
ELACTRLINULAR	
TOOTSYKELCEN	
TATYF	
PHEEPRALIR	
GRAINLET	
SCIVSOU	

Snap shot

Intravenous electrolyte administration

Hypokalaemia and hyperkalaemia can be life threating, as can other electrolyte disturbances. Some patients require electrolyte replacement; this can be administered in a number of ways. Discuss some of the issues related to intravenous electrolyte administration.

Word search

F	O	J	M	W	V	P	R	O	K	A	R	Y	O	T	I	C	S	Z	X
B	G	I	A	E	U	H	B	X	S	J	W	N	X	V	X	E	C	H	O
G	N	M	E	D	T	I	S	U	W	V	H	C	N	H	M	K	U	M	J
A	S	V	O	L	L	A	E	V	E	A	N	Y	P	O	R	L	S	T	Q
Q	I	C	K	A	B	L	B	M	F	Y	O	I	S	Z	O	I	Z	K	L
X	T	R	Y	P	C	A	U	O	H	T	O	O	T	R	N	J	P	T	N
E	L	E	E	U	P	L	E	M	L	Y	B	R	E	A	E	B	V	P	D
J	R	O	N	T	U	V	G	M	M	I	D	T	G	Y	M	F	C	Y	N
T	S	I	S	C	C	Q	A	M	R	X	S	R	Q	A	X	O	G	U	M
M	V	N	I	Z	Y	A	L	G	G	E	O	M	O	X	N	Y	R	C	Y
N	F	T	R	S	N	D	B	V	L	O	P	R	F	P	G	I	J	H	F
P	E	H	F	H	K	R	S	O	R	B	H	M	G	R	H	E	S	Z	C
R	A	I	R	D	N	O	H	C	O	T	I	M	I	A	K	I	D	M	X
N	R	Y	T	E	Q	C	I	F	K	R	M	T	G	Z	N	I	L	W	E
L	D	P	O	H	B	M	L	Z	M	N	Z	X	A	N	T	E	W	I	J
E	N	N	T	U	N	I	C	E	L	L	U	L	A	R	T	T	L	Z	C
B	A	U	S	U	L	O	E	L	C	U	N	V	W	L	T	C	S	L	W
Z	C	I	I	O	Y	H	A	K	U	E	S	V	G	H	P	D	E	J	E
P	U	S	N	I	E	T	O	R	P	O	C	Y	L	G	K	B	N	V	E
Z	H	Y	D	R	O	P	H	O	B	I	C	I	R	Q	L	K	N	K	N

MICROORGANISM	HYDROPHILIC	RIBOSOMES
PROKARYOTIC	BILAYER	RETICULUM
UNICELLULAR	GLYCOPROTEINS	EUKARYOTIC
METABOLISM	IMPERMEABLE	NUCLEUS
BACTERIA	MITOCHONDRIA	NUCLEOLUS
ORGANISM	CHOLESTEROL	CHROMATIN
HYDROPHOBIC	ORGANELLE	

Crossword

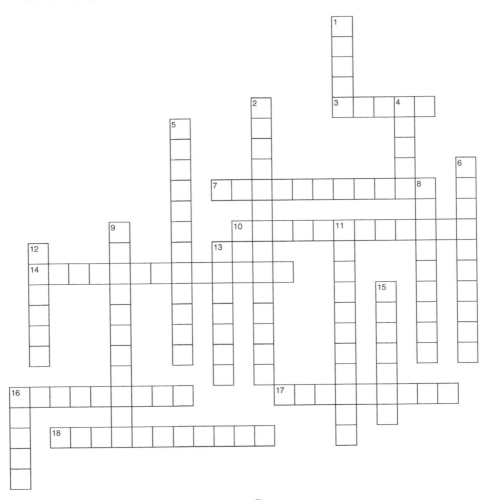

Across

3. This type of endoplasmic reticulum is studded with ribosomes on the cytosolic face

7. Those microorganisms that lack a membrane-bound nucleus

10. The energy-producing site of the cell

14. With regard to cells, humans are said to be this

16. The mitochondria are located here

17. This is found within the cell nucleus

18. Water hating

Down

1. The cytoplasm is composed mainly of this

2. They provide structural support and cell movement

4. This complex packages proteins for secretion

5. This provides support and is a site for specific enzymes

6. Organisms that consist of cells with a membrane-bound nucleus

8. Component which contains genetic information

9. Bacteria, for example

11. Water loving

12. One type of endoplasmic reticulum

13. The genetic information of the cell is packaged here

15. Cytoplasm

16. Basic structural, functional and biological units of all known living organisms

Fill in the blanks

Use the words in the box to complete the sentences:

80%, actively, activities, bacteria, bicarbonate, biological, carbohydrate, cell, cells, cholesterol, chromatin, clear, constant, cytoplasm, cytoplasmic, death, detoxification, division, double, duplication, electrolytes, electrolytes, electrolytes, endoplasmic, energy, energy, eukaryotic, face, fatty, fuel, function, functional, growth, hepatocytes, important, information, information, into, intracellular, lipid, lipids, living, membrane, membrane, membrane-bound, mitochondria, molecules, multicellular, nuclear, nucleus, nutrients, nutrients, organelle, organelle, organelles, out, out, potassium, power, protects, proteins, reproduce, reticulum, retrieval, ribosomes, rough, smooth, storage, suspended, synthesis, thickness, transport, two, without

1. The   basic structural, _____ and _____ units of all known _____ organisms are cells. Humans are _____, this is in comparison to some organisms such as _____ (unicellular). Cells take in _____, convert these nutrients into _____, carry out specialised functions and _____ as necessary.

2. Water, _____ and _____ move in and _____ of a cell through the use of a _____ system. Fluid and _____ are constantly moved between the _____ and extracellular compartments, ensuring that the _____ have a _____ supply of _____, for example, sodium, chloride, _____, magnesium, phosphates, _____ and calcium, required for cellular _____.

3. The cell _____ separates and _____ a cell from its surrounding environment and is primarily made up of a _____ layer of _____ and _____. Within this membrane are embedded a variety of other _____ acting as channels and pumps, transporting different molecules _____ and _____ of the cell. The cell membrane can vary in _____.

4. The cell's _____ producers are the _____, which convert _____ into a form usable by the cell. They also produce _____. The mitochondria are located in the _____; they generate the _____ needed for the cell's various _____. Mitochondria are also concerned with other cell processes, for example cell _____ and _____, and also cell _____.

5. The _____ reticulum is an _____ of cells. The endoplasmic _____ is classified into _____ types, _____ endoplasmic reticulum and _____ endoplasmic reticulum. Rough endoplasmic reticulum is studded with _____ on the cytosolic _____. Rough endoplasmic reticulum is mainly found in _____ where protein _____ occurs _____. Smooth endoplasmic reticulum is a smooth network _____ any ribosomes. The smooth endoplasmic reticulum is associated with _____ and _____ metabolism and _____.

6. The cell _____ is a double _____ _____ and contains the genetic _____ of the cell packaged in the form of _____. The nucleus is a characteristic feature of most _____ cells. The nucleus is said to be one of the most _____ structures of eukaryotic cells. It serves the function of _____ _____, _____ and _____ of genetic information.

7. Cytoplasm is the substance that fills the _____. It is composed of _____ water and is usually _____ in colour. Cytoplasm is the substance of life in which all of the cell's _____ are _____ and held together by a _____ membrane. It is found inside the cell _____, surrounding the _____ envelope and the _____ organelles.

Multiple choice questions

1. What is the spherical organelle that contains the genetic material?

    (a) Ribosomes
    (b) Mitochondria
    (c) Nucleus
    (d) Enzyme

2. What is protoplasm found inside the nucleus known as?

    (a) Riboflavin
    (b) Cytoplasm
    (c) Mitochondria
    (d) Nucleoplasm

3. A prokaryotic genetic system has:

    (a) DNA and but no histones
    (b) Neither DNA nor histones
    (c) Either DNA or histones
    (d) All of the above

4. What does a genophore (nucleoid) consist of?

    (a) RNA and histone
    (b) Histone and non-histone
    (c) A single double strand of DNA
    (d) None of the above

5. Which one of the following organelles digests the old organelles no longer useful to the cell?

    (a) Lysosomes
    (b) Ribosomes
    (c) mDNA
    (d) RNA

6. What do prokaryotic cells lack?

   (a) Cell membrane
   (b) Cell wall
   (c) Membrane-bound nucleolus
   (d) Cytoplasm

7. Humans are

   (a) Unicellular
   (b) Multicellular
   (c) Acellular
   (d) All of the above

8. Centrioles

   (a) Have no role to play in human survival
   (b) Are only present in certain circumstances
   (c) Only associated with cellular destruction
   (d) Associated with cellular reproduction

9. Microfilaments

   (a) Only provide structural support
   (b) Only provide for cell movement
   (c) Provide structural support and cell movement
   (d) Provide cellular nutrition

10. What does hydrophilic mean?

   (a) Water loving
   (b) Water hating
   (c) Water loving and water hating
   (d) Self healing

References

Jenkins, G. and Tortora, G.J. (2013) *Anatomy and Physiology: From Science to Life*, 3rd edn. Hoboken, NJ: John Wiley & Sons, Inc.

Nair, M. and Peate, I. (2009) *Fundamentals of Applied Pathophysiology: An Essential Guide for Nursing Students*. Oxford: John Wiley & Sons, Ltd.

Peate, I. and Nair, M. (2015) *Anatomy and Physiology for Nurses at a Glance*. Oxford: John Wiley & Sons, Ltd.

Tortora, G.J. and Derrickson, B.H. (2009) *Principles of Anatomy and Physiology*, 12th edn. Hoboken, NJ: John Wiley & Sons, Inc.

Chapter 3
Genetics

Genetics is the branch of science dealing with how we inherit physical and behavioural characteristics (traits); these also include medical conditions, and many health problems are linked to genes. Each cell in the human body contains approximately 25 000 to 35 000 genes.

Genes are sections of deoxyribonucleic acid (DNA) that are carried within the chromosomes. Genes contain particular sets of instructions that are related to growth, development, reproduction, functioning and ageing. DNA makes all the basic units of hereditary material, these control cellular structure and direct cellular activities. The ability of the DNA to replicate itself provides the basis of hereditary transmission.

Figure 3.1 provides a representation of a DNA double helix with nucleotides *in situ*.

 Question 1   In Figure 3.1, try the following:
(a) Circle the two strands of the double helix.
(b) Identify the four nucleotides, guanine, cytosine, adenine and thymine.

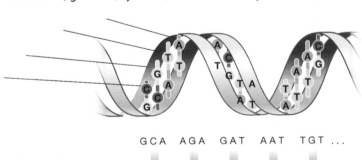

Figure 3.1   A DNA double helix with nucleotides *in situ*. *Source*: Tortora and Derrickson, 2009. Reproduced with permission of John Wiley & Sons.

Fundamentals of Anatomy and Physiology Workbook: A Study Guide for Nursing and Healthcare Students, First Edition. Ian Peate.
© 2017 John Wiley & Sons Ltd. Published 2017 by John Wiley & Sons Ltd.

The four nucleotides (the bases) are very particular as to which other base they pair with. Adenine always pairs with thymine and guanine always pairs with cytosine. Hence, if one half of the DNA has a base sequence AGGCAGTGC then the opposite side of the DNA will have a complementary base sequence, TCCGTCACG (Figure 3.2).

A	G	G	C	A	G	T	G	C
↓	↓	↓	↓	↓	↓	↓	↓	↓
T	C	C	G	T	C	A	C	G

Figure 3.2   Base alignment.

Question 2   In Figure 3.3, identify the bases that will pair, remembering that adenine always pairs with thymine and guanine always pairs with cytosine.

A	G	C	A	G	G	A	T	T
↓	↓	↓	↓	↓	↓	↓	↓	↓

Figure 3.3   Base pairing.

The bases are joined by means of hydrogen/polar bonding. The individual bases are connected to the deoxyribose of the strand (or support of the ladder) by means of covalent bonds.

Question 3   In Figure 3.4, colour in the nucleotides guanine (G), cytosine (C), adenine (A) and thymine (T).

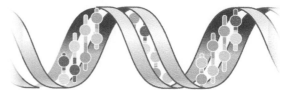

Figure 3.4   DNA double helix with nucleotides *in situ*. *Source*: Peate and Nair, 2015. Reproduced with permission of John Wiley & Sons.

Question 4   Match the pairs.

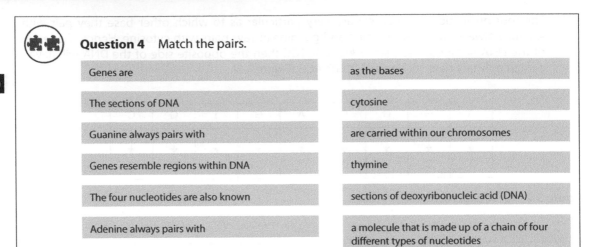

Genes are	as the bases
The sections of DNA	cytosine
Guanine always pairs with	are carried within our chromosomes
Genes resemble regions within DNA	thymine
The four nucleotides are also known	sections of deoxyribonucleic acid (DNA)
Adenine always pairs with	a molecule that is made up of a chain of four different types of nucleotides

Question 5   Time yourself to unscramble these words.

Scrambled	Answer
SEENITGC	
RUEOXIDYBONCLICE	
MULEECOL	
DENISECLOUT	
ELIXH	
SYNITECO	
NINAGUE	
HYMINTE	

Ribonucleic acid (RNA)

RNA is different from DNA: RNA is single-stranded and the sugar is the pentose sugar which contains the pyrimidine base, uracil (U), instead of thymine. Cells have three different RNAs: messenger RNA (mRNA), ribosomal RNA (rRNA) and transfer RNA (tRNA). Figure 3.5 shows the single-stranded RNA.

Question 6   In Figure 3.5:
(a) Circle the single stand of the RNA helix.
(b) Identify the four nucleotides guanine (G), cytosine (C), adenine (A) and uracil (U).

(c) Colour in the nucleotides guanine (G), cytosine (C), adenine (A) and uracil (U).

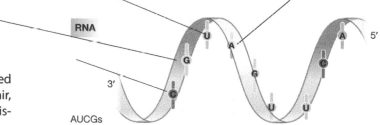

Figure 3.5   The single-stranded RNA. *Source*: Peate and Nair, 2011. Reproduced with permission of John Wiley & Sons.

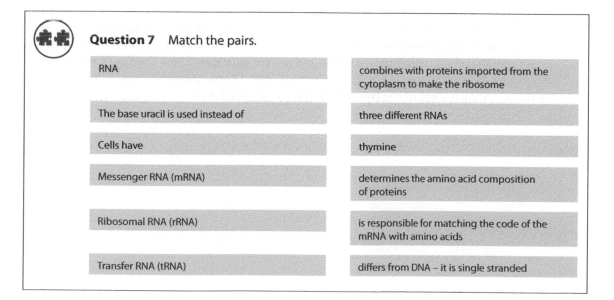

Question 7   Match the pairs.

RNA	combines with proteins imported from the cytoplasm to make the ribosome
The base uracil is used instead of	three different RNAs
Cells have	thymine
Messenger RNA (mRNA)	determines the amino acid composition of proteins
Ribosomal RNA (rRNA)	is responsible for matching the code of the mRNA with amino acids
Transfer RNA (tRNA)	differs from DNA – it is single stranded

Question 8   Time yourself to unscramble these words.

Scrambled	Answer
DANSTR	
CLIECNUBIRO	
LAMBSOOIR	
CLUIAR	
GESSERMEN	
FRANTRES	
DECO	
NOAIM	

Chromosomes

Chromosomes are thread-like structures of DNA that are found inside the nucleus of a cell. Each chromosome is made of protein and a single molecule of DNA. Chromosomes also contain DNA-bound proteins, which package the DNA and control its functions. The unique structure of chromosomes keeps DNA tightly wrapped around spool-like proteins, called histones. Human body cells have 46 chromosomes, 23 inherited from each parent. Each chromosome is a long molecule of DNA, passed from parents to their children; DNA contains the specific instructions that make each type of living creature unique.

Changes in the number or structure of chromosomes in new cells can lead to serious problems. It is also essential that reproductive cells, ova and sperm, contain the right number of chromosomes and that those chromosomes have the correct structure. If not, the resulting offspring may fail to develop properly. For example, those with Down syndrome have three copies of chromosome 21, instead of the two copies found in other people.

Question 9

(a) Identify the component parts of Figure 3.6.

(b) Colour in the various parts of:

- the DNA double helix
- the histones
- the nucleosome
- the chromatids
- the centromere.

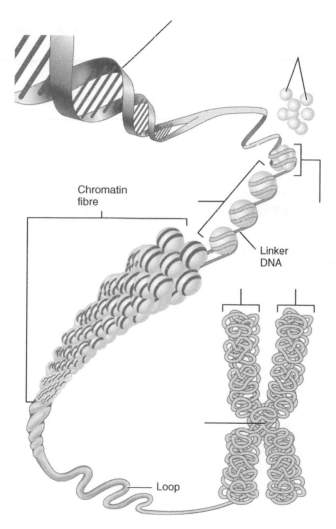

Chromatin
fibre

Linker
DNA

Loop

Figure 3.6 Chromosome formation. *Source*: Tortora and Derrickson, 2009. Reproduced with permission of John Wiley & Sons.

Question 10   Match the pairs.

Chromosomes are thread-like structures of DNA	cells have to constantly divide to produce new cells, replacing old, worn-out cells
Each chromosome is made of	found inside the nucleus of a cell
For organisms to grow and function properly	protein and a single molecule of DNA
Changes in the number or structure of chromosomes in new cells	as the centromere
Those with Down syndrome have	can lead to serious problems
The constricted region of linear chromosomes is known	three copies of chromosome 21

Question 11   Time yourself to unscramble these words.

Scrambled	Answer
CHOOSERMOM	
SCROTEMREEN	
PLACTEIER	
THROMCAID	
THISONES	
XILEH	
DIEPCO	
OWND	

Protein synthesis, transcription and translation

Protein production and all the genetic instructions for making proteins are found in DNA, but in order to synthesise these proteins; the genetic information encoded in the DNA has to be translated first. The first thing that needs to happen in this process is that the DNA has to separate in order to allow for all of the genetic information in a region of DNA to be copied on to RNA.

Question 12

(a) Take a look at Figure 3.7 and identify the bases – adenine, guanine, thymine and cytosine. As the DNA separates, locate the hydrogen bond, phosphate group and deoxyribose sugar.

(b) Colour in the two old DNA strands and then the two new strands.

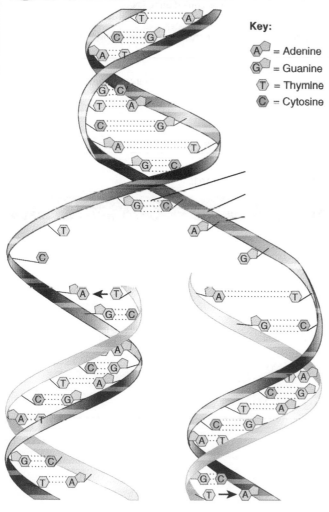

Old strand   New strand   New strand   Old strand

Figure 3.7 The separation of DNA. *Source*: Tortora and Derrickson, 2009. Reproduced with permission of John Wiley & Sons.

Key:

A = Adenine
G = Guanine
T = Thymine
C = Cytosine

Question 13 Match the pairs

In order to synthesise proteins	the RNA attaches to a ribosome where the information contained in the RNA is translated into a corresponding sequence of amino acids, forming a new protein molecule
The first thing that needs to happen during protein production is	the genetic information contained in the DNA is transcribed into the RNA
When the information has been transcribed	the genetic information encoded in the DNA has to be translated
In transcription	that the DNA has to separate in order to allow for all of the genetic information in a region of DNA to be copied on to RNA
The DNA serves as a template for copying the information	two parts, a large subunit and a small subunit
Ribosomes consist of	into a complementary sequence of codons

Question 14 Time yourself to unscramble these words.

Scrambled	Answer
EGENCIT	
THISSENYS	
PRATTSCRINION	
NATIONSRLAT	
MEALPETT	
BUUSTIN	
LIARBOOMS	
DEEDCON	

Gene transference

Genetic information is transferred from cells to new cells and also from parents to their children. In order for the body to grow and for the replacement of body cells that have died, cells have to be able to reproduce themselves. However, to prevent any genetic information from getting lost during reproduction they must be able to reproduce themselves accurately and the cells do this by cloning themselves.

Gene transference can be divided into two stages: mitosis and meiosis.

Mitosis

Mitosis describes the process by which the nucleus of a cell divides to create two new nuclei, each containing an identical copy of DNA.

Question 15   Below identify the four stages of mitosis.

Stage	Name
1.	
2.	
3.	
4.	

Before and after the cells have divided, they enter a stage known as interphase. The interphase is thought to be the resting period of a cell; however, the cell is active in getting ready for replication.

Meiosis

Meiosis is the process by which certain sex cells are created. The spermatozoa of the male and the ova of the female go through the process of meiosis.

Question 16   Identify the two stages of meiosis.

Stage of meiosis	Name
1.	
2.	

During the interphase that precedes meiosis I, the chromosome of the diploid starts to replicate with each chromosome consisting of two identical daughter chromatids. In meiosis II both of the cells produced in meiosis I divide again.

Meiosis I can be further subdivided into four stages.

Question 17 Identify the four subdivided stages associated with meiosis I.

Stage of meiosis I	Name
1.	
2.	
3.	
4.	

Question 18 There are also four stages associated with meiosis II. Can you identify them?

Stage of meiosis II	Name
1.	
2.	
3.	
4.	

Question 19 Match the pairs.

The process of gene transference can be divided into	further divide again
Mitosis describes	the process by which certain sex cells are created
Meiosis is	two stages
The spermatozoa of the male and the ova of the female go through the process of	the chromosome of the diploid starts to replicate
During the interphase that precedes meiosis I	meiosis
In meiosis II both of the cells produced in meiosis I	the process by which the nucleus of a cell divides to create two new nuclei, each containing an identical copy of DNA

Question 20   Time yourself to unscramble these words.

Scrambled	Answer
LIPIDOD	
LICEUN	
HAPENAAS	
STEALHOPE	
STOMACHRID	
FENCESRENTAR	
CLIPARTIONE	
SHAPERENTI	

Snap shot

Cystic fibrosis

This is a well known disease that is inherited as an autosomal recessive disorder and affects 1 in 2500 children born in the UK. A faulty gene causes the condition. The gene is transmitted as an autosomal recessive disorder whereby both parents carry the faulty gene and there is a 1 in 4 chance of each pregnancy leading to a child with cystic fibrosis.

On the diagram label the body systems predominantly affected by cystic fibrosis.

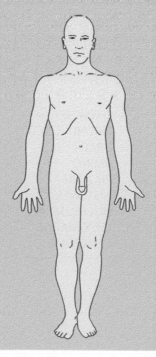

Word search

G	Q	T	H	Y	M	I	N	E	J	E	B	X	R	R	J	E	H	B	J
V	N	J	K	F	I	N	T	E	R	P	H	A	S	E	C	V	P	A	V
R	B	P	F	C	E	N	T	R	O	M	E	E	I	J	Z	K	M	T	D
O	E	B	N	L	T	M	I	T	O	S	I	S	A	M	L	T	N	I	E
U	N	F	N	O	I	T	P	I	R	C	S	N	A	R	T	P	R	N	O
M	I	S	N	L	X	I	L	E	H	H	E	T	A	Z	V	Y	D	U	X
R	S	C	X	C	S	X	D	E	O	X	Y	R	I	B	O	S	E	B	Y
I	O	S	C	I	N	E	B	F	W	B	I	K	M	K	N	S	G	U	R
Z	T	I	T	E	L	V	M	P	C	S	E	N	U	C	H	N	X	S	I
O	Y	S	S	L	S	E	N	O	T	S	I	H	H	L	B	U	S	N	B
E	C	O	C	C	A	B	N	L	S	V	J	C	G	O	J	C	D	K	O
M	P	I	I	U	H	M	B	I	E	O	H	U	P	N	N	L	A	I	N
O	R	E	T	N	X	T	I	O	N	R	M	I	R	E	T	E	S	D	U
S	O	M	E	O	C	G	T	N	O	A	O	O	H	A	I	O	V	T	C
O	T	O	N	B	D	A	Y	M	O	S	U	Q	R	U	C	T	V	P	L
E	E	A	E	I	N	R	A	Q	V	E	F	G	U	H	Y	I	X	Y	E
L	I	P	G	R	Y	T	E	N	I	N	E	D	A	P	C	D	L	E	I
C	N	K	R	G	I	B	A	G	Y	E	K	P	P	D	L	E	B	Y	C
U	Q	Y	U	D	M	P	D	G	N	G	K	V	X	Q	V	S	J	H	D
N	W	R	S	K	A	U	W	F	G	L	A	T	H	W	S	G	A	R	L

GENETICS	THYMINE	CLONE
GENES	RIBONUCLEIC	TRANSCRIPTION
DEOXYRIBONUCLEIC	URACIL	DEOXYRIBOSE
CHROMOSOMES	AMINO	SUBUNIT
NUCLEOTIDES	PROTEIN	MITOSIS
HELIX	HISTONES	MEIOSIS
GUANINE	NUCLEOSOME	INTERPHASE
CYTOSINE	CHROMATIDS	
ADENINE	CENTROME	

Crossword

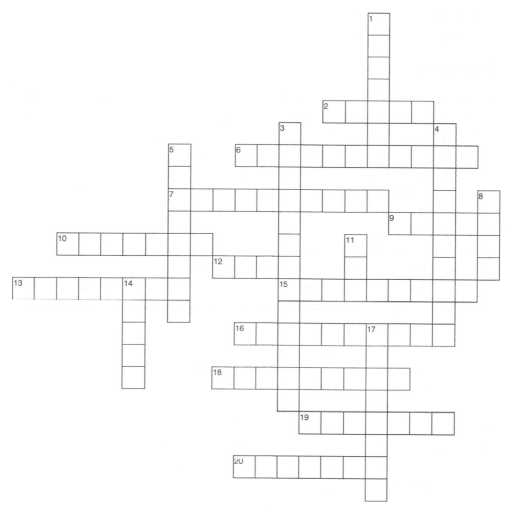

Across

2. The four nucleotides are also known as these
6. Sections of DNA are carried with these
7. Transcription of the DNA ends at a special nucleotide sequence known as what?
9. How many different types of RNA do cells have?
10. The sugar in RNA
12. Number of types of nucleoides in a DNA molecule
13. The bases are joined by this type of bonding
15. What kind of condition is cystic fibrosis?
16. The resting period of a cell
18. Fourth stage of mitosis
19. One of the two processes of gene transference
20. Adenine always pairs with this

Down

1. Process by which the nucleus of a cell divides to create two new nuclei, each containing an identical copy of DNA
3. One of the processes by which information in RNA is translated into a specific sequence of amino acids in a protein molecule
4. The constricted region of linear chromosomes
5. Guanine always pairs with this
8. Chromosomes are thread-like structures of DNA found in the nucleus of what?
11. Number of strands in an RNA molecule
14. Set of instructions for the growth and development of every cell in the body
17. Spool-like protein structure that DNA is tightly wrapped around

Fill in the blanks

Use the words in the box to complete the sentences:

23, 46, accurately, ageing, amino, base, behavioural, cell, cells, cellular, characteristics, children, chromosomes, chromosomes, cloning, cytosine, deoxyribonucleic, died, DNA, DNA, DNA, DNA, DNA, encoded, genes, genes, genes, genes, genetic, grow, growth, hereditary, histones, inherit, inherited, instructions, medical, meiosis, messenger, mitosis, nucleotides, nucleus, pair, parents, parents, pentose, protein, protein, proteins, proteins, pyrimidine, replacement, replicate, reproduce, reproduction, reproduction, ribosomal, RNA, single-stranded, synthesise, thymine, thymine, transcription, transfer, transference, transferred, translated, translated, transmission, unique, unsustainable, uracil

1. Genetics is the branch of science dealing with how we _____ physical and _____ _____ (traits); these also include _____ conditions, and many health problems are linked to _____. Each cell in the human body contains approximately 25 000 to 35 000 _____.

2. Genes are sections of _____ acid (DNA) that are carried within the _____. Genes contain particular sets of instructions that are related functions including _____, development, _____, functioning and _____. Without _____ life would be _____; our genes make us what we are. All of our _____ are inherited from our parents, who in turn _____ theirs from their _____.

3. DNA makes all the basic units of _____ material, these control cellular structure and direct _____ activities. The ability of the _____ to _____ itself provides the basis of hereditary _____.

4. The four _____ (the bases) are very particular as to which other _____ they _____ with. Adenine always pairs with _____ and guanine always pairs with _____.

5. RNA is different from _____. RNA is _____, the sugar is the _____ sugar and contains the _____ base _____ (U) instead of _____. Cells have three different RNAs: _____ RNA (mRNA), _____ RNA (rRNA) and _____ RNA (tRNA).

6. Chromosomes are thread-like structures of _____ found inside the _____ of a _____; each is made of _____ and a single molecule of DNA. The unique structure of _____ keeps DNA tightly wrapped around spool-like _____; these are called _____. Human body cells have _____ chromosomes, _____ inherited from each parent. DNA contains the specific _____ that make each living creature _____.

7. Protein production and all the genetic instructions for making _____ are found in _____. In order to _____ these proteins, the genetic information _____ in the _____ has to be _____ first. A complex series of reactions occurs, information contained in _____ is _____ into a corresponding specific sequence of _____ acids in a newly produced _____ molecule – _____ and translation.

8. Genetic information is _____ from _____ to new cells and also from _____ to their _____. For the body to _____ and for the _____ of body cells that have _____, cells have to _____ themselves. However, to prevent _____ information from getting lost during _____ they must be able to reproduce themselves _____; cells do this by _____ themselves. Gene _____ can be divided into two stages: _____ and _____.

Multiple choice questions

1. How many genes does each cell in the human body contain?

   (a) 2000 to 3000 genes
   (b) 200 to 300 genes
   (c) 250 000 to 350 000 genes
   (d) 25 000 to 35 000 genes

2. What are genes?

   (a) Sections of deoxyribonucleic acid
   (b) Made up only of ribosomes
   (c) Sections of matrix
   (d) None of the above

3. What does guanine always pair with?

   (a) Water
   (b) Cytosine
   (c) Carbon
   (d) Oxygen

4. What are the four nucleotides also known as?

   (a) Excess
   (b) Iodine
   (c) Bases
   (d) All of the above

5. RNA is

(a) Single-stranded
(b) Double-stranded
(c) Has no strands
(d) Has three strands

6. How many chromosomes do human body cells have?

(a) 4 chromosomes
(b) 6 chromosomes
(c) 46 chromosomes
(d) 460 chromosomes

7. In transcription

(a) The genetic information contained in the RNA is transcribed into the DNA
(b) Osmosis occurs
(c) The genetic information contained in the DNA is transcribed into the RNA
(d) The genetic information is destroyed

8. What do ribosomes consist of?

(a) Two parts, a large subunit and a small subunit
(b) Three parts, a large subunit and a small subunit
(c) Two parts, two large subunit and a small subunit
(d) Two parts, a large subunit and three small subunits

9. Gene transference can be divided into:

(a) Osmosis, mitosis and meiosis
(b) Mitosis and meiosis
(c) Osmosis and meiosis
(d) Mitosis and osmosis

10. What is meiosis?

(a) An enzyme
(b) A carbohydrate
(c) The process by which certain sex cells are created
(d) The process by which certain sex cells are destroyed

References

Peate, I. and Nair, M. (2011) *Fundamentals of Anatomy and Physiology for Student Nurses*. 1st edn. Oxford: John Wiley & Sons, Ltd.

Peate, I. and Nair, M. (2015) *Fundamentals of Anatomy and Physiology for Student Nurses*. 2nd edn. Oxford: John Wiley & Sons, Ltd.

Tortora, G.J. and Derrickson, B.H. (2009) *Principles of Anatomy and Physiology*, 12th edn. Hoboken, NJ: John Wiley & Sons, Inc.

Chapter 4

Tissues

There are around 50–106 trillion individual structural working units in the body called cells. Working together, cells ensure that homeostasis is maintained. Cells vary in their shape, size and life span; they can, however, be categorised subject to their structure and functions. Groups of cells that have similar structure and function are known as tissue. There are four main types of tissue within the human body: epithelial tissue, nervous tissue, connective tissue and muscle tissue.

Generally, tissue types are made up of similar cells performing related functions. Consider the epidermis of the face and the lining of the mouth: they are the same tissue type with related functions, however their appearance is very different when observed by the naked eye. Blood and bone are the same type of tissue but they look very different.

Question 1   In Figure 4.1, identify the levels of organisation from atom through to organism.

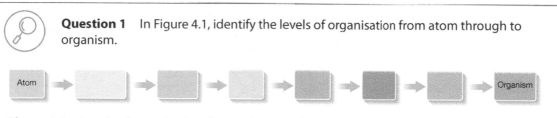

Figure 4.1   Levels of organisation. *Source*: Peate and Nair, 2015. Reproduced with permission of John Wiley & Sons.

Fundamentals of Anatomy and Physiology Workbook: A Study Guide for Nursing and Healthcare Students, First Edition. Ian Peate.
© 2017 John Wiley & Sons Ltd. Published 2017 by John Wiley & Sons Ltd.

Question 2

(a) Identify the various types of tissue in Figure 4.2 from this list:

- skeletal muscle
- cardiac muscle
- nervous tissue
- smooth muscle
- epithelial tissue
- connective tissue.

(b) Now describe the various functions of these types of tissue.

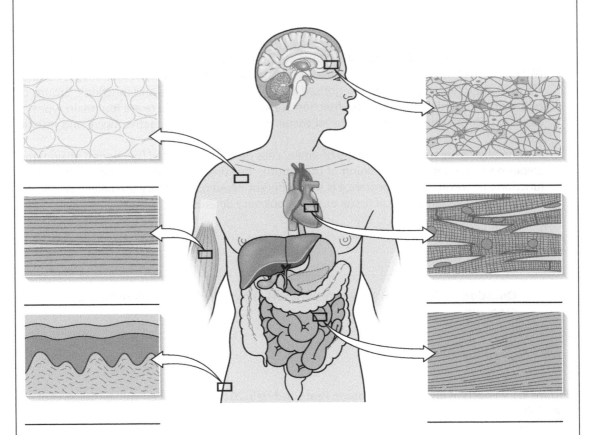

Figure 4.2 Tissues of the human body. *Source*: Peate and Nair, 2015. Reproduced with permission of John Wiley & Sons.

Epithelial tissue

Epithelial tissue is located in the covering of external and internal surfaces of the body, the hollow organs and tubes and also in the glands. The overall function of the epithelium is to provide protection and impermeability (or selective permeability) to the covered structure.

The cells are closely packed and the intracellular substance (the matrix) is minimal. There is usually a basement membrane on which the cells lie. Epithelial tissue may be simple, pseudostratified or stratified, and cell shapes may be squamous, cuboidal or columnar.

Question 3

(a) Identify the simple, pseudostratified and stratified epithelial tissues in Figure 4.3.

(b) Identify and colour in the squamous, cuboidal and columnar cell shapes.

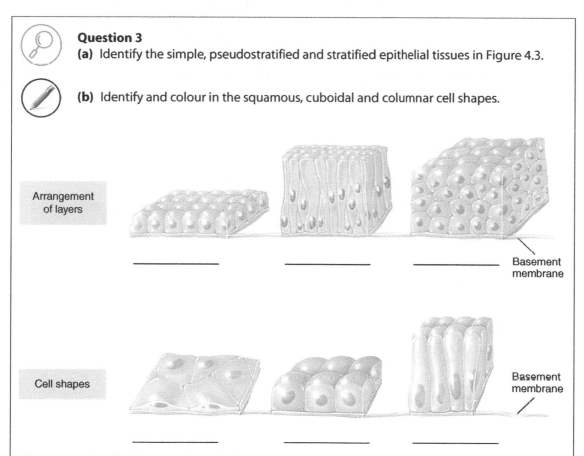

Figure 4.3 Epithelial tissue classified by shape and depth. *Source*: Tortora and Derrickson, 2009. Reproduced with permission of John Wiley & Sons.

Question 4 Match the pairs.

The overall function of the epithelium is	a basement membrane on which the cells lie
Epithelial tissue is classified by	to provide protection and impermeability
In epithelial tissue there is usually	shape and depth
The intracellular substance is minimal and	simple, pseudostratified or stratified
Epithelial tissue may be	covering of external and internal surfaces, the hollow organs, tubes and glands
Epithelial tissue is located in the	the cells are closely packed

(SC^RA-MBLE) **Question 5** Time yourself to unscramble these words.

Scrambled	Answer
DSLANG	
SUESIT	
NAMEBERM	
GROANS	
FAIRTSTIED	
CURATEINLLILAR	
VEINCONECT	
KEELSLAT	

Connective tissue

There are several varieties of connective tissue; this is the most abundant type of tissue. The usual function of connective tissue is to fill empty spaces among other body tissues. Connective tissue is not present on body surfaces, unlike epithelial tissue. Connective tissue is usually highly vascular. Exceptions include cartilage, which is avascular, and tendons, which have a small blood supply.

There are four types of connective tissue:

- connective tissue proper (subdivided into loose and dense connective tissue)
- cartilage
- bone
- blood/lymph (atypical connective tissue).

 Question 6   In Table 4.1 describe the role of the various types of cell.

Table 4.1   The roles of the various types of cell.

Cell	Role
Adipocytes	
Primary blast cells	
Macrophages	
Plasma cells	
Mast cells	
Leucocytes	

Question 7

(a) Label Figure 4.4, you should identify connective tissue and the epithelium.

(b) Colour in the nerve, blood vessel and differentiate between the connective tissue and the epithelium.

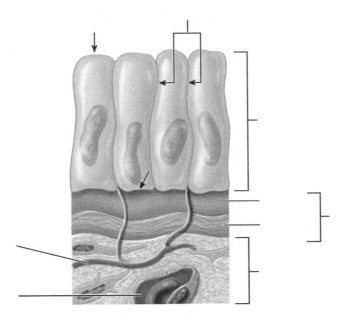

Figure 4.4 Connective tissue. *Source*: Tortora and Derrickson, 2009. Reproduced with permission of John Wiley & Sons.

Question 8 Match the pairs.

This is the most abundant type of tissue	secrete substances composed of extracellular material
The cells of the connective tissue	substance transportation, protection of the organism and insulation
Important biological features of the connective tissues include	connective
The usual function of connective tissue	is not present on body surfaces
The matrix of areolar connective tissue	is to fill empty spaces among other body tissues
Connective tissue	is semi-solid

Question 9   Time yourself to unscramble these words.

Scrambled	Answer
TAILSUNION	
THUMPLEEII	
RAREALO	
ELECTLAXRULAR	
AGENLOLC	
MRTAXI	
NOTICEPROT	
SPORTUP	

Nervous tissue

Nervous tissue is composed of neurones and glial cells. The function of the nervous tissue is to receive and transmit neural impulses (reception and transmission of information). The basic unit of nervous tissue is the neurone. The cell body of the neurone contains the nucleus, cytoplasm and other organelles. Nerve processes are 'finger-like' projections arising from the cell body, they have the ability to conduct and transmit signals. Neurones typically have one axon (this may be branched). Axons frequently terminate at a synapse through which the signal is sent to the next cell, normally through a dendrite.

Question 10
(a) In Figure 4.5, identify the dendrites, nucleus of neurogial cell, nucleus in the cell body and the axon.

(b) Colour in the various components of the neurone, also include the nucleus and the cytoplasm.

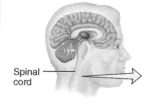
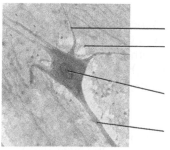
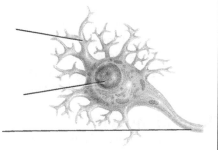

Spinal cord

Neurone of spinal cord

Figure 4.5   An example of nervous tissue. *Source*: Tortora and Derrickson, 2009. Reproduced with permission of John Wiley & Sons.

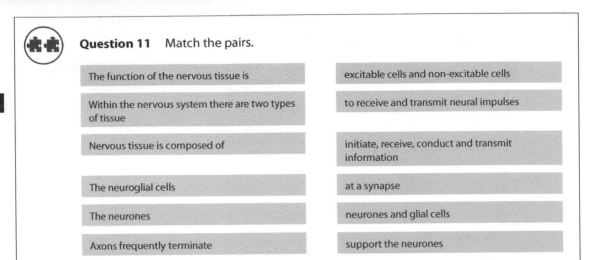

Question 11   Match the pairs.

The function of the nervous tissue is	excitable cells and non-excitable cells
Within the nervous system there are two types of tissue	to receive and transmit neural impulses
Nervous tissue is composed of	initiate, receive, conduct and transmit information
The neuroglial cells	at a synapse
The neurones	neurones and glial cells
Axons frequently terminate	support the neurones

Question 12   Time yourself to unscramble these words.

Scrambled	Answer
PSYNASE	
RENUOGALLI	
SONENURE	
PLUMSEIS	
TINDREED	
ANOX	
MISSISTRANON	
TAXIBLEEC	

Muscle

Muscle tissues are composed of cells that permit contractions and as such they generate movement. The function of the muscle tissue is to pull bones (skeletal striated muscle), to contract and move viscera and vessel walls (smooth muscle) and also to make the heart beat (cardiac striated muscle). Every time we move, each time that our heart beats, every breath we take, when we ingest food or when we micturate, muscle is involved.

Skeletal muscle

Skeletal muscle is also known as striated muscle. It is a voluntary type of muscle, meaning its movement can be consciously controlled. The cells within the skeletal muscle are long and thin and have multiple nuclei. Skeletal muscle is found adjacent to the skeleton and is usually attached to bone by tendons.

Question 13 Label Figure 4.6 to include the following:

- skeletal muscle fibre
- nucleus
- striations.

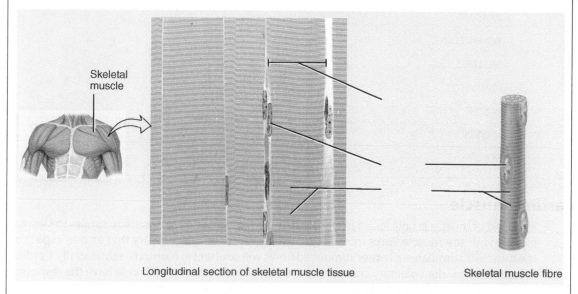

Skeletal
muscle

Longitudinal section of skeletal muscle tissue

Skeletal muscle fibre

Figure 4.6 Skeletal muscle. *Source*: Tortora and Derrickson, 2009. Reproduced with permission of John Wiley & Sons.

Question 14 Match the pairs.

Skeletal muscle is found	by tendons
Skeletal muscle is also known as	permit contractions and as such they generate movement
Muscle tissues are composed of cells that	long muscle fibres
Muscle tissue contains	protective functions
Skeletal muscle also has	striated muscle
Skeletal muscle is usually attached to bone	adjacent to the skeleton

Question 15   Time yourself to unscramble these words.

Scrambled	Answer
SONTEND	
TIRADEST	
TRAINSCONTCO	
NOTLEEKS	
URNAVYLOT	
VASERIC	
SELVESS	
NOBE	

Cardiac muscle

This kind of muscle is only found in the heart. It is a specialised type of muscle similar to skeletal muscle with the muscle fibres interlocking with each other making sure that as one aspect of the muscle is stimulated all other stimulated fibres will contract in harmony, sequentially. Cardiac muscle is not under voluntary control; the special cells of the sino-atrial node have the responsibility for sending out impulses that usually result in cardiac contraction. Cardiac muscle provides the driving force of contraction.

Question 16   Complete the labels for the following:

- nucleus
- cardiac muscle fibre (cell)
- intercalated disc
- striations

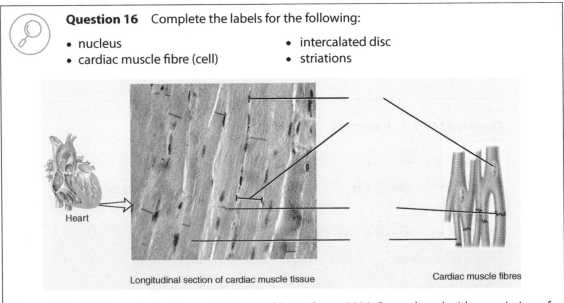

Heart

Longitudinal section of cardiac muscle tissue

Cardiac muscle fibres

Figure 4.7   Cardiac muscle. *Source*: Tortora and Derrickson, 2009. Reproduced with permission of John Wiley & Sons.

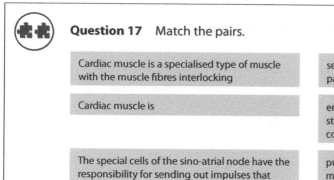

Question 17 Match the pairs.

Cardiac muscle is a specialised type of muscle with the muscle fibres interlocking	set its own contraction rhythm as a result of pacemaker cells
Cardiac muscle is	ensuring as one aspect of the muscle is stimulated all other stimulated fibres will contract sequentially
The special cells of the sino-atrial node have the responsibility for sending out impulses that	pulls the actin filaments together to shrink the muscle cell making it contract
Each cardiac muscle fibre contains	result in cardiac contraction, cardiac muscle provides the driving force of contraction
When the muscle fibres contract, myosin	a single nucleus and is striated
Cardiac muscle tissue is able to	not under voluntary control

Question 18 Time yourself to unscramble these words.

Scrambled	Answer
MAKEPEACR	
SYNIMO	
FAILSNETM	
CINTELOKRING	
DONE	
TRANCCOTION	
LACENDIRATTE	
TINCA	

Smooth muscle

Smooth muscle is non-striated; it is stimulated by involuntary neurogenic impulses and has slow, rhythmical contractions. Contraction of smooth muscle is caused when myosin and actin filaments slide over each other.

It is held together by connective tissue with bands of elastic protein wrapped around them. Smooth muscle is found in the walls of hollow internal structures and vessels, where fluid or solid substances need to be propelled from one area to another.

Question 19 Complete the labels for the following:
- smooth muscle
- smooth muscle fibre (cell)
- nucleus of smooth muscle fibre

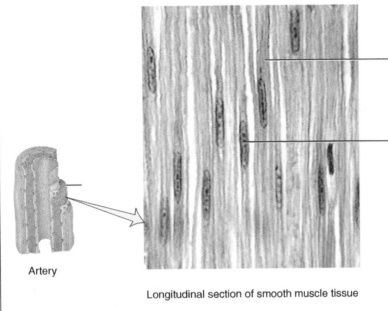

Artery

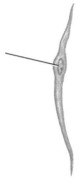

Longitudinal section of smooth muscle tissue

Smooth muscle fibre

Figure 4.8 Smooth muscle. *Source*: Tortora and Derrickson, 2009. Reproduced with permission of John Wiley & Sons.

Question 20 Match the pairs.

Smooth muscle is	it is stimulated by involuntary neurogenic impulses and has slow, rhythmical contractions
Smooth muscle is involuntary	non-striated
It is held together by	in the walls of hollow internal structures and vessels
Smooth muscle is found	connective tissue with bands of elastic protein wrapped around them
Smooth muscle tends to	myosin and actin filaments over each other
Contraction of smooth muscle is caused by the sliding of	have greater elasticity than striated muscle

Question 21   Time yourself to unscramble these words.

Scrambled	Answer
GENIOCRENU	
TRAYVILNOUN	
SPUMESIL	
THOOMS	
SLEVESS	
LICESAT	
NOTICVENCE	
LIDSE	

Summary of tissue types

Question 22
(a) Label the four cell types in Figure 4.9.

(b) Colour in the different parts of the cells.

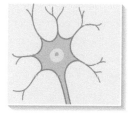

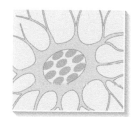

_____

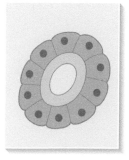

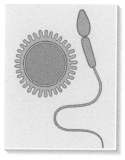

_____

_____

_____

Figure 4.9   Human body cells. _Source_: Peate and Nair, 2015. Reproduced with permission of John Wiley & Sons.

Tissue repair

Tissue repair occurs when cells are damaged, worn out or dead and they need to be replaced. Each of the four tissue types can regenerate and replace cells injured by trauma, disease or other events. The various tissue types have differing success rates. As epithelial cells have to withstand large amounts of wear and tear these have the greatest capacity for renewal. Most connective tissue also has great capacity for renewal but, in some types of connective tissue, healing can take a long time.

Snap shot

Pressure sores are an injury to the skin and underlying tissue. They can range from mild reddening of the skin to severe tissue damage and sometimes infection that can extend into muscle and bone.

Describe the four stages of development of pressure sores.

Word search

R	B	J	H	K	N	Z	E	H	E	G	A	L	I	T	R	A	C	V	I
O	E	Y	F	I	Q	U	X	E	R	U	T	C	U	R	T	S	J	I	Q
D	R	X	S	S	L	E	D	B	P	R	R	Y	Y	V	C	E	E	P
A	T	O	T	T	U	R	A	E	O	X	X	D	O	U	Z	C	P	G	O
T	Y	U	A	R	R	O	Z	D	X	O	Z	K	J	K	B	U	I	R	S
M	V	G	L	C	A	A	M	K	I	M	L	S	O	M	P	Z	T	R	T
B	M	R	A	L	T	C	T	A	O	O	I	B	G	U	S	N	H	D	N
D	K	A	T	A	G	I	E	I	U	C	B	N	B	I	O	E	E	E	E
X	S	N	Y	I	N	N	N	L	F	Q	O	U	M	L	C	R	L	N	M
R	T	M	T	L	E	S	D	N	L	I	S	G	C	E	A	V	I	D	A
N	R	U	I	E	D	K	T	D	T	U	E	V	A	H	I	O	A	R	L
R	I	L	S	H	Q	E	L	A	A	L	L	D	T	T	D	U	L	I	I
C	A	O	S	T	S	L	R	B	E	T	N	A	K	I	R	S	Y	T	F
F	T	C	U	I	T	E	L	V	Y	E	S	I	R	P	A	G	D	E	U
C	E	Q	E	P	N	T	B	M	U	H	T	M	P	E	C	Q	C	S	T
Q	D	U	L	E	Y	A	W	R	P	E	V	I	T	C	E	N	N	O	C
J	N	I	G	E	J	L	O	N	C	B	Z	H	Y	D	M	X	J	R	T
Z	B	E	I	F	D	N	A	Z	O	H	T	O	O	M	S	X	T	R	V
U	R	O	S	J	E	C	K	N	M	A	T	R	I	X	F	C	R	B	I
D	S	Y	U	S	I	M	E	Y	J	W	A	C	W	J	T	X	O	F	F

TISSUE	STRATIFIED	DENDRITES
EPITHELIAL	SQUAMOUS	NEURONES
STRUCTURE	CUBOIDAL	STRIATED
CONNECTIVE	COLUMNAR	MYOSIN
SKELETAL	EXTRACELLULAR	ACTIN
CARDIAC	BLOOD	FILAMENTS
NERVOUS	BONE	REGENERATION
SMOOTH	CARTILAGE	
EPITHELIUM	MATRIX	

Crossword

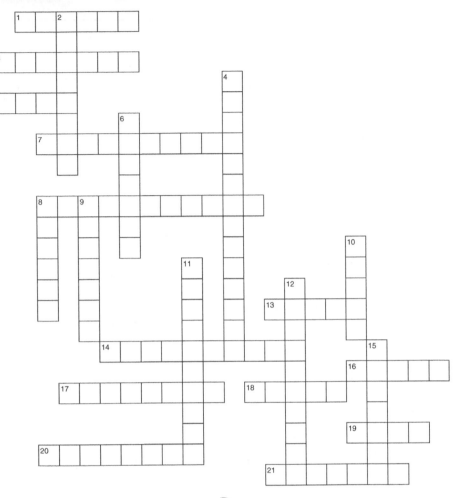

Across

1. Groups of cells that have similar structure and function are known as this
3. Most connective tissue also has great capacity for this
5. Generated by long muscle fibres
7. The most abundant type of tissue
8. These form part of the body's immune system
13. This fluid substance is also a type of connective tissue
14. Fat cells
16. One of the criteria for classification of epithelial tissue
17. The appearance of cardiac muscle fibres
18. One of the cell types in nervous tissue
19. The number of separate types of tissue in the human body
20. Neuroglial cells support these
21. Frequently at the termination of an axon

Down

2. Skeletal muscle is found adjacent to this structure
4. One of the functions of the epithelium
6. Cells that assist in controlling homeostasis
8. Cells governing body movement
9. This kind of muscle is only found in the heart
10. Movement of myosin and actin filaments over each other
11. Basic functional units of striated muscle fibres
12. Feature of smooth muscle
15. Structures that attach skeletal muscle to bone

Fill in the blanks

Use the words in the box to complete the sentences.

abundant, beat, categorised, cell, cells, cells, columnar, composed, conduct, connective, contract, contractions, covering, cuboidal, cytoplasm, empty, excitable, four, function, functions, glands, glial, hollow, impermeability, impulses, initiate, internal, intracellular, life, located, maintenance, material, membrane, minimal, movement, movement, muscle, nerve, neuroglial, neuron, neurons, organelles, packed, permeability, posture, provide, pull, receive, response, secrete, shape, shapes, simple, smooth, spacing, stimulation, stratified, striated, striated, structure, structure, support, tissue, tissue, transmit, tubes, two, two, varieties, vessel, viscera

1. Cells vary in their _____, size and _____ span; they can, however, be _____ subject to their _____ and _____. Groups of _____ that have similar structure and _____ are known as _____; there are _____ separate types of tissue within the human body.

2. Epithelial tissue is _____ in the _____ of external and _____ surfaces of the body, _____ organs and _____ and also in the _____. The overall function of the epithelium is to _____ protection and _____ or selective _____ to the covered _____. The cells are closely _____ and the _____ substance is _____. There is usually a basement _____ on which the cells lie. Epithelial tissue may be _____, pseudostratified or _____, with cell _____ squamous, _____ and _____.

3. There are a number of _____ of connective tissue; it is the most _____ type of tissue. The usual function of _____ tissue is to fill _____ spaces among other body tissues. The cells of connective tissue _____ substances _____ of extracellular _____, providing significant _____ between these _____.

4. Nervous _____ is composed of _____ and _____ cells. The function is to _____ and to also _____ neural _____. Within the nervous system there are _____ types of cell: _____ cells, which _____, receive, _____ and transmit information, and non-excitable cells, the _____ cells, which _____ the neurones. The basic unit of nervous tissue is the neurone, made up of _____ main parts, the _____ body, that contains the neurone's nucleus, _____ and other _____, and the axon.

5. Muscle tissues are composed of cells that permit _____ and as such they generate _____. The function of the _____ tissue is to _____ bones (skeletal _____ muscle); to _____ and move _____ and _____ walls (_____ muscle) and also to make the heart _____ (cardiac _____ muscle). Muscle tissue is found where there is a need for _____ and _____ of _____. Muscle tissues contract in _____ to nerve, _____-like or hormonal _____.

Multiple choice questions

1. Which of the following is not typical of epithelial tissue?

    (a) Arranged like paving
    (b) Simple, cuboidal or columnar
    (c) Large amount of mineral-containing intercellular matrix
    (d) Gives rise to endocrine and exocrine glands

2. Adipose tissue is

    (a) A type of connective tissue storing fat
    (b) Described as pulsatile and voluntary
    (c) Classified as exocrine
    (d) Classified as cardiac and smooth

3. Osseous tissue

    (a) Contains hard mineral-containing intercellular matrix
    (b) Contains osteocytes
    (c) Is a kind of connective tissue
    (d) All of the above

4. With regard to the pleural membranes

    (a) There is a visceral and parietal pleural membrane
    (b) They are connective tissue membranes
    (c) They are also known as adenoids
    (d) They are located in the small intestine

5. The pleura and peritoneum

    (a) Are serous membranes
    (b) Are located within the cranium
    (c) Are located within the urinary bladder
    (d) Surround the appendix

6. Epithelial tissue is avascular, meaning that it

    (a) Has an excessive amount of adipose tissue
    (b) Contains no blood vessels
    (c) Is made of blood vessels
    (d) Cannot repair itself

7. Epithelial tissue is classified by

    (a) Shape, colour and depth
    (b) Shape, vascularity and depth
    (c) Shape, weight and depth
    (d) Shape and depth

8. Connective tissue is

(a) Present on body surfaces, it is highly vascular
(b) Not present on body surfaces
(c) Not present on body surfaces, it is always avascular
(d) None of the above

9. Nervous tissue is composed of

(a) Mainly water
(b) No water
(c) Neurones and glial cells
(d) Only glial cells

10. Cardiac muscle is

(a) Composed of mainly water
(b) Not under voluntary control
(c) Under voluntary control
(d) Made of cardiocytes

References

Peate, I. and Nair, M. (2015) *Anatomy and Physiology for Nurses at a Glance*. Oxford: John Wiley & Sons, Ltd.
Tortora, G.J. and Derrickson, B.H. (2009) *Principles of Anatomy and Physiology*, 12th edn. Hoboken, NJ: John Wiley & Sons, Inc.

Chapter 5

Skeletal system

Bone is a complex living organism; despite that it seems to be a solid, dry, inert material. It is being recreated continually; bone is metabolically active. When old bone dies, new bone is being reconstructed.

The axial and appendicular skeleton

In the adult human skeleton there are 206 named bones. The skeleton is divided into two parts for classification purposes. These are the axial skeleton and the appendicular skeleton; both have their own purposes.

Fundamentals of Anatomy and Physiology Workbook: A Study Guide for Nursing and Healthcare Students, First Edition. Ian Peate.
© 2017 John Wiley & Sons Ltd. Published 2017 by John Wiley & Sons Ltd.

Question 1

(a) Complete the number of bones in each division of the skeleton.

(b) Colour in the appendicular and axial skeleton.

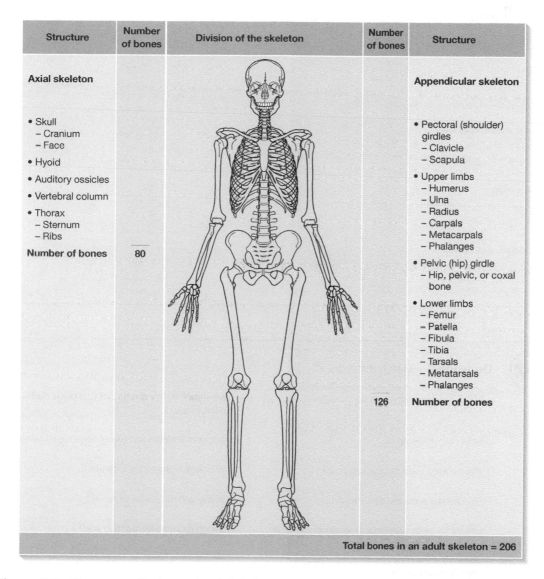

Structure	Number of bones	Division of the skeleton	Number of bones	Structure
Axial skeleton • Skull – Cranium – Face • Hyoid • Auditory ossicles • Vertebral column • Thorax – Sternum – Ribs **Number of bones**	 80		 126	**Appendicular skeleton** • Pectoral (shoulder) girdles – Clavicle – Scapula • Upper limbs – Humerus – Ulna – Radius – Carpals – Metacarpals – Phalanges • Pelvic (hip) girdle – Hip, pelvic, or coxal bone • Lower limbs – Femur – Patella – Fibula – Tibia – Tarsals – Metatarsals – Phalanges **Number of bones**
		Total bones in an adult skeleton = 206		

Figure 5.1 The appendicular and axial skeleton. *Source*: Peate *et al.,* 2014. Reproduced with permission of John Wiley & Sons.

Question 2 In Table 5.1 write notes about the function of bone.

Table 5.1 Bone function.

Function	Description
Support	
Movement	
Minerals and lipid store	
Protection	
Blood cell production	

Question 3 Match the pairs.

When old bone dies	a number of different tissues and this includes bone tissue
Bones are made up of	the axial skeleton and the appendicular skeleton
The skeleton provides the body with	of bones, ligaments and tendons
The skeletal system is comprised	shape and the power to move
Infants are born with large amounts of cartilage	they have more bones than adults
The skeleton is divided into two parts for classification purposes	new bone is being reconstructed

Question 4   Time yourself to unscramble these words.

Scrambled	Answer
CILOBATEM	
NOTJIS	
CIRULATETA	
NILGASTEM	
NODESNT	
IIMERANS	
SIFISOOTCAIN	
USEF	

Bone growth

The process of bone formation is known as ossification.

Bone strength comes from the protein matrix, providing it with resilience and elasticity, permitting bone to give a little as it is comes under pressure. Minerals deposited in bone add to the strength.

Intramembranous and endochondral ossification

Intramembranous and endochondral ossification are embryonic processes of bone formation.

Intramembranous ossification

Intramembranous ossification occurs primarily during the initial formation of the flat bones of the skull, mandible and clavicles. The bone is formed from mesenchyme connective tissue.

Question 5   Label the features of Figure 5.2 that are associated with intramembranous ossification.

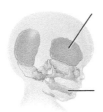

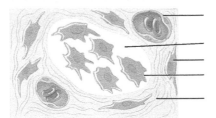

❶ Development of ossification centre

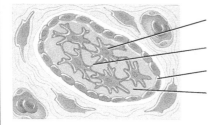

❷ Calcification

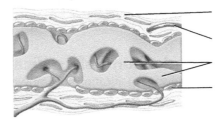

❸ Formation of trabeculae

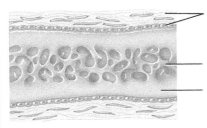

❹ Development of the periosteum

Figure 5.2   Intramembranous ossification. *Source*: Tortora and Derrickson, 2009. Reproduced with permission of John Wiley & Sons.

Question 6 In Table 5.2 identify the activity that takes places during the four stages of bone formation throughout a person's life.

Table 5.2 Bone formation throughout a person's life.

Stage	Activity
One	
Two	
Three	
Four	

Endochondral ossification

Endochondral ossification is key for the formation of long and short bones, and forms the ends of flat and irregular bones (such as ribs and irregular bones).

Question 7 In Figure 5.3, label the features that are associated with endochondral ossification, beginning with the development of cartilage model through to the formation of articular cartilage and epiphyseal plate.

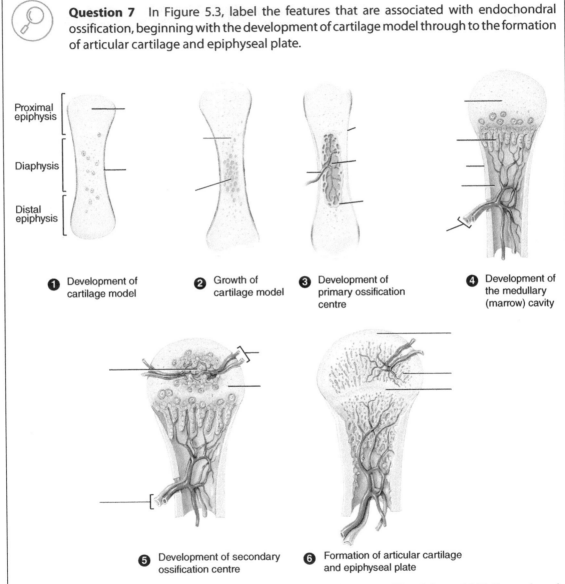

Proximal epiphysis

Diaphysis

Distal epiphysis

① Development of cartilage model

② Growth of cartilage model

③ Development of primary ossification centre

④ Development of the medullary (marrow) cavity

⑤ Development of secondary ossification centre

⑥ Formation of articular cartilage and epiphyseal plate

Figure 5.3   Endochondral ossification of the tibia. *Source*: Tortora and Derrickson, 2009. Reproduced with permission of John Wiley & Sons.

Question 8 Match the pairs.

Intramembranous and endochondral ossification are	mesenchyme connective tissue
Intramembranous ossification occurs	is key for the formation of long and short bones
In intramembranous ossification the bone is formed from	primarily during the initial formation of the flat bones of the skull, mandible and clavicles
Endochondral ossification	embryonic processes of bone formation
Natural healing of small bone fractures	bone growth during infancy, childhood and adolescence
The second stage of bone formation is associated with	is associated with endochondral ossification

Question 9 Time yourself to unscramble these words.

Scrambled	Answer
NOODLEDRANCH	
FOSISIACTION	
INTROREMABAMNUS	
BRICYOMEN	
SYPHIPEALE	
MYCHEMESEN	
BRUTALEACE	
SYPHISAID	

Bone remodelling and bone growth

Bone is a dynamic tissue, continuously being built, broken down and rebuilt in a process known as bone remodelling.

Question 10

(a) Label the component parts to include:

- bone lining cells
- macrophages
- osteoclast
- osteocyte

(b) Complete and colour in the process of bone remodelling.

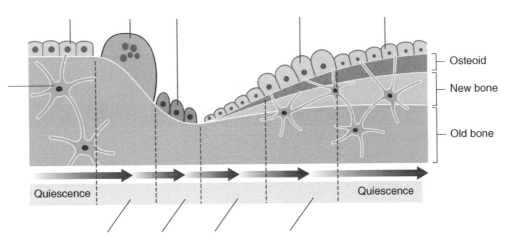

Figure 5.4   Bone remodelling. *Source*: Peate *et al.*, 2014. Reproduced with permission of John Wiley & Sons.

The interior of bone is made up of bone marrow, surrounded by cortical bone and trabecular bone. The basic unit of structure of compact bone is an osteon, comprising a Haversian canal and its concentrically arranged lamellae.

Question 11
(a) In Figure 5.5, label the various aspects of the Haversian canal.

(b) Colour in the blood vessels, trabeculae and other components.

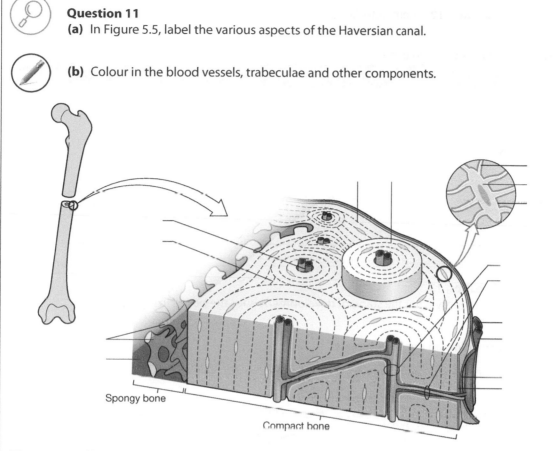

Spongy bone

Compact bone

Figure 5.5 Haversian canal. *Source*: Peate *et al.*, 2014. Reproduced with permission of John Wiley & Sons.

A fine balance exists between the breakdown and build up of bone; if bone is built up too quickly it forms thick and heavy bone. Weak bone or bone tissue loss may result in bone that breaks easily.

There are three types of cell present in bone: osteoblasts, osteocytes and osteoclasts.

Question 12 Complete Table 5.3.

Table 5.3 Types of cell in bone.

Cell	Description	Responsible for
Osteoblasts		
Osteocytes		
Osteoclasts		

 Question 13
(a) Identify what the stage of development is for the bones in Figure 5.6.

 (b) Colour in the growth plates.

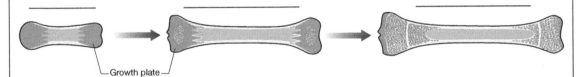

Growth plate

Figure 5.6 Bone growth. *Source*: Peate and Nair, 2015. Reproduced with permission of John Wiley & Sons.

 Question 14 Match the pairs.

Remodelling takes place	it is continuously built, broken down and rebuilt
Bone is dynamic	at different rates in different parts of the body
A fine balance must exist between	the breakdown and build up of bone
If bone is built up too quickly	remodelling
Weak bone, as a result of too much calcium or bone tissue loss, can result in	an abnormally thick and heavy bone will be formed
Bone resorption and formation is known as	bone that breaks easily

Question 15   Time yourself to unscramble these words.

Scrambled	Answer
GOLDLEMINER	
SORPITONER	
STOOLESTABS	
STOOLSTACES	
MALCUIC	
LOCLAGEN	
SHIVERAAN	
SEVERRAL	

Bone fractures

A fracture is the breakage of bone caused by injury or disease. The repair of a bone that has been fractured goes through a number of stages. Whilst bone has a good blood supply, healing may take many months to occur. The break in the bone interferes with blood supply to the bone temporarily, resulting in delayed healing.

Question 16   In Figure 5.7, identify the missing stages associated with bone fracture repair.

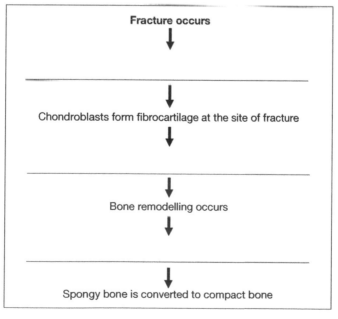

Figure 5.7   The stages of fracture repair.

Bone types, bone shapes

Bone types are classified according to shape and size of the bone; the shapes reflect their functions. When describing specific bones state the type of bone in relation to its shape: the scapula, for example, is a large, flat, triangular bone. Categories of bone include:

- long
- short
- flat
- irregular
- sesamoid

 Question 17 In Table 5.4 describe the bone and provide examples.

Table 5.4 Types of bone.

Type of bone	Description	Example
Long		
Short		
Flat		
Irregular		
Sesamoid		

Question 18

(a) Complete the captions for Figures 5.8, 5.9, 5.10, 5.11 and 5.12.

(b) Complete the labels for each of the bones.

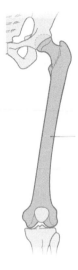

Figure 5.8 A _____ bone. *Source*: Peate and Nair, 2015. Reproduced with permission of John Wiley & Sons.

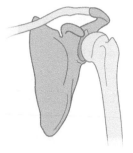

Figure 5.10 A _____ bone. *Source*: Peate and Nair, 2015. Reproduced with permission of John Wiley & Sons.

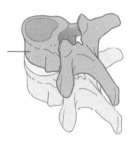

Figure 5.11 An _____ bone. *Source*: Peate 2015. Reproduced with permission of John Wiley & Sons.

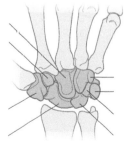

Figure 5.9 A _____ bone. *Source*: Peate and Nair, 2015. Reproduced with permission of John Wiley & Sons.

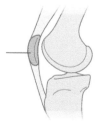

Figure 5.12 A _____ bone. *Source*: Peate and Nair, 2015. Reproduced with permission of John Wiley & Sons.

Question 19 Match the pairs.

Name of bone	Bone
Long bone	
Short bone	
Flat bone	
Irregular bone	
Sesamoid bone	

SCRAMBLE

Question 20   Time yourself to unscramble these words.

Scrambled	Answer
MACAPRETALS	
SOSIMADE	
DOBLASTSCROHN	
IBROCLEARAFITG	
FURCREAT	
PYONGS	
MOCAPCT	
DIHYO	

Joints

The skeleton permits movement; bones act as levers providing the transmission of muscular forces that are generated by skeletal muscles, through the work of the tendons and the ligaments. Movement becomes possible through articulation.

Question 21   In Table 5.5 describe the main types of movement.

Table 5.5   Joint movement.

Movement	Description
Flexion	
Extension	
Adduction	
Abduction	
Rotation	

Fibrous joints

These are also known as synarthrodial joints. They are held together by a ligament only. In this type of joint there is no synovial cavity.

Cartilaginous joints

These are also known as synchondroses. These are found where the connection between the articulating bones is made up of cartilage with no synovial cavity, such as those joints occurring between vertebrae in the spine.

Synovial joints

Also called diarthrosis joints, these are the most common types of joint. There are six types of freely moveable or synovial joints.

Question 22   Identify where in Figure 5.13 the following types of joint may be found:

- hinge
- pivot
- ball and socket
- saddle
- condyloid
- gliding.

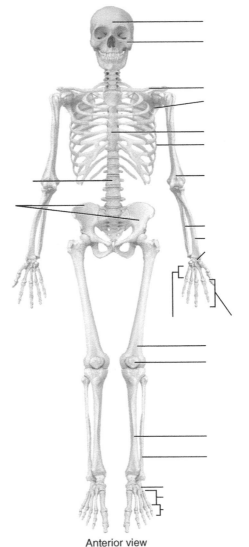

Anterior view

Figure 5.13   The skeleton (anterior view). *Source*: Tortora and Derrickson, 2009. Reproduced with permission of John Wiley & Sons.

Question 23   Match the pairs.

Type of joint	Examples		Structure
Hinge	The carpometacarpal joints of the thumb	Radius — Ulna, Trapezium, Metacarpal of thumb	
Pivot	Elbow, knee	Humerus, Trochlea, Trochlear notch, Ulna	
Ball and socket	Intertarsal and intercarpal joints of the hands and feet	Navicular, Second cuneiform, Third cuneiform	
Saddle	The radiocarpal and metacarpophalangeal joints of the hand	Radius — Ulna, Scaphoid — Lunate	
Condyloid	Radius and ulna, the atlas and axis	Radial notch, Head of radius, Annular ligament, Radius — Ulna	
Gliding	Hip, shoulder	Acetabulum of hip bone, Head of femur	

Source: Peate and Nair, 2015. Reproduced with permission of John Wiley & Sons.

Question 24   Time yourself to unscramble these words.

Scrambled	Answer
SEXTONIEN	
SOURFIB	
NOILSAVY	
MASSDOIE	
TOESCK	
HONEYSDROSSCN	
GEHIN	
LADDES	

Snap shot

Preventing osteoporosis

Lifestyle factors such as diet and exercise influence how healthy the bones are.

   Regular exercise is an essential activity in helping people to prevent osteoporosis. The role of the nurse is multifaceted and one aspect of this role is to help people live healthy lives and prevent potential problems. What advice would you give to an adult with regards to taking exercise?

Word search

H	Z	N	X	U	O	M	U	S	C	L	E	S	E	L	J	N	S	M	L
F	T	K	F	N	H	O	F	G	S	D	I	P	I	L	M	O	E	G	T
Y	X	Y	U	S	C	C	G	P	G	W	J	K	O	P	L	I	T	R	T
S	L	G	S	E	A	G	J	X	A	N	T	R	K	F	O	T	Y	X	S
S	W	L	I	T	R	D	O	N	P	S	N	Z	V	X	M	A	C	E	G
T	J	B	S	Y	T	H	W	T	D	U	O	S	E	H	J	C	O	N	C
S	F	W	A	C	I	A	P	Z	H	O	T	C	V	O	D	I	E	D	P
A	U	P	T	O	L	E	K	W	P	N	E	L	J	E	B	F	T	O	X
L	J	L	S	E	A	M	A	V	R	A	L	E	P	T	Y	I	S	C	U
B	E	I	O	T	G	A	L	Q	R	R	E	V	S	A	B	S	O	H	T
O	X	G	E	S	E	T	T	Z	U	B	K	E	M	L	S	S	J	O	Y
E	Z	A	M	O	W	O	O	Z	U	M	S	R	M	U	C	O	R	N	A
T	Y	M	O	L	S	P	V	U	Z	E	M	A	B	C	K	L	N	D	N
S	M	E	H	A	E	O	W	A	N	M	U	G	A	I	M	A	S	R	M
O	J	N	R	I	S	I	C	G	S	A	I	E	G	T	I	R	J	A	J
Q	S	T	R	X	A	E	I	H	Q	R	C	S	C	R	S	E	G	L	C
A	N	S	A	A	M	S	A	E	V	T	L	Z	Y	A	H	N	T	C	H
D	U	N	D	K	O	I	L	W	W	N	A	D	B	S	E	I	W	N	S
U	S	I	E	N	I	S	P	L	M	I	C	W	Z	L	Q	M	X	E	C
E	D	V	G	S	D	G	Q	A	P	P	E	N	D	I	C	U	L	A	R

SKELETON
MUSCLES
ARTICULATE
CARTILAGE
OSSIFICATION
APPENDICULAR
AXIAL

LEVERAGE
CALCIUM
HOMEOSTASIS
LIPIDS
HAEMATOPOIESIS
LIGAMENTS
MINERAL

INTRAMEMBRANOUS
ENDOCHONDRAL
OSTEOBLASTS
OSTEOCYTES
SESAMOID

Crossword

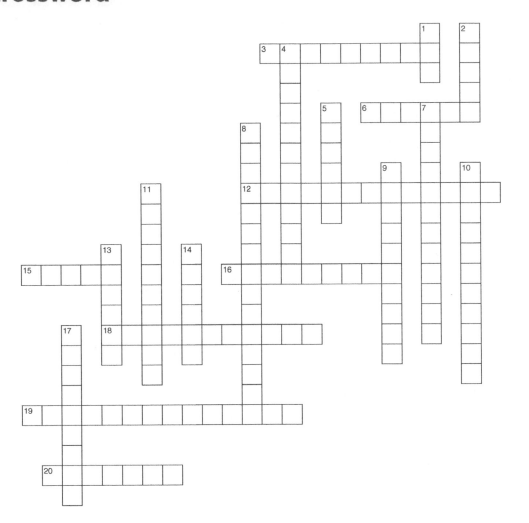

Across

3. Infants are born with large amounts of this
6. The skeletal system supports the body, providing a bony framework for the attachment of soft tissues and what else?
12. When old bone dies, other bone is being what?
15. Number of types of cell present in bone
16. Process of bone formation
18. Cells responsible for building new bone tissue
19. Activity which occurs mainly in red bone marrow
20. The most abundant mineral in the body

Down

1. The periosteum protects this bone marrow
2. These provide the body with its shape/form
4. One of the parts the skeleton is divided into for classification purposes
5. The stage of bone formation associated with bone growth during infancy, childhood and adolescence
7. Movement becomes possible through this
8. Type of ossification that occurs during the initial formation of the flat bones
9. Type of bone
10. Bone resorption and formation
11. Cells with responsibility for maintenance of bone
13. Lipids are stored in this colour bone marrow
14. The basic unit of structure of compact bone
17. Bones which protect the spinal cord

Fill in the blanks

Use the words in the box to complete the sentences:

abduction, adduction, angle, anti-clockwise, articulation, away, bending, body, bone, bone, bones, centre, elbow, extension, fibrous, fibrous, flexion, forces, generated, increasing, joints, knee, knee, leg, leg, levers, ligaments, movement, movement, muscle, muscles, rotation, shoulder, skeleton, stable, straightening, tendons, tissue, tissues, toes, towards, towards, transmission, turning, turning, twisting, types, work

1. The _____ permits _____ ; bones act as _____ providing the _____ of muscular _____ that are _____ by skeletal _____ , through the _____ of the _____ and the _____ . Movement becomes possible through _____ .

2. Tendons are _____ connective _____ attaching _____ to _____ ; they help to move the _____ or structure. Ligaments are _____ connective _____ attaching _____ to bones, holding structures together and keeping them _____ .

3. Different types of _____ provide different _____ of _____ ; the _____ joint, for example, moves in more ways than the _____ does.

4. Reducing the _____ at the joint, _____ the knee or _____ , is _____ . _____ the angle at the joint, for example, _____ the _____ or elbow, is _____ . Moving the _____ part _____ the centre of the body, for example bringing one leg in _____ the other, is _____ . Moving the body part _____ from the _____ of the body, taking one _____ away from the other, is _____ . _____ or _____ a body part, either clockwise or _____ , for example, _____ the _____ to point the _____ outwards, is _____ .

Multiple choice questions

1. What is an osteophyte?

(a) A bone cell
(b) A small bony outgrowth
(c) A bone cancer cell
(d) A lymph cell

2. Where is the medial malleolus located?

(a) The hip
(b) In the thoracic cavity
(c) The fibula
(d) The cranium

3. What is the clavicle is also known as?

(a) The rib
(b) The breast bone
(c) The collar bone
(d) The pelvis

4. What does kinesiology mean?

(a) The study of light
(b) The study of brain
(c) The study of art
(d) The study of movement of the body

5. What are joints that permit free movement known as?

(a) Diarthroses
(b) Haemathroses
(c) Synarthroses
(d) Amphiarthroses

6. When do muscle cells use the anaerobic process of glycolysis?

(a) The mitrochondria lack sufficient oxygen to meet ATP demands
(b) At moderate levels of physical activity
(c) When muscle fatigue occurs
(d) For producing lactic acid

7. How do cardiac muscles differ from skeletal muscle fibres?

(a) They have a greater reliance on anaerobic metabolism
(b) They are larger than skeletal muscles
(c) They can undergo tetanus
(d) They do not require neural stimulation to contract

8. The muscular system

(a) Can work independently of other body systems
(b) Contains approximately 700 muscles that can be voluntarily controlled
(c) Will hypertrophy if not used regularly
(d) Does not play a role in controlling body temperature

9. What are the three types of muscles tissue?

(a) Fibrous, elastic, collagen
(b) Endomysium, epimysium, perimysium
(c) Resting, involuntary, voluntary
(d) Cardiac, smooth, skeletal

10. Cardiac muscle can contract without neural stimulation because it has the following property

(a) Plasticity
(b) Excitability
(c) Pacesetting
(d) Automacity

References

Peate, I. and Nair, M. (2015) *Anatomy and Physiology for Nurses at a Glance*. Oxford: John Wiley & Sons, Ltd.
Peate, I, Wild, K. and Nair, M. (eds) (2014) *Nursing Practice: Knowledge and Care*. Oxford: John Wiley & Sons, Ltd.
Tortora, G.J. and Derrickson, B.H. (2009) *Principles of Anatomy and Physiology*, 12th edn. Hoboken, NJ: John Wiley & Sons, Inc.

Chapter 6

The muscular system

Muscular activity is required for the body to undertake all physical function; all body movement is a result of muscular activity. This chapter concentrates predominantly on skeletal muscle.

Whilst it is the bones that provide the framework and leverage for the body, it is the muscles that pull the bones. Muscles can only pull, they cannot push. Bones cannot move body parts. Muscles contract and move the walls of the viscera and of blood vessels; cardiac muscle makes the heart beat. Energy is turned into locomotion by the muscles, helping to drive the body. If we did not have muscles we would not be able to do anything; without muscles we would not be able to move, we would be unable to blink, unable to swallow, inhale and exhale, we could not smile or frown.

Muscle tissue

The body contains three types of muscle tissue:

1. smooth
2. cardiac
3. skeletal.

Fundamentals of Anatomy and Physiology Workbook: A Study Guide for Nursing and Healthcare Students, First Edition. Ian Peate.
© 2017 John Wiley & Sons Ltd. Published 2017 by John Wiley & Sons Ltd.

Question 1   Identify the types of muscle and label the component parts.

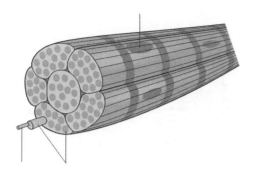

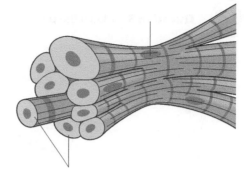

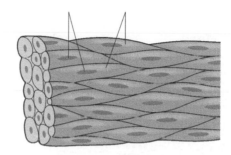

Figure 6.1 Types of muscle. *Source*: Peate and Nair, 2015. Reproduced with permission of John Wiley & Sons.

Question 2   Complete Table 6.1 with regard to the three types of muscle. For each muscle describe where the muscle is located, the type of cell, if the muscle is striated or non-striated and how it is controlled.

Table 6.1   Types of muscle tissue.

	Skeletal muscle	Smooth muscle	Cardiac muscle
Location			
Cell type			
Striation/non-striation			
Control			

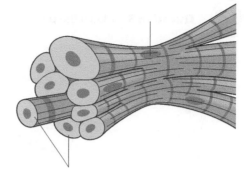

Question 3   Match the pairs.

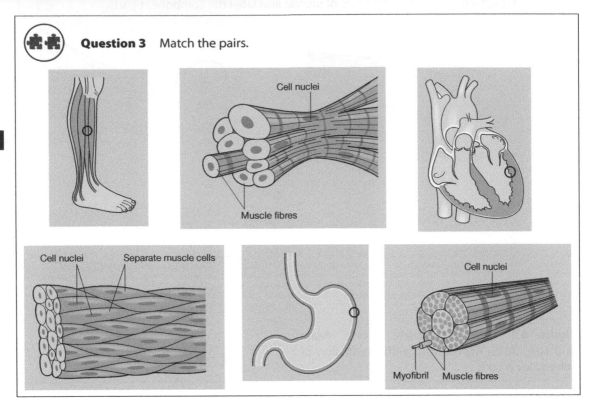

Functions of the muscular system

The muscular system has five important roles to play:

1. maintains posture
2. produces movement
3. stabilises joints
4. protection of internal structures
5. generates heat as it contracts

Maintenance of body posture

Notwithstanding the continuous downward pull of gravity, the body maintains an erect or seated posture as a result of the continuous small adjustments made by the skeletal muscles.

Production of movement

The ability to mobilise is a result of skeletal muscle activity and muscle contraction. When muscles contract they pull on the tendons and bones of the skeleton, producing movement.

Stabilisation of joints

Muscle tendons play a key role in stabilising and reinforcing the joints of the body. During movement, skeletal muscles pull on bones stabilising the joints of the skeleton.

Protection and control of internal tissue structures/organs

Skeletal muscle plays an essential part in protecting the internal organs as the visceral organs and internal tissues in the abdominal cavity are protected by layers of skeletal tissue in the abdominal wall and floor of the pelvic cavity.

Generation of heat

Heat generation is key in maintaining normal body temperature. Skeletal muscles account for 40% of the body's mass. They are the muscle type mainly responsible for the generation of body heat.

Properties of muscle tissue

 Question 4   There are four properties of muscle tissue. Describe them in Table 6.2.

Table 6.2   Muscle properties.

Property	Description
Excitability (irritability)	
Contractility	
Extensibility	
Elasticity	

 Question 5   Time yourself to unscramble these words.

Scrambled	Answer
LICROE	
GENERY	
TEENSTIBLIXIY	
BRITRIITILAY	
NATIONCORTC	
COMINTOLOO	
VOMMENTE	
LYNDACIRCIL	

Skeletal muscle

The most abundant type of muscle tissue in the body is skeletal.

Muscles contain other types of tissues, for example, blood vessels, connective and nervous tissue, and as such they are considered to be organs. Each cell in skeletal muscle tissue is a single muscle fibre; due to their large size they contain hundreds of nuclei.

Gross anatomy of skeletal muscle

Muscle is separated from skin by the hypodermis consisting of adipose tissue and a dense, broad band of connective tissues (fascia) supporting and surrounding muscle tissue, providing a pathway for nerves, lymphatic and blood vessels to enter and exit a muscle. Extending from the fascia are three layers of connective tissue, playing a role in supporting and protecting the muscle. These ensure that the force of contraction from each muscle cell is transmitted to its points of attachment to the skeleton. The three layers of connective tissue are:

1. epimysium: wrapped around the whole muscle
2. perimysium: surrounds bundles of muscle fibres (fascicles)
3. endomysium: covers each individual muscle cell.

Question 6
(a) Identify the gross component parts of the skeletal muscle in Figure 6.2.

(b) Colour in the bone, tendon, epimysium, periosteum; also colour in the fascicle.

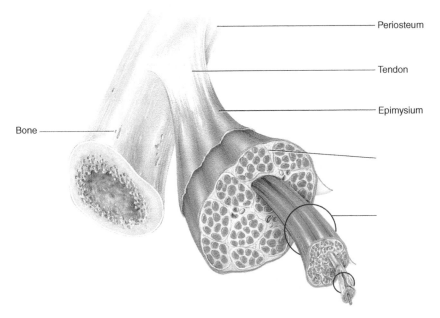

Periosteum

Tendon

Epimysium

Bone

Figure 6.2 Gross anatomy of a skeletal muscle. *Source*: Tortora and Derrickson, 2009. Reproduced with permission of John Wiley & Sons.

Microanatomy of skeletal muscle

Microscopically, skeletal muscle cells appear cylindrical in shape, have a distinctive banded appearance of alternate light and dark stripes and lie parallel to each other.

The sarcolemma and transverse tubules

Each muscle fibre is covered by a plasma membrane, the sarcolemma. Openings in the sarcolemma are connected to transverse tubules filled with extracellular fluid.

The sarcoplasm

This contains multiple mitochondria producing large amounts of ATP during muscle contraction. It is here that the transverse tubules make contact with the sarcoplasmic reticulum (SR). The SR stores calcium ions (in cisternae) and myoglobin, which holds oxygen until needed to generate ATP.

The myofibrils

Myofibrils (bundles of myofilaments) are thread-like structures found in abundance in the sarcoplasm. The myofibrils play a central role in the muscle contraction mechanism. They contain two types of protein filaments – thick filaments composed of myosin, and thin filaments composed of actin and the proteins, tropomyosin and troponin.

Sarcomeres

These are the basic functional units of striated muscle fibres. Extending across each of the thick filaments within the sarcomere is a dark area known as the A band, in the centre of which is a narrow H zone. On either side of the A band is a lighter coloured area consisting of thin filaments known as the I band. The alternating A and I bands give skeletal muscles their striated appearance.

Question 7   Identify the microscopic parts of the skeletal muscle in Figure 6.3.

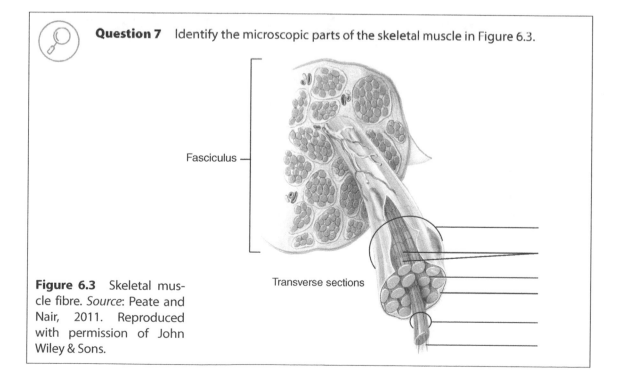

Fasciculus

Transverse sections

Figure 6.3   Skeletal muscle fibre. *Source*: Peate and Nair, 2011. Reproduced with permission of John Wiley & Sons.

Question 8   Match the pairs.

Muscles contain other types of tissues, for example, blood vessels, connective and nervous tissue	they contain hundreds of nuclei
Each cell in skeletal muscle tissue is a single muscle fibre	they have a distinctive banded appearance and lie parallel to each other
Microscopically, skeletal muscle cells appear cylindrical in shape	they are considered to be organs
Each muscle fibre is covered by a plasma membrane, the sarcolemma, and contain cylindrical structures. the myofibrils. These are	the A band in the centre of which is a narrow H zone
The myofibrils play a central role in the muscle contraction mechanism	they contain two types of protein filaments
Extending across each of the thick filaments within the sarcomere is a dark area known as	suspended inside the muscle fibre, extending along its length

Question 9   Time yourself to unscramble these words.

Scrambled	Answer
SELFICCAS	
FOYLISBRIM	
CAROLEMMAS	
SYDNEMOMIU	
MUISYMIPE	
PURIMSMIEY	
TRAINCSEE	
BOYGOMLIN	

Types of muscle fibre

Three types of muscle fibre are found in skeletal muscles, in varying amounts throughout the body.

Question 10 The three fibres are listed In Table 6.3. Provide a description of the fibres and their functions.

Table 6.3 Types of muscle fibre.

Fibre	Description
Slow oxidative (SO)	
Fast oxidative–glycolytic (FOG)	
Fast glycolytic (FG)	

Skeletal muscle contraction and relaxation

Contraction of skeletal muscle is controlled by the nervous system. Each muscle fibre is controlled by a motor neurone that can stimulate a few muscle cells or several hundred, depending on the muscle and the work it does. Skeletal muscle contracts in response to stimulation by a muscle action potential delivered by the motor neurone. The motor neurone connects to the muscle cell at the neuromuscular junction, where the muscle fibre membrane is specialised to form a motor end plate.

A muscle fibre normally has a single motor end plate, the densely branched motor neurone axons mean that one motor neurone axon can connect and control many muscle fibres. The motor neurone and the muscle fibres it controls are known as a motor unit.

Question 11

(a) In Figure 6.4, identify the nine phases of muscle contraction and relaxation. Two phases (4 and 7) have already been completed for you.

(b) Colour in the component parts of the contraction and relaxation cycle.

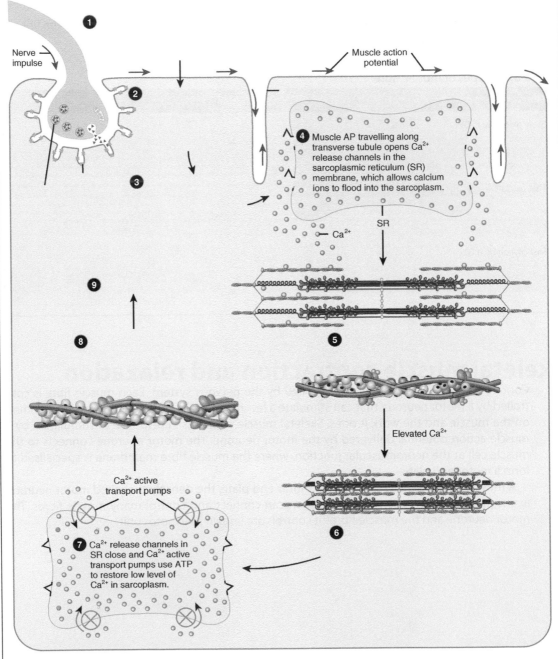

Figure 6.4 Muscle contraction and relaxation. *Source*: Tortora and Derrickson, 2009. Reproduced with permission of John Wiley & Sons.

Question 12   Match the pairs.

Acetylcholine when released	a motor unit
As a nerve impulse reaches the axon terminals	and motor end plate contain acetylcholinesterase
The synaptic cleft	acetylcholine is released into the synaptic cleft
The motor neurone and the muscle fibres it controls are known as	causes changes to the sarcolemma, triggering contraction of the muscle fibre
The densely branched motor neurone axons mean that	stimulation by muscle action potential
Skeletal muscle contracts in response to	one motor neurone axon can connect and control many muscle fibres

 Question 13   Time yourself to unscramble these words.

Scrambled	Answer
SLUMPIE	
PSYICTAN	
FELTC	
ACEHYLINECOLT	
TOONCRACTIN	
LATENTPOI	
UJONCITO	
SLITMANER	

Organisation of the skeletal muscular system

All skeletal muscles are attached at a minimum of two points to bone or other connective tissue. When one part of the skeleton is moved by muscle contraction, related parts are steadied by other muscles for movement to be effective.

Muscles can be named according to size, shape, location and number of origins, associated bones and the action of the muscle.

Question 14 Table 6.4 provides examples of the criteria used to name muscles. Complete the table. Some elements of the table have been completed. The character/term column is fully complete.

Table 6.4

Character/Term	Definition	Example
DIRECTION Transverse Oblique Rectus		Transversus abdominis External oblique Rectus abdominis
SHAPE Trapezius Deltoid Obicularis Rhomboid Platys	Trapezoid Triangular Circular Diamond-shaped Flat	
SIZE Major Minor Maximus Minimus Longus Latissimus		Pectoralis major Pectoralis minor Gluteus maximus Gluteus minimus Adductor longus Latissimus dorsi
NUMBER OF ORIGINS Biceps Triceps Quadriceps	Two origins Three origins Four origins	

The skeletal muscles can be divided into four areas:

1. head and neck muscles
2. muscles of the upper limbs (shoulder, arm, forearm)
3. trunk (thorax and abdomen)
4. muscles of the lower limbs (hip, pelvis/thigh, leg).

Question 15   The body's skeletal muscles can be divided into four areas. List these below:

_____

_____

_____

_____

(b) Indicate these areas on the anterior and posterior views of the body in Figure 6.5.

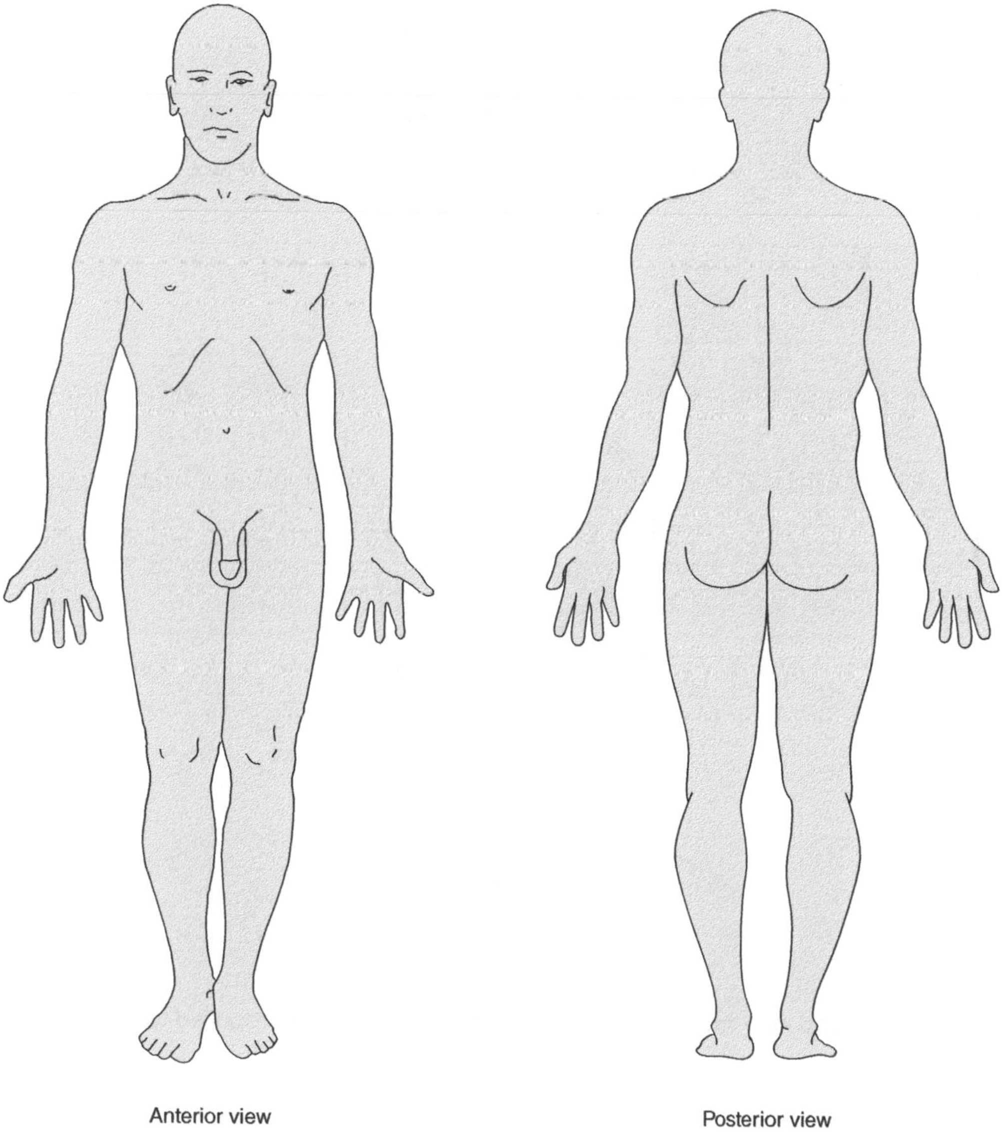

Anterior view   Posterior view

Figure 6.5   The four muscle areas.

Question 16 In Figures 6.6, 6.7, 6.8 and 6.9, identify the various muscles.

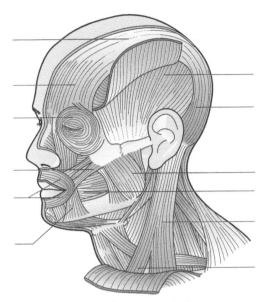

An anterior and lateral view

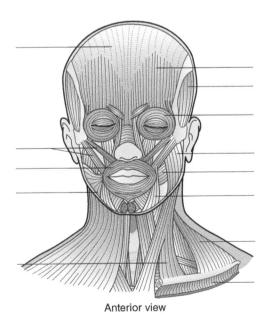

Anterior view

Figure 6.6 Head and neck muscles. *Source*: Peate and Nair, 2011. Reproduced with permission of John Wiley & Sons.

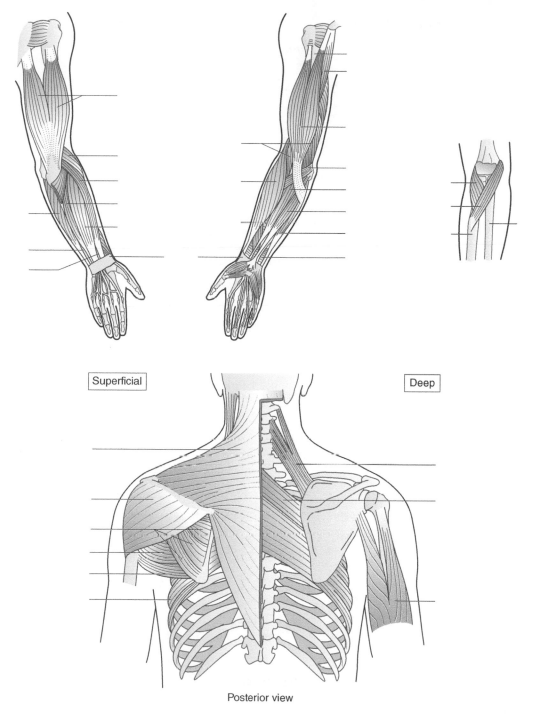

Superficial

Deep

Posterior view

Figure 6.7   Muscles of the upper limbs (shoulder, arm and hand). *Source*: Peate and Nair, 2011. Reproduced with permission of John Wiley & Sons.

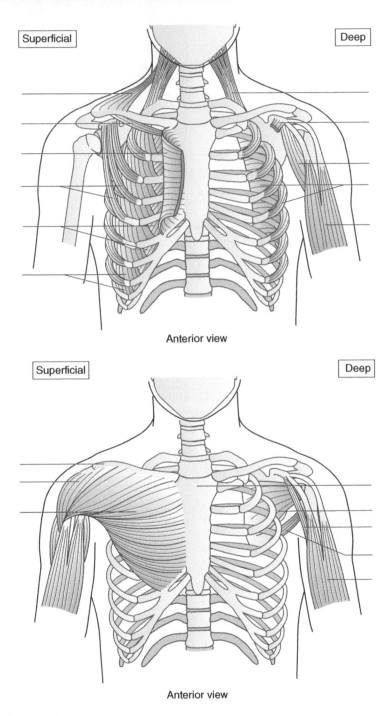

Figure 6.7 (*Continued*)

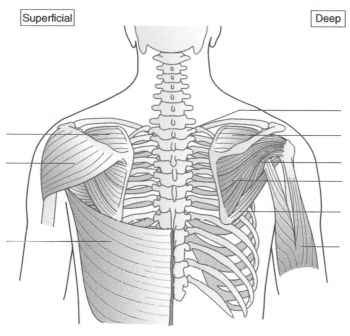

Posterior view

Figure 6.7   (*Continued*)

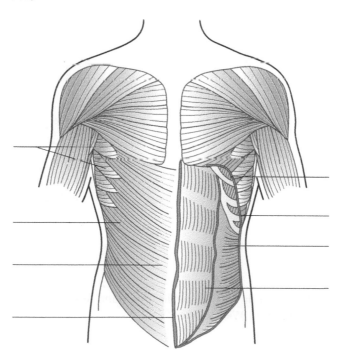

Figure 6.8   Trunk (thorax and abdomen). *Source*: Peate and Nair, 2011. Reproduced with permission of John Wiley & Sons.

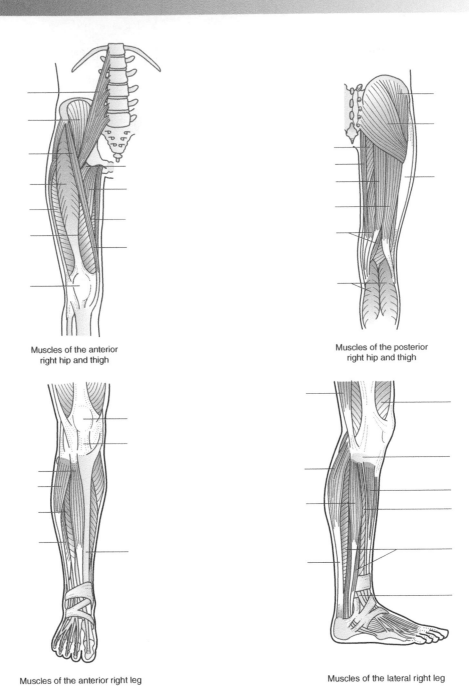

Muscles of the anterior
right hip and thigh

Muscles of the posterior
right hip and thigh

Muscles of the anterior right leg

Muscles of the lateral right leg

Figure 6.9 Muscles of the lower limbs (hip, pelvis, thigh and leg). *Source*: Peate and Nair, 2011. Reproduced with permission of John Wiley & Sons.

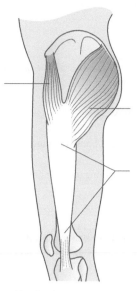

Muscles that move the thigh

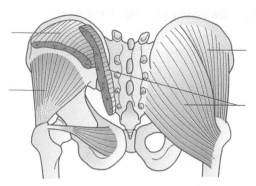

The gluteal muscle group

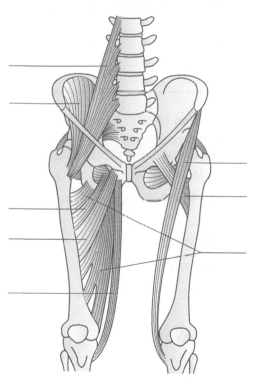

The iliopsoas muscle and the adductor group

Figure 6.9   (*Continued*)

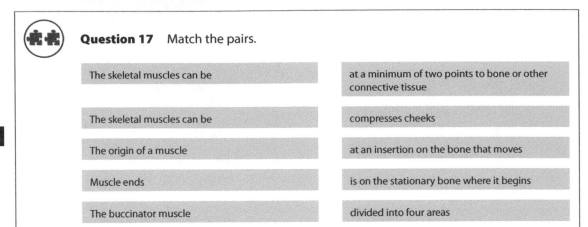

Question 17   Match the pairs.

The skeletal muscles can be	at a minimum of two points to bone or other connective tissue
The skeletal muscles can be	compresses cheeks
The origin of a muscle	at an insertion on the bone that moves
Muscle ends	is on the stationary bone where it begins
The buccinator muscle	divided into four areas
All skeletal muscles are attached	named according to size, shape, location and number of origins, associated bones and the action of the muscle

Question 18   Time yourself to unscramble these words.

Scrambled	Answer
CUBARINCTO	
ALANACOMIT	
LUGALTE	
STRAVENSER	
LARCRUCI	
PECSTRI	
CIBEPS	
TRACODDU	

Skeletal muscle movement

Common types of body movements are detailed in Table 6.5.

 Question 19   Complete Table 6.5, defining the different actions of muscle movement.

Table 6.5   Types of muscle movement.

Action	Definition
Extension	
Flexion	
Abduction	
Adduction	
Circumduction	
Supination	
Pronation	
Plantar flexion	
Dorsiflexion	
Rotation	

Question 20   Match the pairs.

Two opposing muscles are called	may cause an arm to bend
An agonist is also called	will cause an arm to straighten
Prime movers are	causes muscle movement in the opposite direction
An antagonist of a prime mover	mainly responsible for producing an action
An agonist	agonist and antagonist
The antagonist	a prime mover

Question 21   Time yourself to unscramble these words.

Scrambled	Answer
GNATOIS	
RIPEM	
GIANTASTON	
TRAITOON	
ELFIXON	
STENEXION	
DIMNILE	
PARTNAL	

Snap shot

Intramuscular injection

You have been asked to administer an intramuscular injection under supervision. Your mentor has explained to you that an intramuscular injection is given directly into a selected muscle and you are being asked to administer it into the gluteus medius (ventrogluteal site) muscle which runs beneath the gluteus maximus from the ilium to the femur.

The injection is given into the upper outer quadrant of the buttock. Where on this diagram would you inject?

Why is this?

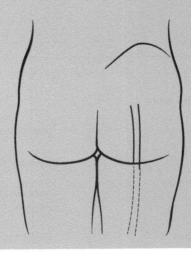

Word search

Z	R	B	N	K	M	A	B	N	H	P	I	Q	O	X	V	Y	Z	H	S
K	R	O	T	A	N	I	C	C	U	B	E	E	D	J	Q	U	E	D	E
O	A	C	A	I	D	R	A	C	M	N	W	R	O	C	T	F	Y	G	G
T	W	C	S	R	S	M	O	O	T	H	Z	I	I	E	Y	J	Q	T	J
F	W	H	E	L	W	Z	P	R	W	P	N	M	C	M	N	G	S	X	U
H	A	E	L	T	R	V	H	L	F	T	Y	T	D	S	Y	I	P	L	N
Y	A	S	C	H	Y	I	E	L	S	O	J	M	J	G	N	S	Z	P	G
T	F	N	S	C	F	L	Q	Q	F	N	P	E	R	O	L	L	I	B	V
I	K	O	U	K	O	T	C	I	A	J	N	E	G	P	Z	O	X	U	B
L	E	D	M	W	V	N	B	H	Q	D	N	A	A	P	T	C	J	F	M
I	P	N	K	Q	J	R	D	C	O	E	D	J	S	X	K	O	M	E	I
T	I	E	H	D	I	A	J	M	M	L	W	P	I	Q	I	M	C	R	L
C	M	T	P	L	L	R	Y	E	O	H	I	J	X	S	W	O	C	E	A
A	Y	Z	S	R	W	S	K	T	B	V	C	N	J	X	Y	T	X	M	T
R	S	N	D	S	I	T	R	G	F	N	E	T	E	K	Z	I	N	O	E
T	I	C	D	U	D	U	B	O	C	M	H	M	X	G	T	O	S	C	L
N	U	E	M	P	E	P	R	K	T	L	A	A	E	A	I	N	M	R	E
O	M	A	B	L	E	Q	S	N	U	C	L	F	I	N	A	T	C	A	K
C	J	D	E	J	T	S	I	N	O	G	A	T	N	A	T	R	V	S	S
N	O	D	M	S	Y	N	A	P	T	I	C	Y	Q	E	P	J	H	U	S

MUSCLES	TENDONS	PERIMYSIUM
ENERGY	ACETYLCHOLINE	ENDOMYSIUM
SMOOTH	SYNAPTIC	MYOFIBRILS
CARDIAC	CONTRACTILITY	SARCOMERE
SKELETAL	LOCOMOTION	BUCCINATOR
JOINTS	NUCLEI	ANTAGONIST
MOVEMENT	EPIMYSIUM	AGONIST

Crossword

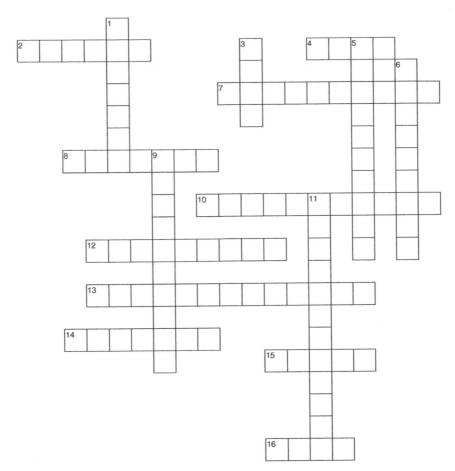

Across

2. Each cell in skeletal muscle tissue contains hundreds of these

4. Muscles generate this as they contract

7. Turning up the palm of the hand

8. These pull the bones

10. Microscopically, skeletal muscle cells appear to be this shape

12. This is wrapped around the whole muscle

13. The ability of muscle to shorten

14. Intramuscular injections can be given into the upper outer quadrant of what aspect of the body?

15. The buccinator muscle compresses what part of the body?

16. All skeletal muscles are attached at a minimum of two points to other connective tissue and what else?

Down

1. When muscles contract they pull on the bones and what else?

3. Number of areas the skeletal muscles can be divided into

5. There are usually at least two opposing muscles acting on a joint; one is an agonist, what is the other?

6. Skeletal muscle is under this type of control

9. Energy is turned into this by the muscles

11. Elevation of the foot

Fill in the blanks

Use the words in the box to complete the sentences.

abdominal, action, adenosine, adjustments, agonist, antagonist, antagonist, attached, blood, body, body, bone, bone, bones, bones, bones, bones, cavity, continuous, contract, contract, contraction, contraction, contraction, contraction, direction, downward, drive, ends, energy, erect, framework, generation, generation, gravity, heart, heat, joint, joints, layers, location, locomotion, maintaining, mobilise, move, movement, movement, movement, mover, muscle, muscle, muscles, opposite, organs, origin, pelvic, points, posture, prime, protecting, pull, push, release, size, skeletal, skeletal, stabilising, stationary, steadied, temperature, tendons, tendons, tissue, tissues, two

1. It is the _____ that provide the _____ and leverage for the _____ . The muscles _____ the bones; they can only pull, they cannot _____ . Bones cannot _____ body parts. Muscles _____ and move the walls of viscera and _____ vessels, cardiac _____ makes the _____ beat. Energy is turned into _____ by the muscles, helping to _____ the body.

2. Notwithstanding the continuous _____ pull of _____ , the body maintains an _____ or seated _____ as a result of the _____ small _____ made by the skeletal muscles. The ability to _____ occurs as a result of skeletal muscle activity and muscle _____ . When muscles _____ they pull on the _____ and _____ of the skeleton producing _____ .

3. Muscle _____ play a role in _____ and reinforcing the joints. During movement _____ muscles pull on _____ stabilising the _____ of the skeleton. Skeletal muscle plays a key part in _____ the internal _____ , as the visceral organs and internal _____ in the abdominal _____ are protected by _____ of skeletal tissue inside the _____ wall and floor of the _____ cavity.

4. Heat _____ is essential in _____ normal body _____ . Skeletal _____ account for 40% of _____ mass, they are the _____ type primarily responsible for the generation of body heat. During muscle _____ , _____ triphosphate is used to _____ the energy, with about 75% of its _____ escaping as _____ .

5. All _____ muscles are _____ at a minimum of two _____ to _____ or other connective _____ . When one part of the skeleton is moved by muscle _____ , related parts are _____ by other muscles for _____ to be effective. The _____ of a muscle is on the _____ bone where it begins, and the muscle _____ at an insertion on the _____ that moves. Muscles can be named according to _____ , shape, _____ and number of origins, associated _____ and the action of the muscle.

6. There are usually at least _____ opposing muscles, _____ and _____ , acting on a _____ bringing about movement in _____ directions. An agonist or _____ _____ is a muscle mainly responsible for producing an _____ ; an _____ of a prime mover causes muscle _____ in the opposite _____ .

Multiple choice questions

1. Which of the following is a function of the muscular system?

   (a) Produces movement
   (b) Provides enzymes
   (c) Decreases bone build up
   (d) Reduces movement

2. Which of the following is NOT a trait of muscle cells?

   (a) Reactivation
   (b) Deactivation
   (c) Motility
   (d) Osmosis

3. By what are muscles are attached to bones?

   (a) Osteophytes
   (b) Tendons
   (c) Spurs
   (d) Ligaments

4. Choose the term that describes muscles that oppose one another.

   (a) Synergistic
   (b) Dependable
   (c) Reliable
   (d) Antagonistic

5. What is the term for the end of the muscle that is attached to the bone that moves?

   (a) Point of origin
   (b) Insertion
   (c) Detraction
   (d) Deduction

6. What is the contractile unit of skeletal muscle called?

   (a) Sarcomere
   (b) Glia
   (c) Neuron
   (d) Actin

7. The striated, or striped, appearance of skeletal muscles is caused by which of the following?

   (a) Heat
   (b) Myofibrils
   (c) Actin
   (d) ATP

8. What is the first energy source for muscle contraction at the molecular level?

(a) Vitamin D
(b) Calcium
(c) ATP
(d) None of the above

9. What is the junction between a motor neurone and a muscle cell called?

(a) Neuromuscular junction
(b) Sinus
(c) Fistula
(d) All of the above

10. The strength of a contraction depends upon the number of what?

(a) Motor units
(b) Twitch
(c) ATP
(d) Anaerobes

References

Peate, I. and Nair, M. (2011) *Fundamentals of Anatomy and Physiology for Student Nurses*. Oxford: John Wiley & Sons, Ltd.

Peate, I. and Nair, M. (2015) *Anatomy and Physiology for Nurses at a Glance*. Oxford: John Wiley & Sons, Ltd.

Tortora, G.J. and Derrickson, B.H. (2009) *Principles of Anatomy and Physiology*, 12th edn. Hoboken, NJ: John Wiley & Sons, Inc.

Chapter 7

Circulatory system

The circulatory system includes the heart, the blood, the blood vessels and the lymphatic system. The blood vessels transport blood throughout the body. Blood consists of formed elements and a fluid portion – plasma. The blood vessels form a network permitting blood to flow from the heart to all living cells and back to the heart. Blood has many functions, including transportation of nutrients, respiratory gases such as oxygen and carbon dioxide, metabolic waste such as urea and uric acid, hormones, electrolytes and antibodies. Circulation of blood occurs through a network of blood vessels leading away from and returning to the heart.

Question 1
(a) Identify the formed elements of blood in Figure 7.1.

(b) Colour in the formed elements of blood.

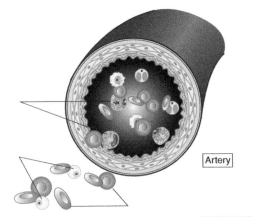

Artery

Figure 7.1 The formed elements of blood. *Source*: Peate and Nair, 2011. Reproduced with permission of John Wiley & Sons.

Fundamentals of Anatomy and Physiology Workbook: A Study Guide for Nursing and Healthcare Students, First Edition. Ian Peate.
© 2017 John Wiley & Sons Ltd. Published 2017 by John Wiley & Sons Ltd.

Blood

Blood is a fluid connective tissue consisting of formed elements such as red blood cells (RBC), white blood cells (WBC) and platelets, and a fluid portion, plasma.

When a sample of blood is centrifuged, the formed elements account for 45% of the blood, plasma makes up 55% of the total blood volume. Unless a person has a physiological problem, for example haemorrhage, the volume of blood is constant.

Question 2

(a) Look at Figure 7.2 and identify the components of blood including percentages.

(b) Colour in the formed elements of the blood.

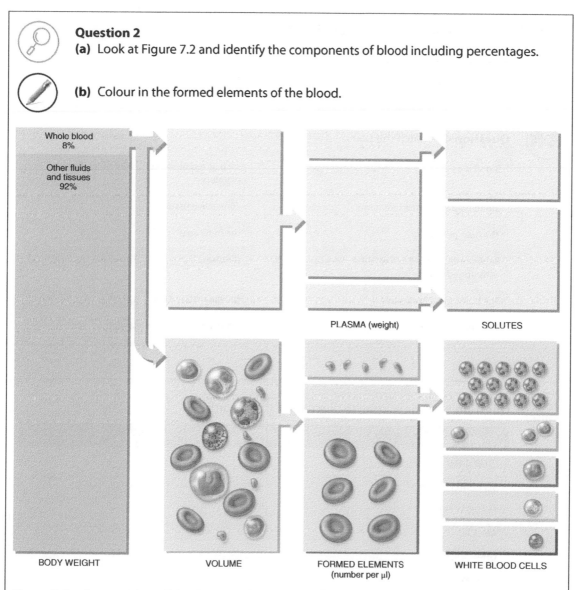

Whole blood
8%

Other fluids
and tissues
92%

PLASMA (weight)

SOLUTES

BODY WEIGHT

VOLUME

FORMED ELEMENTS
(number per μl)

WHITE BLOOD CELLS

Figure 7.2 Composition of blood. *Source*: Tortora and Derrickson, 2009. Reproduced with permission of John Wiley & Sons.

Question 3
(a) In Figure 7.3, identify the elements of the test tube, also attach percentage values.

(b) Colour in the elements of the test tube.

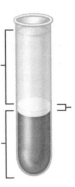

Figure 7.3 The appearance of centrifuged blood.
Source: Tortora and Derrickson, 2009. Reproduced with permission of John Wiley & Sons.

Question 4 Match the pairs.

Blood is a fluid	such as red blood cells, white blood cells, platelets
Blood contains formed elements	connective tissue
The fluid portion is	the buffy coat
Between the plasma and erythrocytes in a centrifuged sample lies	plasma
The buffy coat consists of	the haematocrit
The percentage of the formed elements is	white blood cells and platelets

Question 5 Time yourself to unscramble these words.

Scrambled	Answer
CHATTIAMORE	
SLEEPTALT	
EYESTRYCORTH	
AMSLAP	
GHARAHOREEM	
STEELMEN	
PHYML	
CLLES	

The functions of blood

 Question 6   Blood has a number of functions. Describe these functions in Table 7.1.

Table 7.1   The functions of blood.

Function	Description
Transportation	
Maintaining body temperature	
Maintaining the acid–base balance	
Regulation of fluid balance	
Removal of waste products	
Blood clotting	
Defence action	

The formation of blood cells

The process by which formed elements of blood develop is known as haemopoiesis. In the last 3 months of gestation and throughout life the red bone marrow is the primary centre for haemopoiesis.

Question 7

(a) In Figure 7.4, identify the blood cells that have been developed from the initial multipotent stem cell.

(b) Colour in the final layer of cells, the red cells, the granular leucocytes and the agranular leucocytes.

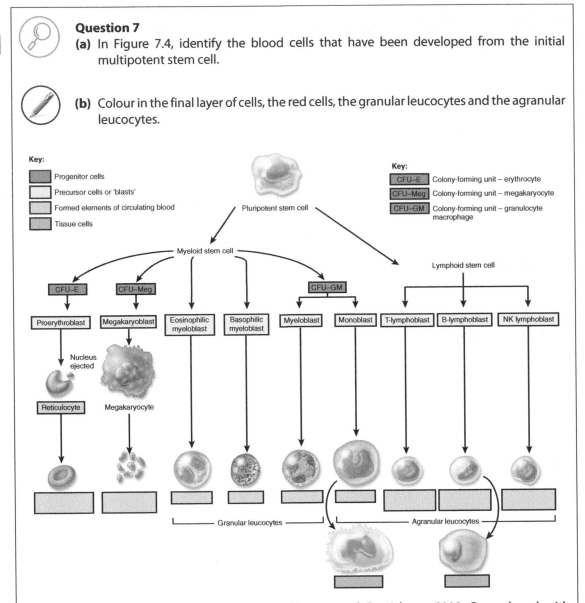

Figure 7.4 Blood cell development. *Source*: Tortora and Derrickson, 2009. Reproduced with permission of John Wiley & Sons.

Question 8   Match the pairs.

Blood helps to maintain the body temperature by	erythrocytes
By the mechanism of clotting	in order to produce blood cells
The process by which formed elements of blood develop is known as	haemopoiesis
Multipotent stem cells divide into myeloid and lymphoid stem cells in the bone marrow	loss of blood cells and body fluids is prevented
Myeloid stem cells further subdivide in the bone marrow producing	in the thymus and may then migrate to other lymph tissues
T-lymphocytes continue their development	distributing heat produced by chemical activity of cells evenly, throughout the body

Question 9   Time yourself to unscramble these words.

Scrambled	Answer
TIPTOENUTML	
METS	
ORWARM	
DIMELOY	
PHYMODIL	
GCLINTTO	
NOIS	

Red blood cells

The most abundant blood cells are the erythrocytes; they are biconcave discs containing the oxygen-carrying protein, haemoglobin. They live for around 120 days. Young red blood cells contain a nucleus; however, in a mature red blood cell the nucleus is absent, increasing the oxygen-carrying capacity of the red blood cell.

Question 10

(a) Identify the surface view and the sectioned view in Figure 7.5.

(b) Colour in the cell.

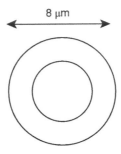

8 µm

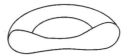

Figure 7.5 The bi-concave red cell. *Source*: Tortora and Derrickson, 2009. Reproduced with permission of John Wiley & Sons.

Question 11   Identify the missing words in Figure 7.6.

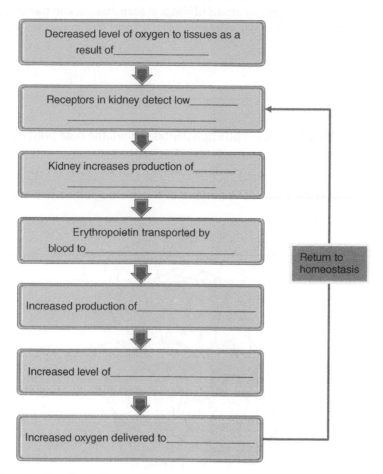

Figure 7.6   Negative feedback for erythropoiesis. *Source*: Peate and Nair, 2011. Reproduced with permission of John Wiley & Sons.

Haemoglobin

Haemoglobin is composed of the protein, globin, bound to iron-containing pigments called haem. Each globin molecule has four polypeptide chains consisting of two alpha and two beta chains. Each haemoglobin molecule has four atoms of iron and each atom of iron transports one molecule of oxygen, hence one molecule of haemoglobin will transport four molecules of oxygen.

Question 12
(a) In Figure 7.7, identify the alpha polypeptide chain, the beta polypeptide chain, iron molecules and the oxygen molecules attached to iron.

(b) Now colour in the various components of the haemoglobin molecule.

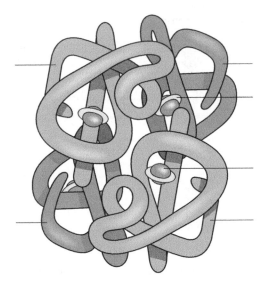

Figure 7.7   The haemoglobin molecule. *Source*: Peate and Nair, 2015. Reproduced with permission of John Wiley & Sons.

White blood cells

The white blood cells, also called leucocytes, only circulate for a short portion of their life span, spending most of their life migrating through dense and loose connective tissues. Some of the white blood cells are capable of phagocytosis – the neutrophils, eosinophils and monocytes.

Neutrophils

The most abundant white blood cells are neutrophils, which play an important role in immunity.

Question 13

(a) In Figure 7.8, identify the granules in the cytoplasm and the multi-lobed nucleus.

(b) Colour in the granules in the cytoplasm and the multi-lobed nucleus.

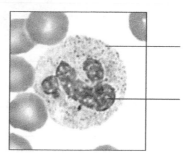

Figure 7.8 Neutophil. *Source*: Tortora and Derrickson, 2009. Reproduced with permission of John Wiley & Sons.

Eosinophils

These cells have B-shaped nuclei; they also migrate from blood vessels and are 10–12 μm in diameter. They are phagocytes and contain lysosomal enzymes and peroxidase in their granules.

Question 14

(a) In Figure 7.9, identify the B-shaped nucleus.

(b) Colour in the B-shaped nucleus.

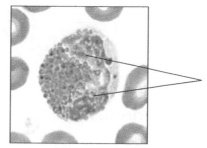

Figure 7.9 Eospinophil. *Source*: Tortora and Derrickson, 2009. Reproduced with permission of John Wiley & Sons.

Basophils

These are the least abundant white blood cells. They have elongated lobed nuclei, and are 8–10 µm in diameter. In inflamed tissue they become mast cells secreting granules containing heparin, histamine and other proteins, promoting inflammation.

Question 15

(a) In Figure 7.10, identify the large granules (the nucleus has been obscured by the granules).

(b) Colour in the large granules.

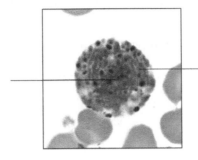

Figure 7.10 Basophil. *Source*: Tortora and Derrickson, 2009. Reproduced with permission of John Wiley & Sons.

Monocytes

These are circulating leucocytes and develop in the bone marrow, spreading through the body in 1–3 days. They are approximately 12–20 µm in diameter, and play a vital role in immunity and inflammation by destroying specific antigens.

Question 16

(a) In Figure 7.11, identify the kidney- or horseshoe-shaped nucleus.

(b) Colour in the nucleus.

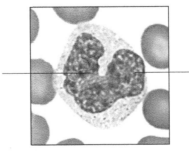

Figure 7.11 Monocyte. *Source*: Tortora and Derrickson, 2009. Reproduced with permission of John Wiley & Sons.

Lymphocytes

These are mostly found in the lymphatic tissue such as lymph nodes and spleen. The life span of lymphocytes ranges from a few hours to years.

Question 17

(a) In Figure 7.12, identify the large nucleus.

(b) Colour in the nucleus.

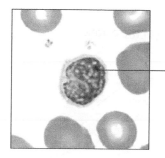

Figure 7.12   Lymphocyte. *Source*: Tortora and Derrickson, 2009. Reproduced with permission of John Wiley & Sons.

Question 18

(a) In Figure 7.13, identify the white blood cells.

(b) Colour in the various types of white blood cells.

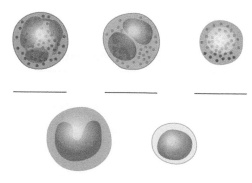

Figure 7.13   White blood cells. *Source*: Peate and Nair, 2011. Reproduced with permission of John Wiley & Sons.

Platelets

These are small blood cells consisting of some cytoplasm surrounded by a plasma membrane. They are produced in the bone marrow from megakaryocytes: fragments of megakaryocytes break off to form platelets. Platelets have a key role to play in preventing blood loss by the formation of platelet plugs, sealing holes in blood vessels, releasing chemicals and aiding blood clotting.

Question 19

(a) In Figure 7.14, identify the component parts of the platelet.

(b) Colour in the various elements of the platelet.

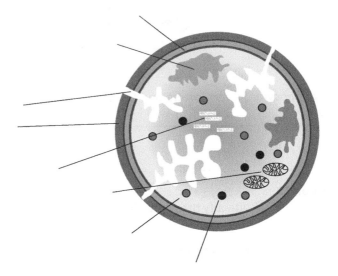

Figure 7.14   Platelet. *Source*: https://commons.wikimedia.org/wiki/File:Platelet_structure.png

Haemostasis

This is a sequence of responses that stops bleeding and can prevent haemorrhage from smaller blood vessels. Haemostasis plays an important part in maintaining homeostasis.

Question 20   In Table 7.2 identify the common names for the various clotting factors.

Table 7.2   Blood clotting factors.

Factor	Common name
I	
II	
V	
VII	
VIII	
IX	
X	
XI	
XII	
XIII	

Blood groups

The red blood cells define which blood group a person belongs to. On the surface of the red cells are markers called antigens. The ABO system is the structure used for defining blood groups. If an individual has blood group A, then they have A antigens covering their red cells. Group B has B antigens on their red blood cell, while group O has neither antigens, and group AB has both antigens.

The ABO system also covers antibodies in the plasma, the body's natural defence against foreign antigens. Blood group A, for example, has anti-B in the plasma, B has anti-A, and so on. Group AB however, has no antibodies and group O has both.

Question 21

(a) In Figure 7.15, identify the antigens and antibodies.

(b) Colour in the various components of the red blood cells and the plasma.

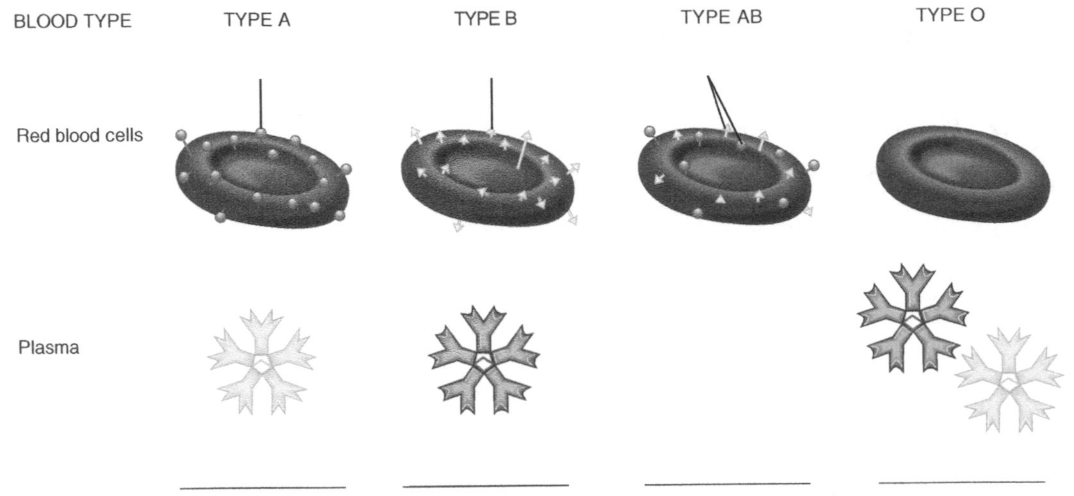

BLOOD TYPE	TYPE A	TYPE B	TYPE AB	TYPE O

Red blood cells

Plasma

Figure 7.15   ABO blood groups. *Source*: Tortora and Derrickson, 2009. Reproduced with permission of John Wiley & Sons.

Another factor (factor D) also has to be considered – the Rhesus factor (Rh) system.

Question 22   Complete Table 7.3, identifying the antigens and antibodies. Also complete who could safely receive blood and who would make suitable donor.

Table 7.3   Blood groups.

Blood type	Antigens	Antibodies	Can donate blood to	Can receive blood from
A				
B				
AB				
O				

Question 23 Match the pairs.

The most abundant blood cells are the	antigens
Blood cells are produced in the	megakaryocytes
Haemoglobin is composed of the protein, globin, bound to the iron-containing pigment called	emigration
All white blood cells migrate from the blood vessel by a process known as	erythrocytes
Platelets are produced in the bone marrow from	bone marrow
On the surface of the red cells are markers called	haem

Question 24 Time yourself to unscramble these words.

Scrambled	Answer
SNIGENTA	
STEELLTAP	
COMSTONEY	
DOILSPHAS	
BIACEVONC	
RAGURANL	
LOGANUCOATI	
RUSHES	

Blood vessels

These are part of the circulatory system transporting blood throughout the body. There are three major types of blood vessels:

1. arteries, which carry the blood away from the heart
2. capillaries, which enable the actual exchange of water, nutrients and chemicals between the blood and the tissues
3. veins, which carry blood from the capillaries back towards the heart.

Question 25

(a) In Figure 7.16, identify the blood vessels.

(b) Colour in the various components of the blood vessels.

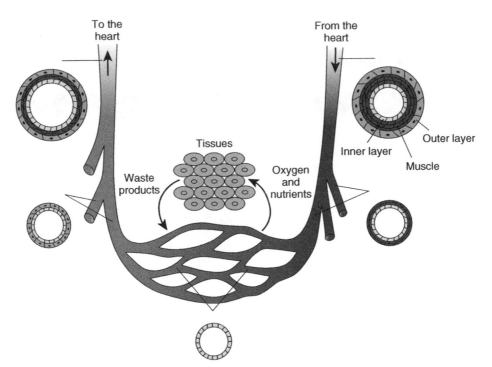

Figure 7.16 Blood vessels. *Source*: Peate and Nair, 2011. Reproduced with permission of John Wiley & Sons.

Question 26 In Figure 7.17, identify the vein and the artery and label the features of both.

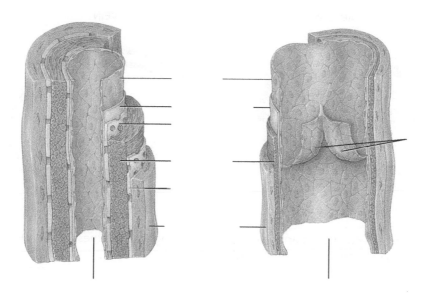

Figure 7.17 An artery and a vein. *Source*: Tortora and Derrickson, 2009. Reproduced with permission of John Wiley & Sons.

Question 27

(a) In Figure 7.18, identify the various features of the capillary.

(b) Colour in Figure 7.18.

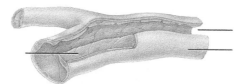

Figure 7.18 A capillary. *Source*: Tortora and Derrickson, 2009. Reproduced with permission of John Wiley & Sons.

The walls of the blood vessels differ:

- arteries have thick walls
- veins have thinner walls
- capillaries are very delicate

Question 28 In Figure 7.19, identify the parts of the blood vessel walls.

ARTERY   VEIN

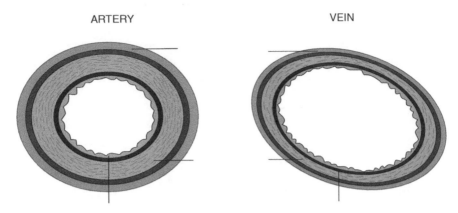

Figure 7.19 Cross-section of an artery and a vein showing wall thickness. *Source*: Peate and Nair, 2011. Reproduced with permission of John Wiley & Sons.

 Question 29 List the differences in structure and function between arteries and veins in Table 7.4.

Table 7.4 The differences between arteries and veins.

Arteries	Veins

Capillaries

Capillaries are very small blood vessels, around 5–20 μm in diameter. In most of the organs and tissues of the body there are networks of capillaries.

Lymphatic system

This is part of the circulatory system, and transports a clear fluid called lymph. The lymphatic system begins with very small, closed-end vessels called lymphatic capillaries, which are in contact with the surrounding tissues and the interstitial fluid.

Question 30

(a) In the image below identify the following features:

- Blood capillarities
- Arteriole
- Venule
- Lymphatic capillaries

(b) Now colour in the components.

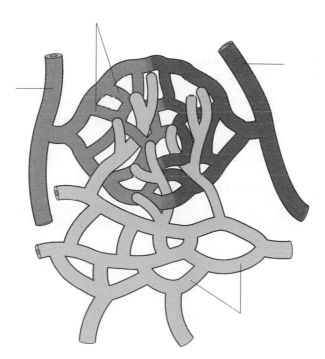

Figure 7.20 Lymphatic capillaries. *Source*: Peate and Nair, 2011. Reproduced with permission of John Wiley & Sons.

Lymph

This is a clear fluid found inside the lymphatic capillaries. Similar to plasma, it is the ultra-filtrate of the blood produced at the capillary ends of the blood vessels. Blood pressure in the blood vessel forces fluid and other substances such as albumin from the capillaries into the tissue space as interstitial fluid; this then enters the lymphatic capillaries as lymph.

Lymph nodes

Lymph nodes are bean-shaped organs located along the lymphatic vessels, found in the largest numbers in the neck, axillae, thorax, abdomen and the groin. The lymphocytes in lymph nodes filter out harmful substances from lymph and are sites for specific defences of the immune system.

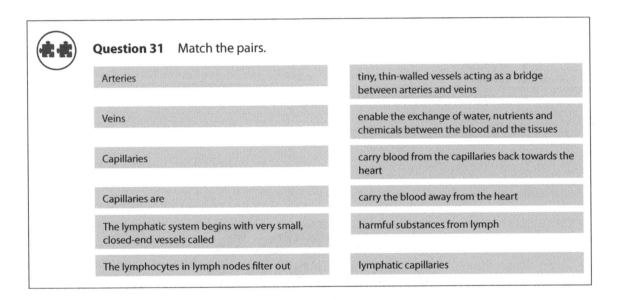

Question 31   Match the pairs.

Arteries	tiny, thin-walled vessels acting as a bridge between arteries and veins
Veins	enable the exchange of water, nutrients and chemicals between the blood and the tissues
Capillaries	carry blood from the capillaries back towards the heart
Capillaries are	carry the blood away from the heart
The lymphatic system begins with very small, closed-end vessels called	harmful substances from lymph
The lymphocytes in lymph nodes filter out	lymphatic capillaries

Question 32   Time yourself to unscramble these words.

Scrambled	Answer
PARCELSILIA	
RATERY	
NEIV	
PHYLM	
NOXGATEDEY	
SALVEV	
SLAPAM	
TRIFLATE	

Snap shot

Varicosities

Usually blood collected from superficial venous capillaries is directed upward and inward via one-way valves into superficial veins. They then drain via perforator veins that pass through muscle fascia into veins that are deep under the fascia. Leakage in a valve allows a retrograde flow back into the vein. Unlike deep veins (these are thick-walled and confined by fascia), the superficial veins cannot withstand high pressure and they eventually become dilated and tortuous. When one valve fails this puts pressure on its neighbours and this in turn can result in retrograde flow, and then varicosity, of the whole local superficial venous network.

On the diagram identify where varicosities can occur.

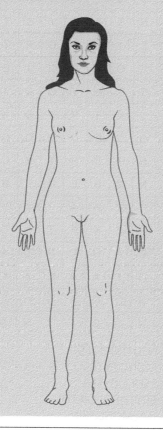

Word search

R	N	F	J	Q	T	N	I	T	E	I	O	P	O	R	H	T	Y	R	E
Y	S	E	S	L	I	H	P	O	S	A	B	M	I	K	S	G	I	C	B
B	Z	Q	S	I	S	E	I	O	P	O	M	E	A	H	L	B	P	J	Q
X	I	H	P	M	Y	L	E	L	L	E	U	C	O	C	Y	T	E	S	B
P	L	A	S	M	A	I	S	E	T	Y	C	O	B	M	O	R	H	T	E
E	E	U	O	G	F	Q	G	N	T	I	R	C	O	T	A	M	E	A	H
O	V	A	S	O	C	O	N	S	T	R	I	C	T	I	O	N	N	S	Z
S	M	R	E	Y	H	S	L	I	H	P	O	R	T	U	E	N	E	N	L
I	H	H	T	C	W	S	F	O	O	F	G	I	E	L	U	T	N	S	M
N	A	B	Y	A	N	N	C	S	W	Y	O	O	J	P	Y	S	E	L	I
O	E	I	C	P	A	I	L	L	I	V	S	D	X	C	Z	I	X	Q	T
P	M	C	O	I	R	F	Q	Q	E	U	Q	C	O	S	D	U	S	I	E
H	O	O	R	L	T	Z	S	I	S	O	T	Y	C	O	G	A	H	P	Y
I	G	N	H	L	E	E	N	E	B	L	R	E	B	B	S	V	X	X	B
L	L	C	T	A	R	C	H	Y	X	A	I	I	H	U	Y	T	J	L	S
S	O	A	Y	R	Y	R	P	Z	K	R	T	P	O	Q	L	T	F	G	M
Y	B	V	R	I	R	C	E	A	H	N	P	L	A	T	E	L	E	T	S
T	I	E	E	E	P	X	G	Y	A	A	S	E	T	Y	C	O	N	O	M
E	N	R	C	S	X	E	N	C	O	A	G	U	L	A	T	I	O	N	I
O	I	P	B	J	M	S	N	E	G	I	T	N	A	D	K	W	M	Q	E

PLASMA
LYMPH
PLATELETS
ERYTHROCYTES
HAEMATOCRIT
THROMBOCYTES
HAEMOPOIESIS
BASOPHILS
EOSINOPHILS

NEUTROPHILS
MONOCYTES
LEUCOCYTES
ERYTHROPOIETIN
HAEMOGLOBIN
PHAGOCYTOSIS
ANTIGENS
ANTIBODIES
MEGAKARYOCYTES

COAGULATION
VASOCONSTRICTION
RHESUS
BICONCAVE
CAPILLARIES
ARTERY
VEIN

Crossword

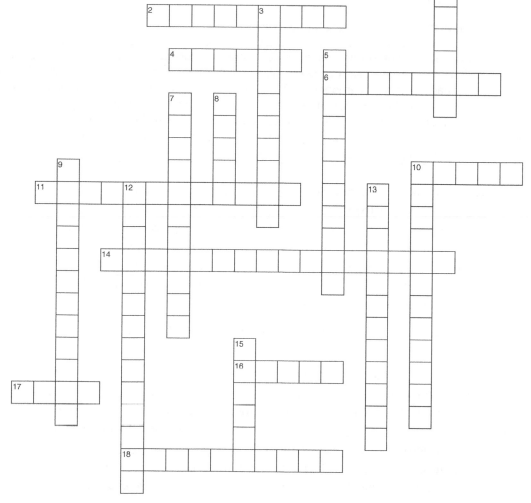

Across

2. One of the components of the buffy coat
4. The T-lymphocytes continue their development here
6. Markers located on the surface of the red cells
10. Arteries transport blood away from this organ
11. Platelets
14. Contraction of smooth muscle of the vessel wall
16. The lymphatic system drains this
17. Iron-containing pigment in haemoglobin
18. Process of white blood cells migrating from the blood vessel

Down

1. Organ containing lymphatic tissue
3. White blood cells
5. Percentage of the formed elements of blood
7. Oxygen-carrying protein
8. 'Coat' between the plasma and erythrocytes in a centrifuged sample
9. Platelets release these vasoconstrictors
10. Process by which formed elements of blood are developed
12. Platelets are produced in the bone marrow from these
13. Cells produced from myeloid stem cells in the bone marrow
15. The fluid portion of blood

Fill in the blanks

Use the words in the box to complete the sentences:

120, 5–9, A, AB, ABO, absent, antigens, antigen, B, basophils, biconcave, blood, blood, body, bone, both, cell, cells, clotting, connective, cytoplasm, diameter, elements, emigration, erythrocytes, fluid, formed, group, haemoglobin, haemopoiesis, heart, heart, holes, hormones, leucocytes, life, loss, lymph, lymphatic, lymphoid, marrow, mature, membrane, metabolic, migrate, migrating, monocytes, monocytes, multipotent, myeloid, nucleus, nucleus, nutrients, O, organelles, oxygen, phagocytosis, plasma, platelets, platelets, plugs, portion, releasing, short, stem, surface, T-lymphocytes, thymus, transport, transportation, types, urea, vessels, vessels

1. The circulatory system includes the _____, the _____, the blood _____ and the _____ system. The blood vessels _____ blood throughout the _____. Blood consists of _____ elements and a fluid _____, plasma. Blood has many functions, including _____ of _____, respiratory gases such as _____ and carbon dioxide, _____ waste such as _____ and uric acid, _____, electrolytes and antibodies. Circulation of blood occurs through a network of blood _____ leading away from and returning to the _____.

2. Blood is a _____ connective tissue, consisting of formed _____ such red blood _____, white _____ cells, _____, and a fluid portion, _____.

3. The process by which formed elements of blood develop is called _____. In the last three months of gestation and throughout _____, the red bone _____ is the primary centre for haemopoiesis. In order to produce blood cells, _____ stem cells divide into _____ and _____ stem cells in the bone marrow. Myeloid stem cells further subdivide in the bone marrow producing red blood cells, _____ (thrombocytes), _____, eosinophils, neutrophils and _____. Lymphoid _____ cells begin the development in the _____ marrow as B- and _____. B-lymphocytes continue development in bone marrow, prior to migrating to _____ nodes, spleen or tonsils. T-lymphocytes continue their development in the _____ and may then _____ to other lymph tissues.

4. The most abundant blood cells are the _____; they are _____ discs containing oxygen-carrying protein, _____. They live for around _____ days. Young red blood cells contain a _____; however, in a _____ red blood cell the nucleus is _____ and the cell has no _____, this increases the _____-carrying capacity of the red blood cell.

5. White blood cells, also called _____, only circulate for a _____ portion of their life span, spending most of their life span _____ through dense and loose _____ tissues. All white blood cells migrate from the blood vessel by a process known as _____. Some of the white blood cells are capable of _____ – the neutrophils, eosinophils and _____.

6. Platelets are small blood cells, consisting of some _____ surrounded by a plasma _____, produced in the bone marrow from _____; fragments break off to form platelets. They are around 2–4 μm in _____ without a _____, living for approximately _____ days. Platelets have a role to play in preventing blood _____ by the formation of platelet _____, sealing _____ in blood vessels, _____ chemicals and aiding blood _____.

7. The red blood cells define which blood _____ a person belongs to. On the _____ of the red cells are antigens. Apart from identical twins, each person has different _____, these identify blood _____. The _____ system is the system used for defining blood groups. If an individual has blood group A, then they have _____ antigens covering their red cells. Group B has _____ antigens on their red blood _____; while group _____ has neither _____ and group _____ has _____ antigens.

Multiple choice questions

1. The erythrocyte

   (a) Is phagocytic
   (b) Contains haemoglobin, transports oxygen
   (c) Prevents blood coagulation
   (d) Destroys antibodies that are involved in the immune response

2. The neutrophil

   (a) Is a cytotoxic T-cell
   (b) Is a granulocytic phagocyte
   (c) Secretes chyme
   (d) Deactivates plasmin

3. Thrombin

   (a) Activates fibrinogen
   (b) Is responsible for the formation of the complement
   (c) Is inactivated by vitamin B12
   (d) Is inactivated by prothrombin

4. What statement is true regarding the administration of type A+ blood to a type O− recipient?

   (a) The blood types are compatible; no haemolytic reaction is expected
   (b) People with O− blood are allergic to type A+ blood
   (c) The administration of type A+ blood to a type O− recipient causes haemolysis
   (d) Those with type O− blood can safety receive type A+ blood

5. Erythropoietin

   (a) Is synthesised by the kidneys
   (b) Stimulates the bone marrow to make RBCs
   (c) Is released by the kidney in response to hypoxaemia
   (d) All of the above are true

6. What is most likely to cause jaundice?

   (a) Anaemia
   (b) An increase of erythropoietin
   (c) A deficiency of the extrinsic factor
   (d) Haemolysis

7. Which of the following is a true statement?

   (a) The reticulocyte is an undeveloped thrombocyte
   (b) The neutrophil is a phagocytic granulocyte
   (c) The neutrophil, basophil and eosinophil are elements of the megakaryocyte
   (d) A deficiency of reticulocytes causes hypoprothrombinaemia

8. Hypoprothrombinaemia along with a prolonged prothrombin time is

   (a) Related to bleeding
   (b) Indicative of pernicious anemia
   (c) A result of heparin therapy
   (d) A consequence of thrombocytopenia

9. Hyperbilirubinaemia

   (a) Can be caused by haemolysis
   (b) Causes jaundice
   (c) Can cause kernicterus
   (d) All of the above are true

10. Which of the following is least related to haem?

   (a) Oxygen
   (b) Phagocytosis
   (c) RBC
   (d) Iron

References

Peate, I. and Nair, M. (2011) *Fundamentals of Anatomy and Physiology for Student Nurses*. Oxford: John Wiley & Sons, Ltd.

Peate, I. and Nair, M. (2015) *Anatomy and Physiology for Nurses at a Glance*. Oxford: John Wiley & Sons, Ltd.

Tortora, G.J. and Derrickson, B.H. (2009) *Principles of Anatomy and Physiology*, 12th edn. Hoboken, NJ: John Wiley & Sons, Inc.

Chapter 8

The cardiac system

The heart is a little larger than the owner's closed fist. It is located in the thoracic cavity in the mediastinum, behind and to the left of the sternum. The heart is a muscular organ with four chambers; its main function is to pump blood around the circulatory system of the lungs and the systemic circulation of the rest of the body.

 Question 1   In Figure 8.1, identify the contents of the thoracic cavity.

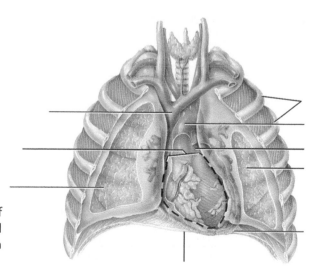

Figure 8.1 The location of the heart. *Source*: Tortora and Derrickson, 2009. Reproduced with permission of John Wiley & Sons.

Fundamentals of Anatomy and Physiology Workbook: A Study Guide for Nursing and Healthcare Students, First Edition. Ian Peate.
© 2017 John Wiley & Sons Ltd. Published 2017 by John Wiley & Sons Ltd.

The structure of the heart

Heart wall

Pericardium

The heart is surrounded by the pericardium, made up of the fibrous pericardium and the serous pericardium which are closely connected to each other. Between the parietal and visceral pericardium is a thin film of pericardial fluid, reducing friction between the membranes as the heart moves during its cycle of contraction and relaxation.

Myocardium

Underlying the pericardium is the heart muscle known as the myocardium. It makes up the bulk of the heart.

Endocardium

The endocardium is a layer of smooth simple epithelium that lines the inside of the heart chambers and the heart valves.

Question 2

(a) In Figure 8.2, identify the layers of the heart wall.

(b) Colour in the layers of the heart wall.

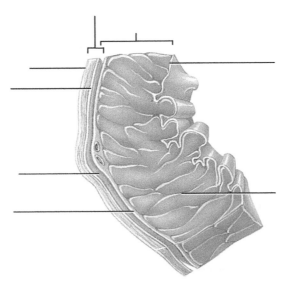

Figure 8.2 The heart wall. *Source*: Tortora and Derrickson, 2009. Reproduced with permission of John Wiley & Sons.

The chambers of the heart

The heart has four chambers: the atria and the ventricles. Whilst the heart is referred to as a pump, thinking of it as two pumps may be more helpful.

- **Right heart pump**. The right heart pump receives deoxygenated blood from the tissues and pumps it out into the pulmonary circulation.
- **Left heart pump**. The left heart pump receives oxygenated blood from the pulmonary circulation and pumps it out to the systemic circulation.

Atria

The atria are the smaller chambers of the heart and lie superior to the ventricles. There are two atria. A thin wall divides the atria, the interatrial septum. There are two valves between the atria and the ventricles (the atrioventricular valves) the tricuspid valve and the bicuspid valve. The atrioventricular valves prevent the backward flow of blood from the ventricles into the atria.

Ventricles

There are two ventricles (right and left ventricles), each pumps the same amount of blood per beat but they have very different pressures. The interventicular septum divides the ventricles.

Question 3

(a) In Figure 8.3, identify the chambers of the heart, the associated blood vessels and the interventricular septum.

(b) Colour in the various components.

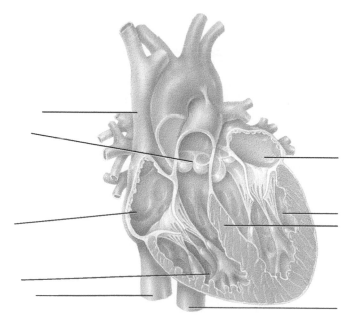

Figure 8.3   The chambers of the heart. *Source*: Tortora and Derrickson, 2009. Reproduced with permission of John Wiley & Sons.

Question 4 Match the pairs.

The apex of the heart is below	this reduces friction as the heart moves during its cycle of contraction and relaxation
Between the parietal and visceral pericardium is a thin film of pericardial fluid	the base of the heart, lying on the diaphragm
The bulk of muscle in the heart is	prevent the backward flow of blood from the ventricles into the atria.
The atria are	divides the ventricles
The atrioventricular valves	the myocardium
The interventicular septum	the smaller chambers of the heart

SCRAMBLE **Question 5** Time yourself to unscramble these words.

Scrambled	Answer
RATIONEXAL	
ARATI	
SERVENTICL	
DECARUMRIPI	
DECORUMNADI	
DACOMRUMIY	
DISCUTRIP	
DISCUBIP	

Blood supply to the heart

The heart receives approximately 5% of the body's blood supply. The plentiful supply of blood ensures the constant supply of oxygen and nutrients and the efficient removal of waste products.

 Question 6 Each artery and branch supplies different areas of the heart muscle. In Table 8.1 there is a summary of the main arteries and their branches. Identify the areas of the heart they supply.

Table 8.1 Names of the coronary arteries and their major branches.

Artery	Major branches	Area of the heart supplied
Left anterior descending (LAD)	Diagonals Septals	
Circumflex artery	Oblique marginal	
Right coronary artery (RCA)	Posterior descending artery	

 Question 7 In Figure 8.4, identify the coronary arteries and the associated anatomy of the heart.

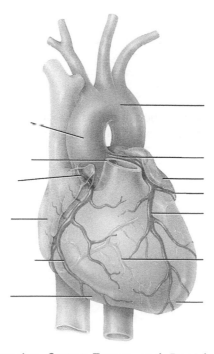

Figure 8.4 The coronary arteries. *Source*: Tortora and Derrickson, 2009. Reproduced with permission of John Wiley & Sons.

Flow of blood through the heart

The heart is best thought of as two pumps, the right and the left pumps. The pumps are both made up of two chambers, the atria and the ventricles, along with their associated valves.

Question 8

(a) In Figure 8.5, identify the boxes representing the lungs, the body, right atrium, left atrium, right ventricle and left ventricle.

(b) In Figure 8.5, using two different colours (red arrows for oxygenated blood and blue dotted arrows for deoxygenated blood), indicate the flow of blood through the heart.

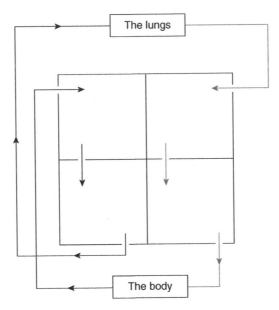

Figure 8.5   A diagrammatic representation of the flow of blood through the heart. *Source*: Peate and Nair, 2011. Reproduced with permission of John Wiley & Sons.

Question 9

(a) In Figure 8.6, identify the anatomy of the heart in relation to flow of blood.

(b) Using two different colours (red for oxygenated blood and blue for deoxygenated blood) outline the flow of blood through the heart.

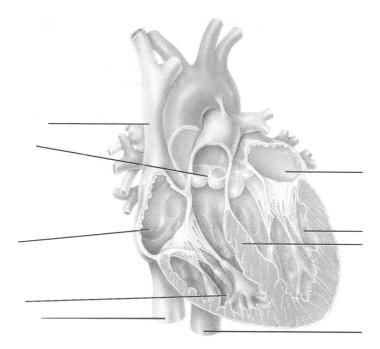

Figure 8.6 The anatomical flow of blood through the heart. *Source*: Tortora and Derrickson, 2009. Reproduced with permission of John Wiley & Sons.

Question 10 Time yourself to unscramble these words.

Scrambled	Answer
CRUFMECLIX	
YARNCROO	
SANCHBRE	
LACTIONCURI	
MYSTICES	
YONEXTAGED	
SEVONU	
TRAILARE	

Question 11 Match the pairs.

The heart receives	the atrium and the ventricle, as well as their associated valves
The heart receives a plentiful supply of blood ensuring the constant supply of	approximately 5% of the body's blood supply
The inner part of the endocardium is	oxygen and nutrients and the efficient removal of waste products
The circumflex artery supplies the	supplied with blood directly from the inside of the heart chambers
The heart is best thought of as two pumps	back and side of the left ventricle
The pumps are made up of two chambers	the right and the left pumps

The conduction system of the heart

There is a specialised network of electrical pathways within the heart dedicated to ensuring rapid transmission of electrical impulses.

Question 12
(a) In Figure 8.7, identify the sino-atrial node and the atrioventricular node and draw in the normal electrical pathways.

(b) Colour in the septum and the chambers of the heart.

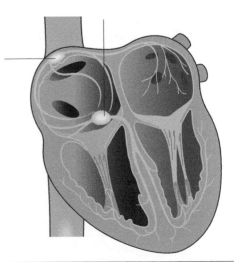

Figure 8.7 The conducting system of the heart. *Source*: Peate *et al.*, 2014. Reproduced with permission of John Wiley & Sons.

Cardiac cycle

This is the sequence of events that occurs when the heart beats. There are two phases, diastole (relaxation) and systole (contraction). One cardiac cycle is completed when the heart fills with blood and the blood is pumped out.

The cardiac cycle refers to the mechanical action of the heart; electrical activity stimulates this action and can be seen by the use of an electrocardiogram (ECG). The changes from the baseline on the ECG are labelled with letters of the alphabet.

Question 13   In Figure 8.8, add the letters related to the ECG.

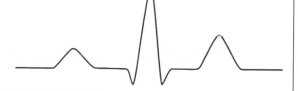

Figure 8.8   The normal ECG of one cycle of the heart.

Question 14   Complete Table 8.2, matching the ECG letters to heart activity and corresponding action.

Table 8.2   The ECG.

ECG letter(s)	Heart electrical activity	Corresponding action
P		Atrial contraction
QRS		
T	Ventricular repolarisation	

Hormones

Question 15   Complete Table 8.3, describing the action of the hormones listed in relation to cardiac activity.

Table 8.3   Hormones and their action on the heart.

Hormones	Action
Epinephrine	
Norepinephrine	
Thyroxine	

Question 16 Match the pairs.

The cardiac cycle refers to	in the carotid sinus and the aortic arch, sensitive to the amount of stretch in these blood vessels
Systole corresponds to	the autonomic nervous system and hormone activity
Diastole corresponds to	the amount of blood the heart pumps out in 1 minute
'Cardiac output' is a term relating to	the relaxation of a heart chamber (atrium or ventricle)
Heart rate is controlled by two main mechanisms:	the contraction of a heart chamber (atrium or ventricle)
Baroreceptors are specialised mechanical receptors located	the mechanical activity of the heart

 Question 17 Time yourself to unscramble these words.

Scrambled	Answer
REALTICCLE	
TUPTUO	
ROTACID	
LAIDPOORSATINE	
SADLIETO	
YESLSTO	
CAUTIONMO	

Snap shot

Taking a patient's pulse

Pulse rate assessment is an essential activity that requires a skilled, competent and confident person to undertake the task safely and effectively. The nurse needs to understand how the pulse rate is maintained, factors impacting upon the pulse and how to measure the pulse rate effectively and safely. Having taken a pulse the nurse must also understand what the various measurements may mean, how to record the pulse rate and how to report any abnormality, ensuring that the person is provided with care that is safe and responsive to their needs.

In this diagram identify the sites that may be used to assess a person's pulse.

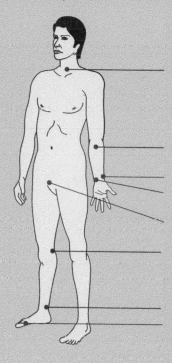

Define the following terms

Term	Definition
Asystole	

Term	Definition
Bradycardia	
Tachycardia	
Arrhythmia	
Sinus rhythm	
Fibrillation	

Word search

D	S	E	P	T	U	M	M	U	I	D	R	A	C	I	R	E	P	H	Q
H	I	M	R	G	N	R	M	R	J	G	C	X	K	A	P	E	F	W	D
O	W	P	G	M	X	J	Y	R	M	E	D	I	A	S	T	I	N	U	M
R	S	G	S	K	X	I	L	X	L	D	T	F	I	E	I	D	L	S	V
W	T	L	V	U	G	T	Q	L	E	X	M	R	P	T	C	I	J	T	O
C	N	W	J	A	C	R	A	T	K	T	D	I	I	O	G	Q	L	S	R
P	L	K	A	N	Z	I	A	Z	S	E	N	F	R	C	D	V	E	Y	D
S	L	H	J	O	R	N	B	F	N	F	X	O	A	H	U	N	C	F	Z
V	Z	E	K	E	E	W	L	D	P	L	N	I	O	H	O	S	K	J	N
L	Q	H	T	G	S	C	O	H	D	A	K	F	F	M	K	A	P	N	X
B	I	R	Y	G	I	C	R	H	R	Q	Q	I	R	D	A	T	R	I	A
W	A	X	C	R	A	I	O	Y	W	K	I	O	L	K	U	I	V	K	D
I	O	A	T	R	N	F	L	Z	X	W	H	H	X	A	V	X	C	R	I
G	N	N	D	E	T	A	N	E	G	Y	X	O	E	D	H	E	E	U	E
Q	E	I	B	D	V	E	N	O	U	S	G	A	Y	W	I	S	P	P	D
V	U	S	Y	B	M	M	M	Y	O	C	A	R	D	I	U	M	B	F	A
M	G	F	H	U	Q	Y	S	X	C	D	Y	I	X	V	G	T	Z	A	M
O	M	M	X	D	E	P	O	L	A	R	I	S	A	T	I	O	N	X	B
O	E	N	I	X	O	R	Y	H	T	N	T	H	E	M	A	R	L	W	M
D	S	I	H	U	E	N	Z	M	J	J	D	C	S	N	J	L	Y	B	B

DEOXYGENATED	VENTRICLES	THYROXINE
OXYGENATED	ATRIA	VENOUS
MYOCARDIUM	SEPTUM	ARTERIAL
ENDOCARDIUM	BICUSPID	HIS
PERICARDIUM	TRICUSPID	PURKINJE
MEDIASTINUM	APEX	DEPOLARISATION
CORONARY	EPINEPHRINE	HORMONES

163

Crossword

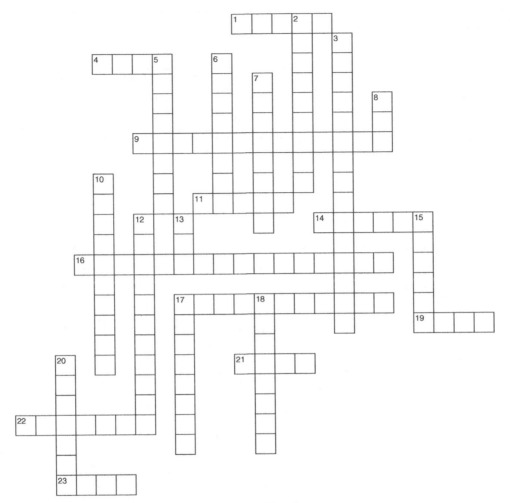

Across

1. The largest blood vessel in the body
4. The heart is said to be the size of this
9. Specialised mechanical receptors located in the carotid sinus and the aortic arch
11. The plural of atrium
14. The dividing wall between the ventricles
16. Nervous system regulation of the heart originates in this centre located in the medulla oblongata
17. Membrane surrounding the heart
19. This side of the heart is more muscular than the other
21. The number of chambers in the heart
22. The breast bone
23. Where blood travels to after it has gone through the pulmonary valve

Down

2. Valve with three cusps
3. Usually cardiac veins are free of this type of plaque
5. Body cavity where the heart is located
6. Shorten
7. Type of stimulus released by the sino-atrial node
8. The bundle is a collection of heart muscle cells specialised for electrical conduction
10. A muscle mass that makes up most of the heart
12. The smooth lining of the heart
13. Number of phases in the cardiac cycle
15. The bicuspid valve
17. Fibres located in the inner ventricular walls of the heart
18. Arteries which come directly off the aorta, just after the aortic valve
20. Gland which secretes epinephrine and norepinephrine

Fill in the blanks

Use the words in the box to complete the sentences:

anger, aorta, atrio-ventricular, atrium, blood, bloodstream, cardiac, circulation, conduction, dioxide, electrical, emotions, epinephrine, five, four, glands, His, hormone, impulses, increase, increasing, left, lungs, medulla, metabolism, oxygen, pressure, pumped, Purkinje, rate, released, right, sino-atrial, stimulant, strength, thyroxine, two, venous, ventricle, ventricle,

1. The heart is made up of _____ chambers, two atria and _____ ventricles. Deoxygenated _____ returns to the _____ side of the heart via the _____ circulation. It is _____ into the right _____ and then to the _____ where carbon _____ is _____ and _____ is absorbed. The oxygenated blood then travels back to the _____ side of the heart into the left _____, then into the left _____ from where it is pumped into the _____ and arterial _____.

2. The heart creates its own _____ impulses and controls the route the _____ take through a specialised _____ pathway made up of _____ elements, the _____ node, the _____ node, the bundle of _____, the left and right _____ branches and the _____ fibres.

3. Epinephrine is a _____ secreted by the _____ of the adrenal _____. Strong _____, such as fear or _____, cause _____ to be released into the _____, which causes an _____ in heart rate, muscle _____, blood _____ and sugar _____. Epinephrine is used chiefly as a _____ in _____ arrest. _____ released in large quantities has the effect of _____ the heart _____.

Multiple choice questions

1. Which of the following is NOT true of the heart?

   (a) The heart is situated within the mediastinum
   (b) The apex is sited to the left of the sternal midline at the level of the fifth intercostal space
   (c) The base of the heart is located at the level of the second rib
   (d) The cardiac sphincter is composed of cardiac muscle

2. Which of the following statements is correct about cardiac output?

   (a) Cardiac output is determined by the heart rate and pulse
   (b) Stimulation of the sympathetic nerves decreases cardiac output
   (c) Vagal discharge increases cardiac output
   (d) Cardiac output is determined by heart rate and stroke volume

3. Which statement is true of ventricle diastole?

   (a) Blood is ejected from the ventricles
   (b) The semilunar valves are open
   (c) The atrioventricular valves are closed
   (d) Blood fills the ventricles

4. Which of the following is the function of a valve?

   (a) Controls the direction of the flow of blood through the heart
   (b) Regulates the amount of carbon dioxide bound to haemoglobin
   (c) Regulates strength of heart
   (d) Directs the progression of the cardiac impulse

5. Which of the following is true concerning the structures of the electrical conduction system?

   (a) The AVF node is the pacemaker
   (b) In normal sinus rhythm, the electrical signal arises within the SA node
   (c) The Purkinje fibres spreads the electrical signal from the right atrium to the left atrium
   (d) The purpose of the AV node is to severely reduce heart rate

6. Which of the following is bradycardia?

   (a) Heart rate below 60 beats per minute
   (b) No cardiac output
   (c) Heart rate over 100 beats per minute
   (d) None of the above

7. Pacemaker cells fire at a faster rate in the

   (a) Left coronary artery
   (b) SA node
   (c) Ventricular myocardium
   (d) AV node

8. The coronary arteries

   (a) Exit the aorta at a point immediately distal to the aortic semilunar valve
   (b) Prevent the right atrium from filling with blood
   (c) Provide cardiac electrical stimulation
   (d) Deliver most O_2 and nutrients while the myocardium is contracted

9. What does ventricular systole refer to?

(a) Arial depolarisation
(b) Cardiac stand still
(c) Ventricular filling
(d) Contraction of the ventricular myocardium

10. Which of the following is least related to the vagus nerve?

(a) Parasympathetic
(b) Slows heart rate
(c) Positive inotropic effect
(d) Autonomic nerve

References

Peate, I. and Nair, M. (2011) *Fundamentals of Anatomy and Physiology for Student Nurses*. Oxford: John Wiley & Sons, Ltd.

Peate, I, Wild, K. and Nair, M. (eds) (2014) *Nursing Practice: Knowledge and Care*. Oxford: John Wiley & Sons, Ltd.

Tortora, G.J. and Derrickson, B.H. (2009) *Principles of Anatomy and Physiology*, 12th edn. Hoboken, NJ: John Wiley & Sons, Inc.

Chapter 9

The gastrointestinal system

The gastrointestinal system is also called the digestive system or the alimentary canal. It travels the length of the body from the mouth through the thoracic, abdominal and pelvic cavities, and ends at the anus; it is about 10 m long. Its key role is to convert food from the diet into a form that can be utilised by the cells of the body.

 Question 1 Complete Table 9.1, describing the five key functions of the gastrointestinal tract.

Table 9.1 The five key functions of the gastrointestinal tract.

Function	Description
Ingestion	
Propulsion	
Digestion	
Absorption	
Elimination	

Fundamentals of Anatomy and Physiology Workbook: A Study Guide for Nursing and Healthcare Students, First Edition. Ian Peate.
© 2017 John Wiley & Sons Ltd. Published 2017 by John Wiley & Sons Ltd.

Question 2

(a) In Figure 9.1, identify the various components of the gastrointestinal tract from the mouth to the anus.

(b) Colour in the oesophagus, stomach, small intestine, large intestine and anus.

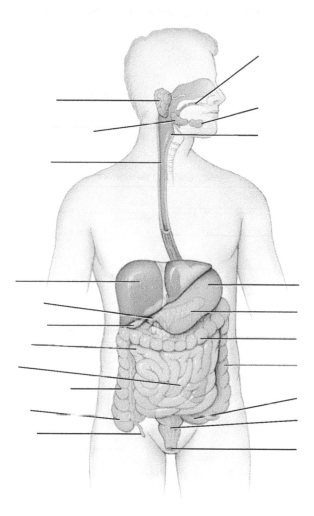

Figure 9.1   The gastrointestinal system. *Source*: Tortora and Derrickson, 2009. Reproduced with permission of John Wiley & Sons.

The oral cavity

Food enters the mouth or oral cavity where the process of digestion begins. The oral cavity consists of several structures.

Question 3

(a) In Figure 9.2, identify the various structures in the mouth.

(b) Colour in the structures.

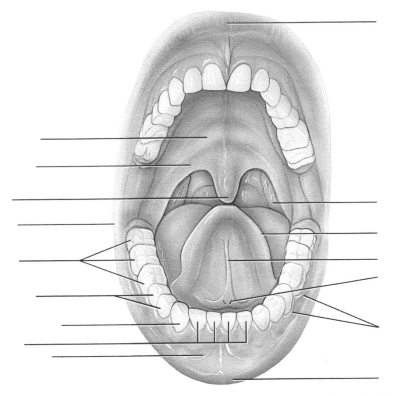

Figure 9.2 The oral cavity. *Source*: Tortora and Derrickson, 2009. Reproduced with permission of John Wiley & Sons.

The teeth

There are 32 permanent teeth. Sixteen are in the maxilla arch (upper) and 16 are in the mandible (lower).

Question 4

(a) In Figure 9.3, identify and number the teeth.

(b) Colour in the different types of teeth.

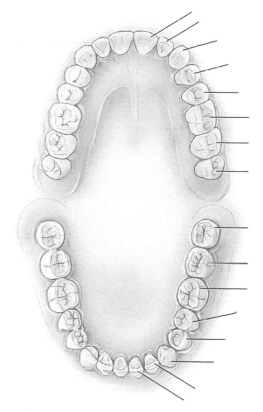

Figure 9.3 Permanent dentition. *Source*: Tortora and Derrickson, 2009. Reproduced with permission of John Wiley & Sons.

Salivary glands

There are three main pairs of salivary glands:

- parotid
- submandibular
- sublingual

Question 5

(a) In Figure 9.4, identify the three main salivary glands.

(b) Colour in the three main salivary glands.

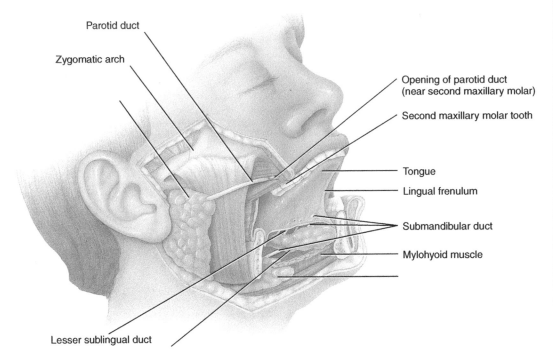

Figure 9.4 The salivary glands. *Source*: Tortora and Derrickson, 2009. Reproduced with permission of John Wiley & Sons.

Question 6 Complete Table 9.2 concerning saliva.

Table 9.2 Saliva.

1.	What does saliva contain?
2.	What are the functions of saliva?
3.	What is the pH of saliva?
4.	In health what volume of saliva is produced daily?

Swallowing

Swallowing is also known as deglutition. It occurs in three phases:

1. voluntary phase
2. pharyngeal phase
3. oesophageal phase.

Question 7
(a) Identify the structures in Figure 9.5.

(b) Colour in the structures.

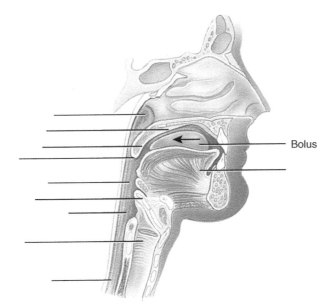

Bolus

Figure 9.5 The position of structures prior to swallowing. *Source*: Tortora and Derrickson, 2009. Reproduced with permission of John Wiley & Sons.

Question 8

(a) In Figure 9.6, identify the bolus and the direction in which food travels when in the oesophagus.

(b) Colour in the bolus.

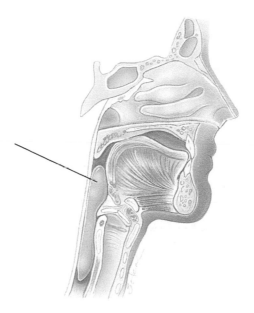

Figure 9.6 The position of structures post swallowing. *Source*: Tortora and Derrickson, 2009. Reproduced with permission of John Wiley & Sons.

Question 9 Match the pairs.

The tongue is a large	located anterior to the ears
The palate	leads to an increased production of saliva in response to the sight, smell or taste of food
The parotid glands are the largest of the salivary glands and are	and enters the oesophagus
The activity of the parasympathetic fibres	three parts
The pharynx consists of	forms the roof of the mouth and consists of two parts: the hard palate and the soft palate
The food bolus leaves the oropharynx	voluntary muscular structure which occupies much of the oral cavity

Question 10 Time yourself to unscramble these words.

Scrambled	Answer
LUPISPORON	
LAXIAML	
VASAIL	
LAMESAY	
YESYMOLZ	
GASHOSOUPE	
XNYRAHP	
USLOB	

Layers of the gastrointestinal tract

There are four layers of tissue existing throughout the length of the gastrointestinal tract.

Question 11
(a) In Figure 9.7, identify the four layers of the gastrointestinal tract.

(b) Colour in the layers.

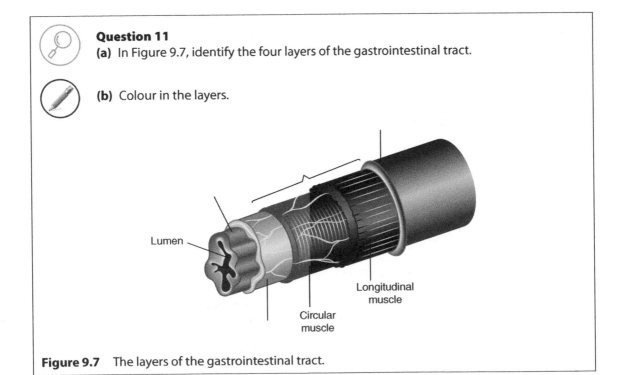

Figure 9.7 The layers of the gastrointestinal tract.

The stomach

The stomach is located in the abdominal cavity, lying between the oesophagus superiorly and the duodenum inferiorly. It is divided into regions.

Question 12

(a) In Figure 9.8, identify the structures and associated structures of the stomach and label the component parts.

(b) Colour in the component parts.

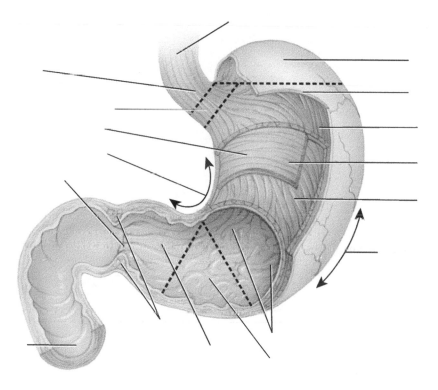

Figure 9.8   The stomach. *Source*: Tortora and Derrickson, 2009. Reproduced with permission of John Wiley & Sons.

The gastric mucosa

Question 13   Complete Table 9.3 concerning the gastric mucosa.

Table 9.3   The gastric mucosa.

Component	Functions
Surface mucous cells	
Mucous neck cells	
Parietal cells	
Chief cells	
Enteroendocrine cells (G cells)	

Question 14 In Figure 9.9, label the diagram and identify the surface mucous cell, mucous neck cells, parietal cell, chief cell and G cell. Then describe the secretion of each cell.

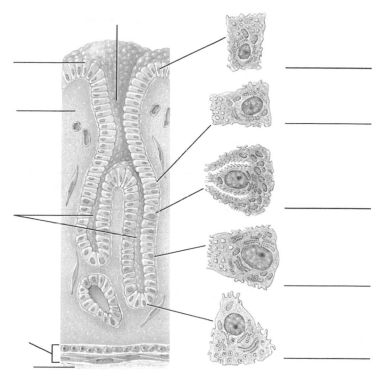

Figure 9.9 Gastric glands and cells. *Source*: Tortora and Derrickson, 2009. Reproduced with permission of John Wiley & Sons.

Question 15 Time yourself to unscramble these words.

Scrambled	Answer
NOSINGPEPE	
SHOTMAC	
LATERPAI	
TIRESONCE	
GSTARIC	
URAGE	
DRCHOOYCHIRL	

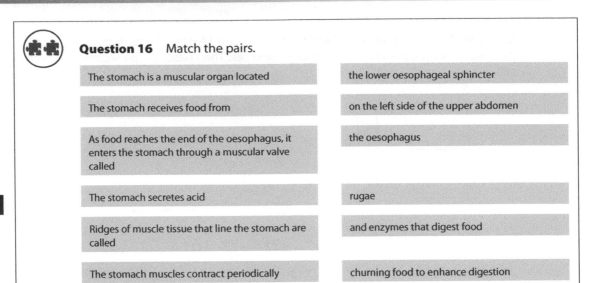

Question 16   Match the pairs.

The stomach is a muscular organ located	the lower oesophageal sphincter
The stomach receives food from	on the left side of the upper abdomen
As food reaches the end of the oesophagus, it enters the stomach through a muscular valve called	the oesophagus
The stomach secretes acid	rugae
Ridges of muscle tissue that line the stomach are called	and enzymes that digest food
The stomach muscles contract periodically	churning food to enhance digestion

Small intestine

The small intestine anatomically follows the stomach; much of the digestion and absorption of food takes place here. There are three sections: the first is the duodenum, the middle portion is the jejunum and the final section is the ileum, which leads to the large intestine.

Question 17
(a) In Figure 9.10, identify the three sections of the small intestine and the adjacent structures.

(b) Colour in the sections of the small intestine.

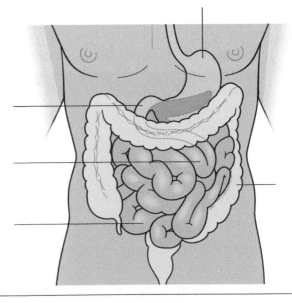

Figure 9.10 Small intestine. *Source*: Peate and Nair, 2014. Reproduced with permission of John Wiley & Sons.

Question 18   Complete Table 9.4, with the description and functions of the sections of the small intestine.

Table 9.4   The sections, functions and description of the three sections of the small intestine.

Section	Function/description
The duodenum	
The jejunum	
The ileum	

Large intestine

The large intestine consists of four regions: the caecum, colon, rectum and anus. It is approximately 1.5 m in length and has a smooth inner wall. In the upper half of the large intestine, enzymes from the small intestine complete the digestive process and bacteria produce B vitamins (B12, thiamin and riboflavin). The primary function of the large intestine is to absorb water and turn the food residue into semi-solid faeces.

Question 19

(a) In Figure 9.11, identify the four regions of the large intestine and label the other elements associated with the large intestine.

(b) Colour in the various features.

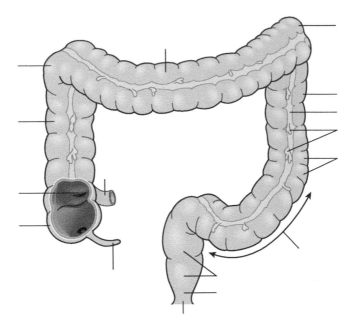

Figure 9.11   Large intestine. *Source*: Peate and Nair, 2014. Reproduced with permission of John Wiley & Sons.

Question 20 Match the pairs.

The small intestine consists of	four sections
The first section of the small intestine is called	anal canal
The large intestine consists of	three sections
The large intestine mucosa contains large numbers of goblet cells that secrete mucus to	some vitamins, minerals, electrolytes and drugs
The simple columnar epithelium changes to stratified squamous epithelium at the	the duodenum
The large intestine absorbs	ease the passage of faeces and protect the walls of the colon

Question 21 Time yourself to unscramble these words.

Scrambled	Answer
MUDDUONE	
MILEU	
NUMEJJU	
TINESCRE	
LIVLI	
AMUCEC	
SAFECE	
BLOGET	

The accessory organs of digestion

There are several organs that contribute to digestion – liver, gall bladder and pancreas. All are located close to the gastrointestinal tract.

Question 22
(a) In Figure 9.12, identify the three organs, liver, gallbladder and pancreas, and their various aspects.

(b) Colour in the three organs.

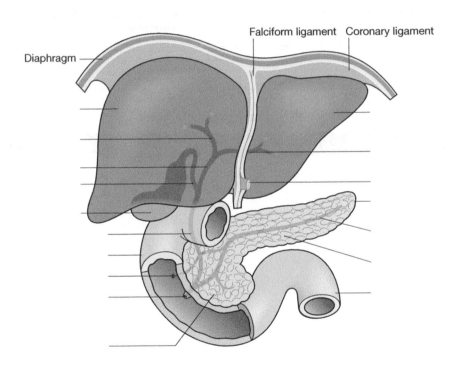

Figure 9.12 The liver, gallbladder and pancreas. *Source*: Peate and Nair, 2014. Reproduced with permission of John Wiley & Sons.

Gallbladder

Question 23   Arrange the boxes using arrows to describe the production and storage of bile.

| Pancreatic duct from pancreas |

| Common hepatic duct from liver |

| Left hepatic duct |

| Cystic duct from gallbladder |

| Common bile duct |

| Right hepatic duct |

Source: Tortora and Derrickson, 2009. Reproduced with permission of John Wiley & Sons.

Liver

The liver is divided into segments these are further divided into lobules. Lobules are usually represented as discrete hexagonal aggregations of hepatocytes.

Question 24   In Figure 9.13, identify the histological components of the liver.

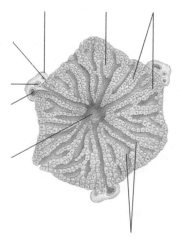

Figure 9.13   Liver lobule. *Source*: Peate and Nair, 2015. Reproduced with permission of John Wiley & Sons.

Pancreas

The pancreas is composed of exocrine and endocrine tissue, consisting of a head, body and tail. The cells of the pancreas are responsible for making the endocrine and exocrine products.

Question 25

(a) In Figure 9.14, identify the component parts.

(b) Colour in the various aspects.

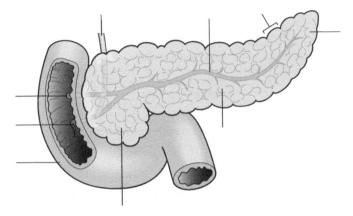

Figure 9.14   The pancreas. *Source*: Peate and Nair, 2015. Reproduced with permission of John Wiley & Sons.

Question 26   Match the pairs.

The liver is located	the release of pancreatic juice
The liver is involved in lipid metabolism, lipogenesis and	the endocrine and exocrine products
The gall bladder functions as a	the synthesis of cholesterol
When the walls of the gallbladder contract, bile is expelled into the cystic duct and down into the common bile duct before entering the duodenum via the	reservoir for bile
The cells of the pancreas are responsible for making	hepatopancreatic ampulla
Parasympathetic vagus nerve stimulation promotes	in the right upper quadrant

Question 27 Time yourself to unscramble these words.

Scrambled	Answer
ELIB	
PONGIISLEES	
APHOTESTYEC	
CHEPATI	
SHOOTCLLEER	
DOCREENIN	
REXONEIC	
ICEJU	

Snap shot

Drug-induced gastric irritation

Whilst medications are given to promote a person's health and well-being there are many types of medication that can cause the patient harm (this is known as iatrogenic).

Elizabeth Hernandez is a 68-year-old lady who has osteoarthritis and has been taking a medication called Arthrotec (diclofenac and misoprostol). The dose is diclofenac 50 mg/misoprostol 200 mg: one tablet orally three times daily. Arthrotec is used to treat osteoarthritis and rheumatoid arthritis in people at high risk for developing stomach or intestinal ulcers.

Diclofenac is a non-steroidal anti-inflammatory drug (NSAID). It works by reducing hormones that cause inflammation and pain in the body.

Misoprostol reduces stomach acid and replaces protective substances in the stomach that are reduced by NSAIDs.

In order to prevent gastric ulcers occurring what advice should the nurse give to Ms Hernandez?

Word search

T	H	H	Z	G	V	I	U	S	U	G	A	H	P	O	S	E	O	C	L
E	L	C	D	K	D	N	A	L	U	C	O	S	J	D	X	N	U	Q	W
L	Y	M	A	F	G	G	S	T	C	Z	E	N	I	R	C	O	X	E	Y
B	S	K	O	M	N	E	D	I	O	M	G	I	S	L	A	U	P	R	R
O	O	R	X	S	O	S	C	C	I	B	I	D	O	B	I	A	A	V	J
G	Z	E	Y	W	T	T	D	D	K	A	E	K	B	M	R	T	O	X	T
B	Y	V	S	S	X	I	S	Z	X	N	L	U	M	O	N	H	F	I	F
Y	M	I	E	X	A	O	O	P	T	J	R	G	T	E	B	W	A	Y	S
V	E	L	N	I	M	N	O	I	T	A	N	I	M	I	L	E	E	Y	V
M	I	Z	A	M	G	O	T	Q	Z	M	D	I	C	I	Y	G	C	F	O
K	O	T	K	Y	M	I	A	T	O	C	L	F	Y	P	N	H	E	S	E
E	R	U	H	M	O	Q	U	G	V	A	O	C	J	U	G	M	S	K	C
Y	A	A	T	N	I	D	I	J	E	J	E	N	I	T	S	E	T	N	I
S	V	Q	D	H	Y	D	R	O	C	H	L	O	R	I	C	F	R	O	Y
U	O	D	G	C	V	P	A	N	C	R	E	A	S	Z	Y	W	M	V	Y
O	O	M	X	I	L	E	O	C	A	E	C	A	L	B	V	K	I	B	E
C	K	B	P	U	X	Q	T	A	V	I	L	A	S	E	A	R	L	G	F
U	Y	P	C	G	U	B	O	L	U	S	N	S	C	W	X	O	I	U	F
M	G	Z	G	V	U	N	B	W	B	R	U	G	A	E	O	X	T	D	K
V	J	E	J	U	N	U	M	B	U	L	N	O	I	T	S	E	G	I	D

ALIMENTARY	OESOPHAGUS	BOLUS
MOUTH	INGESTION	MUCOUS
INTESTINE	DIGESTION	RUGAE
LIVER	ELIMINATION	HYDROCHLORIC
PANCREAS	PAROTID	JEJUNUM
STOMACH	SALIVA	GOBLET
ILEOCAECAL	DENTITION	EXOCRINE
FAECES	LYSOZYME	SIGMOID

Crossword

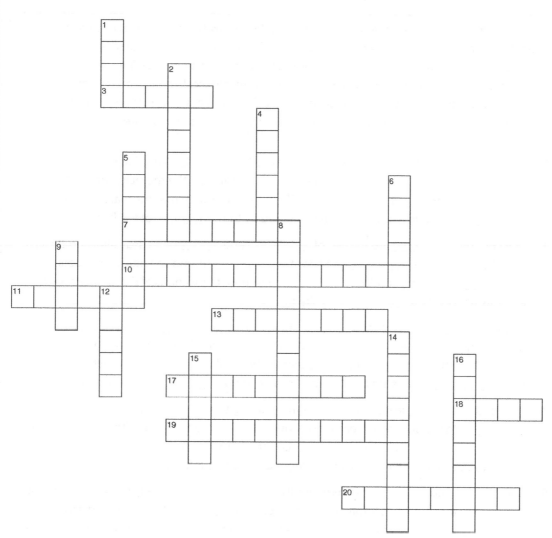

Across

3. Ridges of muscle tissue lining the stomach
7. Constituent of saliva with an antibacterial action
10. Salivary gland located below the mandible
11. Forms the roof of the mouth and consists of two parts
13. Cells that produce hydrochloric acid and intrinsic factor
17. Breaking down food
18. The end of the gastrointestinal tract
19. Liver cells
20. First section of the small intestine

Down

1. Number of sections in the large intestine
2. Accessory organ of digestion which secretes insulin
4. Faecal matter is stored here until defecation
5. Salivary digestive enzyme
6. Absorbed by the large intestine
8. When waste products of digestion are excreted from the body as faeces
9. Substance stored in the gallbladder
12. Number of sections in the small intestine
14. Taking food into the digestive system
15. The largest organ in the body
16. The liver is located in the right upper what?

Fill in the blanks

Use the words in the box to complete the sentences:

> 1.5, 25, 7, abrasion, absorption, anus, bladder, body, bolus, cavity, cells, cheeks, chemical, chemical, churning, connective, convert, digestion, duodenum, ears, eliminated, enzyme, enzymes, expand, floor, fluid, food, ileocaecal, ileum, ileum, intestine, intestine, jaw, large, laryngopharynx, length, liver, mastication, mechanical, mechanical, metres, metres, mouth, mucus, muscle, oesophagus, oesophagus, parotid, pyloric, saliva, saliva, salivary, store, stores, sublingual, submandibular, teeth, three, three, tract, transport, vitamins, water

1. The gastrointestinal _____ is approximately 10 _____ long. Travelling the _____ of the _____ from the _____, through the thoracic, abdominal and pelvic cavities, ending at the _____. The digestive system has one major function: to _____ food into a form that can be utilised by the _____ of the body.

2. The lips and _____ are formed of _____ and _____ tissue allowing the lips and cheeks to move _____ mixed with _____ around the mouth and begin _____ digestion. The _____ contribute to mechanical digestion, chewing and mixing food with _____ is called _____.

3. There are _____ pairs of _____ glands. The _____ glands are the largest, located anterior to the _____; saliva from the parotid glands enters the oral _____. The _____ glands are located below the _____ on each side of the face. _____ glands are the smallest, located in the _____ of the mouth.

4. The food _____ leaves the oropharynx entering the _____; this extends from the _____ to the stomach, measuring about _____ cm in length. The function is to _____ substances. Thick _____ is secreted by the mucosa of the _____, aiding the passage of the bolus, protecting the oesophagus from _____.

5. The stomach can _____ to temporarily _____ food, partially digesting food. The _____ action of the stomach muscles mechanically breaks down the food, acids and _____ are released for _____ breakdown. The _____ pepsin is responsible for protein breakdown. The passage of food from the stomach to the small _____ is controlled by the _____ sphincter.

6. The small _____ is approximately 6 _____ long. Here food is further broken down by _____ and _____ digestion, and _____ of the products of digestion takes place. The small intestine is divided into _____ parts, _____, jejunum and _____. The small intestine joins the large intestine at the _____ valve.

7. Accessory organs of _____ are the _____, gall _____ and pancreas.

8. Once food residue has reached the _____ intestine it cannot flow back into the _____. The large intestine measures _____ m in length and _____ cm in diameter. It reabsorbs _____ and maintains the _____ balance of the body, it absorbs certain _____, processes undigested material and _____ waste before it is _____ via the _____.

Multiple choice questions

1. The oesophagus

   (a) Secretes vitamin D
   (b) Secretes intrinsic factor necessary for the absorption of vitamin B$_{12}$
   (c) Is a hollow tube carrying food from the pharynx to the stomach
   (d) Is where chyme is formed

2. Which of the following is true concerning the stomach?

   (a) It digests all fats
   (b) It is lined with microvilli
   (c) It is attached distally to the jejunum and proximally to the oesophagus
   (d) It delivers chyme to the duodenum

3. Which of the following is NOT descriptive of bile?

   (a) Aids in the digestion of fat
   (b) Acts as an emulsifier
   (c) Is classified as a lipase
   (d) Is stored by the gall bladder

4. How many permanent teeth are there?

   (a) 16
   (b) 20
   (c) 24
   (d) 32

5. Which of the following is not a function of the liver?

   (a) Makes blood-clotting factors
   (b) Produces bile
   (c) Secretes cholecystokinin and secretin
   (d) Stores fat-soluble vitamins

6. Which of the following best describes emulsification?

   (a) A fat is chemically digested into fatty acids and glycerol
   (b) The fatty acids are absorbed into the lacteal, becoming chyme
   (c) A large fat globule is broken down mechanically into smaller fat globules
   (d) A large protein that forms ammonia

7. The pancreas

   (a) Secretes the potent digestive enzymes
   (b) Secretes bile
   (c) Is dependent on the spleen
   (d) Empties its digestive enzymes into the oesophagus

8. The duodenum is most concerned with which of the following?

(a) The secretion of vitamin B12
(b) Digestion and absorption
(c) The production of clotting factors and plasma proteins
(d) None of the above

9. In health how much saliva is produced daily?

(a) None
(b) 100 mL
(c) 200–250 mL
(d) 1–1.5 L

10. The pharynx consists of how many parts?

(a) 2
(b) 3
(c) 4
(d) None of the above

References

Peate, I. and Nair, M. (2015) *Anatomy and Physiology for Nurses at a Glance*. Oxford: John Wiley & Sons, Ltd.
Peate, I., Wild, K. & Nair, M. (eds) (2014) *Nursing Practice: Knowledge and Care*. Oxford: John Wiley & Sons, Ltd.
Tortora, G.J. and Derrickson, B.H. (2009) *Principles of Anatomy and Physiology*, 12th edn. Hoboken, NJ: John Wiley & Sons, Inc.

Chapter 10

The renal system

The renal system is also known as the urinary system. The kidneys play a key role in maintaining homeostasis, removing waste products through the production and excretion of urine, and regulating fluid balance in the body. Kidneys filter essential substances, such as sodium and potassium from the blood, selectively reabsorbing substances necessary to maintain homeostasis, while unneeded substances are excreted in the urine. Urine is formed through the processes of filtration, selective reabsorption and excretion. The kidneys also secrete hormones such as renin and erythropoietin.

The renal system consists of:

- kidneys   • ureters   • urinary bladder   • urethra

   Question 1   In Figure 10.1, identify the parts of the renal system.

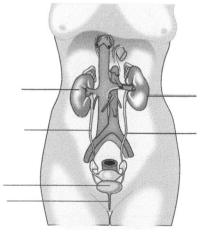

Anterior view

Figure 10.1   The renal system (anterior view). *Source*: Tortora and Derrickson, 2009. Reproduced with permission of John Wiley & Sons.

Fundamentals of Anatomy and Physiology Workbook: A Study Guide for Nursing and Healthcare Students, First Edition. Ian Peate.
© 2017 John Wiley & Sons Ltd. Published 2017 by John Wiley & Sons Ltd.

The kidney: macroscopic

There are usually two kidneys, one on each side of the spinal column, approximately 11 cm long, 5–6 cm wide and 3–4 cm thick. They are bean-shaped organs where the outer border is convex. The inner border is known as the hilum; here the renal arteries, renal veins, nerves and the ureters enter and leave the kidneys.

Question 2
(a) Identify the structures in Figure 10.2.

(b) Colour in the different features.

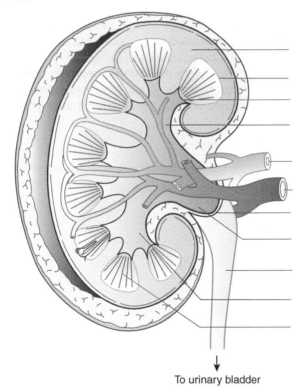

To urinary bladder

Figure 10.2 Macroscopic structure of the kidney. *Source*: Peate and Nair, 2011. Reproduced with permission of John Wiley & Sons.

The kidney: microscopic

Within the kidney there are three distinct regions:

1. renal cortex
2. renal medulla
3. renal pelvis.

 Question 3   Identify and label the structures of the kidney in Figure 10.3.

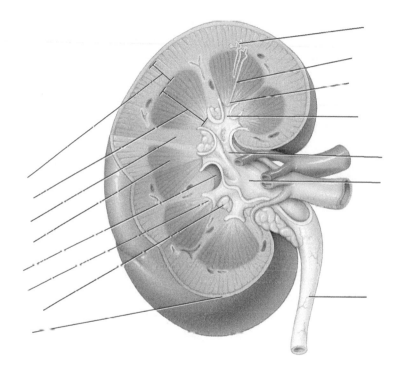

Figure 10.3   The internal structures of the kidney. *Source*: Tortora and Nair, 2009. Reproduced with permission of John Wiley & Sons.

Question 4 Match the pairs.

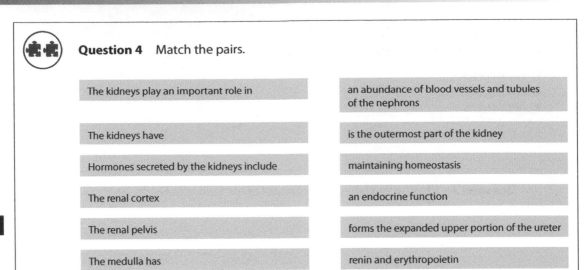

The kidneys play an important role in	an abundance of blood vessels and tubules of the nephrons
The kidneys have	is the outermost part of the kidney
Hormones secreted by the kidneys include	maintaining homeostasis
The renal cortex	an endocrine function
The renal pelvis	forms the expanded upper portion of the ureter
The medulla has	renin and erythropoietin

Question 5 Time yourself to unscramble these words.

Scrambled	Answer
DELLAMU	
SPLIVE	
LIFTRATION	
BAPTISRONREO	
PHOTOTYRERIEIN	
TREEUR	
CASAFI	
SLYCACE	

Nephrons

These are small structures, which form the functional units of the kidney. They consist of a glomerulus and a renal tubule. There are over one million nephrons per kidney. These structures form urine: they filter blood, perform selective reabsorption and excrete unwanted waste products. The nephron is divided into several sections:

- Bowman's capsule
- proximal convoluted tubule
- loop of Henle
- distal convoluted tubule

Question 6

(a) In Figure 10.4, identify the sections of the nephron.

(b) Colour in the various components of the nephron.

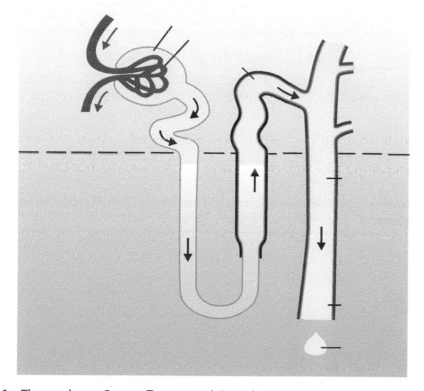

Figure 10.4 The nephron. *Source*: Tortora and Derrickson, 2009. Reproduced with permission of John Wiley & Sons.

Bowman's capsule, also known as glomerular capsule, is a cup-like sac. It is the first portion of the nephron and is part of the filtration system in the kidneys. When blood reaches the kidneys, it enters the Bowman's capsule, and is separated into two components: a filtered blood product and a filtrate that is moved through the nephron.

Question 7   Label Figure 10.5.

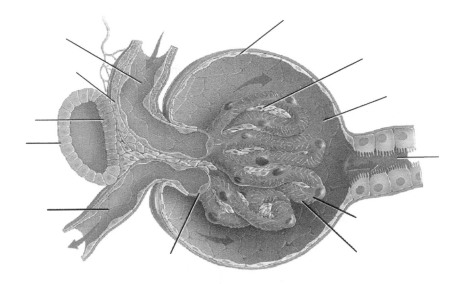

Figure 10.5   Bowman's capsule. *Source*: Tortora and Derrickson, 2009. Reproduced with permission of John Wiley & Sons.

Question 8 In Table 10.1 write notes about the four components of the Bowman's capsule.

Table 10.1 Components of the Bowman's capsule.

Component	Description/function
Proximal convoluted tubule	
Loop of Henle	
Distal convoluted tubule	
Collecting duct	

Question 9 Match the pairs.

These are small structures, forming the functional units of the kidney	one million nephrons per kidney
There are over	proximal convoluted tubule
When blood reaches the kidneys for filtration	it enters the Bowman's capsule
From the Bowman's capsule, the filtrate drains into the	is divided into the descending and ascending loops
The loop of Henle	nephrons
Sodium and water	are reabsorbed in the final stage

Question 10 In Table 10.2 summarise the functions of the kidney. Two functions have already been added.

Table 10.2 A summary of the functions of the kidney.

Function	Description
Regulation of electrolytes	
Secretion	

Question 11 Identify the renal blood vessels in Figure 10.6.

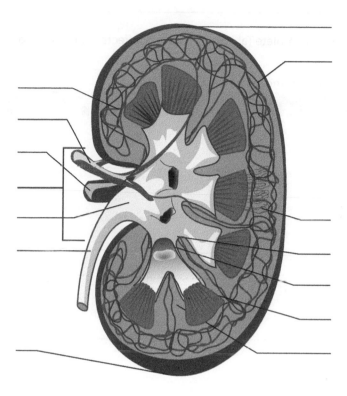

Figure 10.6 The renal blood supply and associated structures.

Hormones working on the kidney

 Question 12 Complete Table 10.3 about the effects of hormones on the kidney.

Table 10.3 The effects of hormones on the kidney.

Hormone	Secreted by	Function
Aldosterone		
Atrial natriuretic peptide	Atria of the heart	
Brain natriuretic peptide	Ventricles of the heart	
Antidiuretic hormone		
	Parathyroid gland	Stimulates the reabsorption of calcium and the excretion of phosphate

Question 13 Match the pairs.

The kidneys	arises from the abdominal aorta at the level of first lumbar vertebra
Kidneys synthesise hormones such as	a hormone that stimulates the production of red blood cells
Kidneys produce erythropoietin, this is	renin and angiotensin
Healthy kidneys keep bones strong by producing	maintain fluid balance, electrolyte balance and the acid–base balance of the blood
Renal artery	water
Urine is 96%	the hormone calcitriol

Question 14 Time yourself to unscramble these words.

Scrambled	Answer
TOADSLERONE	
MORULESLUG	
HORENPN	
TROXEC	
SLIVEP	
DELLAUM	
LUBETU	
SOOTSISHAME	

Ureters and bladder

The ureters are tubular organs running from the renal pelvis to the base of the urinary bladder. They are approximately 25–30 cm in length and 5 mm in diameter.

The urinary bladder is a hollow muscular organ, located in the pelvic cavity posterior to the symphysis pubis. In men the bladder lies anterior to the rectum, in females it is located anterior to the vagina and inferior to the ureters. It is a smooth muscular sac that stores urine. The bladder normally distends to hold approximately 350–750 mL of urine. The inner lining of the urinary bladder is a mucous membrane of transitional epithelium, continuous with that in the ureters. When the bladder is empty, the mucosa has numerous folds called rugae; these permit the bladder to expand as it fills.

The inner floor of the bladder includes a triangular section called the trigone, formed by three openings. Two of the openings are from the ureters, and the third opening, at the apex of the trigone, is into the urethra. A band of the detrusor muscle encircles this opening forming the internal urethral sphincter.

Question 15
(a) In Figure 10.7, identify the urinary bladder and the associated structures.

(b) Colour in the bladder, ureters and other structures.

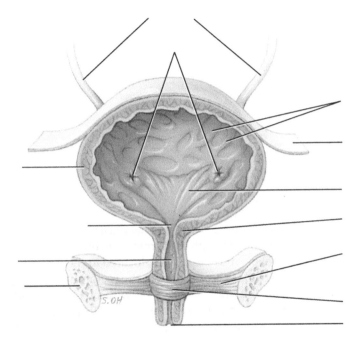

Figure 10.7   The urinary bladder and associated structures. *Source*: Tortora and Derrickson, 2009. Reproduced with permission of John Wiley & Sons.

The urethra

The male urethra is made up of four main segments. The preprostatic urethra that runs anterior to the prostate, while the prostatic urethra courses through that gland. The membranous urethra travels through the external urethral sphincter, and the spongy urethra travels the length of the penis and concludes at the meatus at the tip of the penis. The urethra not only excretes fluid wastes but is also part of the reproductive system.

The female urethra is bound to the anterior vaginal wall and is approximately 4 cm long. It leads out of the body via the urethral orifice. In the female, the urethral orifice is located in the vestibule in the labia minora.

Question 16

(a) Figure 10.8 depicts the male ureters, bladder and urethra. Identify these three structures and adjacent parts.

(b) Colour in the three key structures.

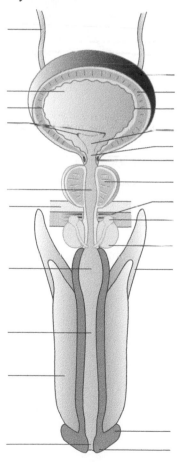

Figure 10.8   The male urethra. *Source*: Peate and Nair, 2011. Reproduced with permission of John Wiley & Sons.

Question 17
(a) Figure 10.9 depicts the female urethra. Identify the structures and adjacent parts.

(b) Colour in the key structures.

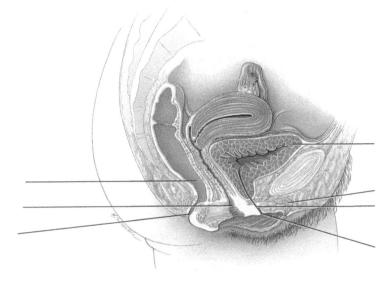

Figure 10.9 The female urethra. *Source*: Peate and Nair, 2011. Reproduced with permission of John Wiley & Sons.

Question 18 Match the pairs.

The urinary bladder is	a muscular tube that drains urine from the bladder and conveys it out of the body
In the male the bladder lies	called the trigone
In the female the bladder lies	anterior to the rectum
The inner floor of the bladder includes a triangular section	anterior to the vagina and inferior to the uterus
The ureters are	tubular organs which run from the renal pelvis to the posterolateral base of the urinary bladder
The urethra is	a hollow muscular organ and is located in the pelvic cavity posterior to the symphysis pubis

Question 19 Time yourself to unscramble these words.

Scrambled	Answer
THERAUR	
TRUERE	
SIPBU	
UAGER	
IGRONTE	
STRUDERO	
CHIPSTERN	
VACYTI	

Snap shot

Urinalysis

Andy Coulston is 38 years of age and has been to the general practice. He was complaining of pain when he 'passed water': he said it is like 'peeing razor blades'. After taking Andy's history and examining him, the practice nurse asked him to provide a urine specimen so she could carry out a dipstick analysis.

What is urinalysis and why was it performed? What might test results reveal?

Word search

B	L	A	D	D	E	R	B	Q	G	F	I	L	T	R	A	T	I	O	N
P	X	O	R	W	N	P	S	L	Q	R	C	S	I	E	K	O	K	M	Y
U	U	B	O	S	O	Y	O	A	T	M	E	B	K	S	I	F	J	E	R
B	S	S	J	A	R	M	E	T	E	P	E	N	M	I	D	P	Y	D	E
O	W	J	R	P	E	J	M	S	H	F	R	S	A	V	N	J	J	U	T
W	L	C	Z	R	T	D	G	I	Y	P	Y	N	H	L	E	B	X	L	E
M	V	G	U	A	S	T	T	D	A	S	T	T	M	E	Y	L	B	L	R
A	K	L	P	B	O	R	G	V	Z	E	H	L	H	P	S	O	E	A	U
N	U	J	T	K	D	G	Q	G	V	T	R	G	U	F	H	J	H	L	M
S	T	Z	P	I	L	W	K	N	C	Y	O	K	R	L	G	K	C	M	B
E	N	L	J	R	A	S	Z	S	E	L	P	U	E	U	K	X	R	C	L
C	M	O	A	Y	O	R	I	J	C	O	O	N	T	R	O	E	E	H	R
U	F	S	R	E	A	X	H	I	Q	R	I	C	H	I	S	T	N	E	T
C	L	K	K	H	H	M	I	H	W	T	E	K	R	N	E	R	I	N	Q
K	I	L	K	I	P	Z	K	M	J	C	T	D	A	E	E	O	N	L	L
R	V	J	N	R	V	E	L	I	A	E	I	Z	U	D	K	C	G	E	K
X	C	L	Z	E	I	E	N	S	Y	L	N	H	H	E	Y	K	Z	I	L
C	P	F	Y	B	B	V	E	O	I	E	E	N	O	G	I	R	T	Z	J
B	Z	D	E	T	U	L	O	V	N	O	C	O	A	R	M	I	V	O	E
M	P	R	O	K	C	Q	L	C	H	N	W	K	Q	P	F	Q	F	U	J

RENAL	RENIN	PROXIMAL
KIDNEYS	ERYTHROPOIETIN	DISTAL
URETHRA	NEPHRONS	CONVOLUTED
URETER	GLOMERULUS	ELECTROLYTES
BLADDER	BOWMANS	ALDOSTERONE
MEDULLA	FILTRATION	TRIGONE
PELVIS	URINE	CORTEXTHENLE

208

Crossword

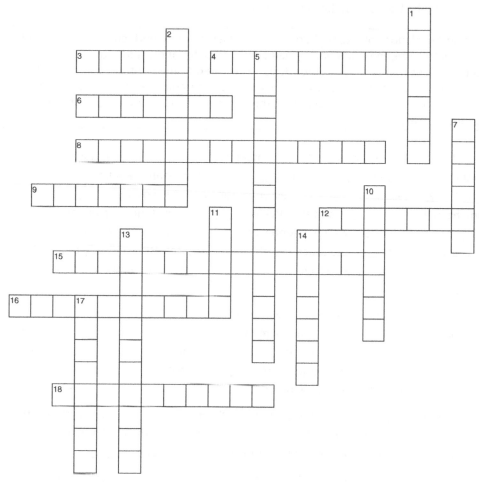

Across

3. The loop of?
4. Blood in the urine
6. Conveys urine to the exterior
8. An infection of kidney tissue
9. They convey urine to the bladder
12. The area of the inner floor of the bladder
15. Hormone precursor produced by the hepatocytes of the liver
16. Hormone that maintains the right levels of calcium and phosphate in the blood and bones
18. One of the three processes involved in the formation of urine

Down

1. Storage organ for urine
2. The small functional units of the kidney
5. One of the hormones that contributes to red cell production
7. The outermost part of the kidney
10. They remove waste products through the production and excretion of urine and regulate fluid balance in the body
11. Artery that carries blood to the kidneys
13. The act of passing urine
14. The glomerular capsule
17. Infection of the bladder

Fill in the blanks

Use the words in the box to complete the sentences:

balance, bladder, bladder, blood, body, detrusor, diameter, drains, endocrine, erythropoietin, excrete, excreted, excretion, excretion, females, filter, filter, filtration, folds, functional, glomerulus, hollow, homeostasis, homeostasis, inner, internal, involuntary, kidney, length, million, mucous, muscles, muscular, muscular, muscular, muscular, pelvic, pelvis, production, pubis, reabsorb, selective, sodium, sphincter, three, tubular, tubule, urinary, urinary, urine, urine, voluntary, wall, walls, waste

1. The kidneys play an important role in maintaining _____. They remove _____ products through the _____ and _____ of urine and regulate fluid _____ in the body. The kidneys _____ essential substances, such as _____ and potassium, from the _____, and selectively _____ substances essential to maintain _____. Any substances not essential are _____ in the urine. The formation of urine is achieved through the processes of _____, selective reabsorption and _____. The kidneys also have an _____ function, secreting hormones such as renin and _____.

2. Nephrons are small structures and they form the _____ units of the _____. The nephron consists of a _____ and a renal _____. There are approximately one _____ nephrons per kidney and it is in these structures where _____ is formed. The nephrons _____ blood, perform _____ reabsorption and _____ unwanted waste products from the blood.

3. The ureters are _____ in shape running from the renal _____ to the base of the _____ bladder. They are approximately 25–30 cm in length and 5 mm in _____. The ureters enter obliquely through the muscle _____ of the _____.

4. The _____ bladder is a _____ muscular organ and is located in the _____ cavity posterior to the symphysis _____; it is a smooth _____ sac which stores _____. When the bladder is empty, the _____ wall of the bladder forms _____, but as the bladder fills with urine the _____ of the _____ become smoother.

5. The urethra is a _____ tube which _____ urine from the bladder and conveys it out of the _____. Its wall has _____ coats: _____, erectile and _____. The _____ coat is the continuation of the bladder muscle layer. The urethra is encompassed by two separate urethral sphincter _____. The _____ urethral sphincter muscle is formed by _____ smooth muscle, while _____ muscles make up the external _____. The internal sphincter is created by the _____ muscle. The urethra is different in _____ in males and _____.

Multiple choice questions

1. What does micturition refer to?

   (a) Excessive vomiting
   (b) Dehydration
   (c) The bladder's ability to store urine
   (d) The act of urinating

2. The filtration of 180 L per day of blood

   (a) Is an abnormal event
   (b) Moves water from the renal tubules into the peritubular capillaries
   (c) Is the rate at which urine flows into ureters
   (d) Occurs across the glomerular membrane

3. Which is the first tubular structure to receive the glomerular ultrafiltrate?

   (a) Collecting duct
   (b) Renal pelvis
   (c) Loop of Henle
   (d) Bowman's capsule

4. The active pumping of Na$^+$ from the proximal convoluted tubule into the peritubular capillaries

   (a) Blocks the micturition reflex
   (b) Prevents diuresis
   (c) Is responsible for the passive reabsorption of water
   (d) Only occurs when the person is dehydrated

5. Which of the following is least true of aldosterone?

   (a) It is a mineralocorticoid
   (b) It is the 'salt-retaining' hormone
   (c) It is a glucocorticoid
   (d) It promotes tubular reabsorption of sodium and water

6. The renal pelvis

   (a) Is found close to the bladder
   (b) Forms the expanded upper portion of the ureter
   (c) Determines the amount of urine passed
   (d) Determines the pore size of the glomeruli

7. What does a drug blocking the renal reabsorption of Na$^+$ cause?

    (a) Death
    (b) Diuresis
    (c) Anuria
    (d) Hypernatraemia

8. Why is glucose not usually excreted in the urine?

    (a) Glucose is not filtered
    (b) All filtered glucose is reabsorbed
    (c) Glucose is used up by the gallbladder
    (d) Glucose is converted to ammonia and excreted as urea

9. Over how many nephrons are there per kidney?

    (a) One hundred
    (b) One thousand
    (c) Ten thousand
    (d) One million

10. Oliguria

    (a) Concerns a lowered serum potassium
    (b) Can develop in response to hypotension
    (c) Is a response to an antiemetic
    (d) Most often accompanies a decline in serum creatinine

References

Peate, I. and Nair, M. (2011) *Fundamentals of Anatomy and Physiology for Student Nurses*. Oxford: John Wiley & Sons, Ltd.

Tortora, G.J. and Derrickson, B.H. (2009) *Principles of Anatomy and Physiology*, 12th edn. Hoboken, NJ: John Wiley & Sons, Inc.

Chapter 11

The respiratory system

The respiratory system is responsible for gaseous exchange between the circulatory system and the atmosphere. Air is taken in via the upper airways (the nasal cavity, pharynx and larynx) through the lower airways (trachea, primary bronchi and bronchial tree) and into the small bronchioles and alveoli within the lung tissue.

 Question 1   In Figure 11.1, identify the major structures of the upper and lower respiratory tract.

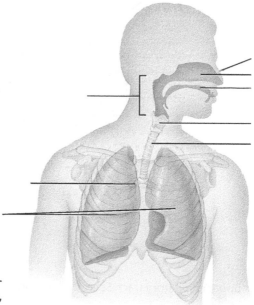

Figure 11.1   Upper and lower respiratory tract. *Source:* Tortora and Derrickson, 2009. Reproduced with permission of John Wiley & Sons.

Fundamentals of Anatomy and Physiology Workbook: A Study Guide for Nursing and Healthcare Students, First Edition. Ian Peate.
© 2017 John Wiley & Sons Ltd. Published 2017 by John Wiley & Sons Ltd.

The upper respiratory tract

The mouth, nose, nasal cavity and pharynx are the organs of the upper respiratory tract. The upper respiratory tract warms, filters and moistens the inhaled air. The nasal cavity is divided by the nasal septum. The nasal cavities are subdivided into three air passages (meatuses), divided by the superior, middle and inferior conchae (turbinates). The pharynx is a chamber shared by the digestive and respiratory systems, connecting the nasal and oral cavity with the larynx. There are three regions of the pharynx:

1. nasopharynx
2. oropharynx
3. laryngopharynx.

Question 2 Label the structures and the associated structures of the upper respiratory tract in Figure 11.2.

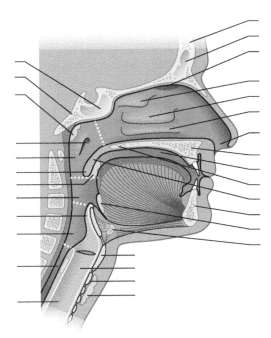

Figure 11.2 The upper respiratory tract. *Source*: Peate and Nair, 2014. Reproduced with permission of John Wiley & Sons.

The larynx

The larynx consists of nine pieces of cartilage tissue, three single pieces and three pairs. The single pieces of cartilage are:

- the thyroid cartilage (commonly known as the Adam's apple), protects the vocal cords
- the epiglottis, protects the airway from food and water
- the cricoid cartilage, provides connectivity for different ligaments, cartilages and muscles.

Question 3
(a) In Figure 11.3, identify the various components of the larynx.

(b) Colour in the components.

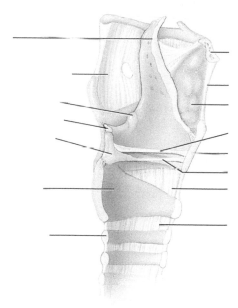

Figure 11.3 The larynx. *Source*: Tortora and Derrickson, 2009. Reproduced with permission of John Wiley & Sons.

The trachea and bronchial tree

The trachea extends from the laryngopharynx at the level of the cricoid cartilage at the top to the carina (tracheal bifurcation). There are 15–20 C-shaped cartilage rings which reinforce and protect the trachea. The carina is a ridge-shaped structure and possesses sensory nerve endings that cause coughing if food or water is inhaled accidentally.

The trachea divides into two main bronchi, the left and the right, at the carina. The right main bronchus is more vertical, wider and shorter, and subdivides into three lobar bronchi; the left main bronchus divides into two. The segmental bronchi divide into many primary bronchioles that divide into terminal bronchioles, several respiratory bronchioles, and terminate in alveoli.

Question 4 Complete Table 11.1 – the branches of the bronchial tree, from the trachea to the terminal bronchioles.

Table 11.1 The branches of the bronchial tree.

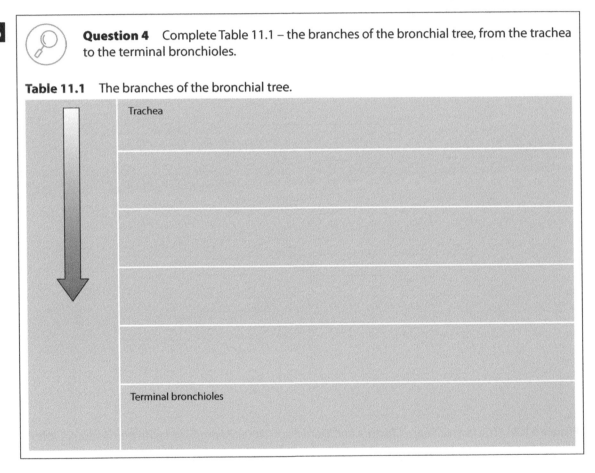

Trachea

Terminal bronchioles

Question 5

(a) In Figure 11.4, identify the parts of the bronchial tree.

(b) Colour in the parts of the bronchial tree.

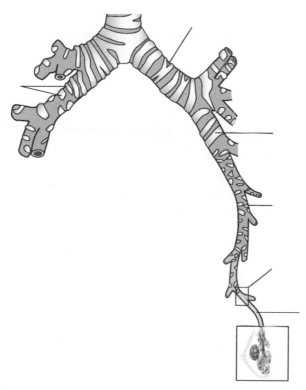

Figure 11.4   The bronchial tree. *Source*: Peate and Nair, 2011. Reproduced with permission of John Wiley & Sons.

The lungs

The lungs are divided into regions – lobes: three lobes in the right lung and two in the left. Two thin protective membranes, the parietal and visceral pleura, surround each lung. The space between the two pleura, the pleural space, contains a thin film of lubricating fluid, reducing friction between the two pleura during breathing. The fluid also helps the visceral and parietal pleura to adhere to each other.

 Question 6   In Figure 11.5, identify the various aspects of the lower respiratory tract.

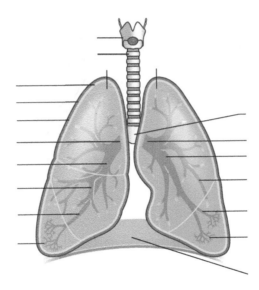

Figure 11.5   The lungs. *Source*: Peate and Nair, 2014. Reproduced with permission of John Wiley & Sons.

 Question 7   Match the pairs.

As cells use oxygen	warms, filters and moistens the inhaled air
The organs of the upper respiratory tract are the	three lobes in the right lung and two in the left
The upper respiratory tract	carbon dioxide is produced as waste
Nine pieces of cartilage tissue, three single pieces and three pairs,	mouth, nose, nasal cavity and pharynx
The trachea	form the larynx
The lungs are divided into lobes,	extends from the laryngopharynx to the carina

Question 8   Time yourself to unscramble these words.

Scrambled	Answer
CHEATAR	
SHURCONB	
NARXYPH	
NARCIA	
RULEAP	
CGARATILE	
SHOENCROBIL	
VEILOLA	

Respiration

This is the process by which oxygen and carbon dioxide are exchanged between the atmosphere and body. There are four distinct phases:

1. pulmonary ventilation
2. external respiration
3. transport of gases
4. internal respiration.

Question 9   In Table 11.2, describe the four distinct phases of respiration.

Table 11.2   The four distinct phases of respiration.

Phase	Description
Pulmonary ventilation	
External respiration	
Transport of gases	
Internal respiration	

Inspiration and expiration

During inspiration the thoracic cavity expands enabling air to be drawn in. The rib cage moves up and out and the diaphragm contracts and moves down. Pressure within the lungs decreases and the air comes rushing in. During expiration the rib cage moves down and in, and the diaphragm relaxes and moves up. The pressure in the lungs increases so air is pushed out.

Question 10 In Figure 11.6, label the diagram.

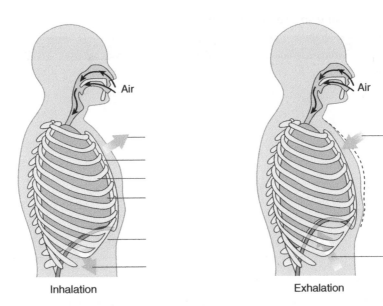

Air

Air

Inhalation

Exhalation

Figure 11.6 Inspiration and expiration. *Source*: Peate and Nair, 2011. Reproduced with permission of John Wiley & Sons.

Question 11 In Figure 11.7, identify the muscles involved in pulmonary ventilation.

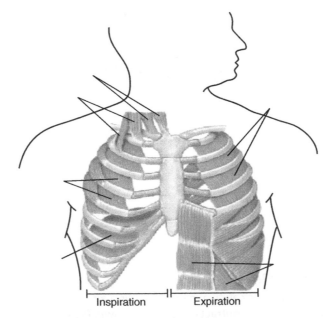

Inspiration

Expiration

Figure 11.7 The muscles associated with pulmonary ventilation. *Source*: Peate 2015. Reproduced with permission of John Wiley & Sons.

The control of breathing

The rate and depth of breathing are controlled by the respiratory centres, which are found in the brain stem, within the areas called the medulla oblongata and pons. The rate of breathing is set by the medulla oblongata; within the medulla oblongata there are specialised chemoreceptors which continually analyse carbon dioxide levels within cerebrospinal fluid.

Question 12

(a) Identify the structures and the various areas of the brain associated with breathing in Figure 11.8. Label the diagram.

(b) Colour in the structures and the areas in the brain stem.

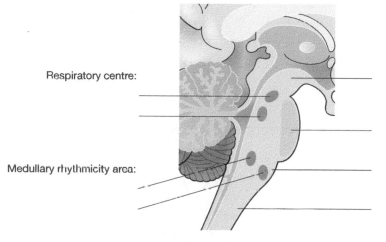

Respiratory centre:

Medullary rhythmicity area:

Figure 11.8 The respiratory centre. *Source*: Peate and Nair, 2014. Reproduced with permission of John Wiley & Sons.

Peripheral chemoreceptors

Chemicals dissolved in the blood also affect breathing. These chemicals are detected by sensory cells called chemoreceptors.

Question 13
(a) Identify the various aspects of Figure 11.9 that are associated with breathing.

(b) Colour in the components.

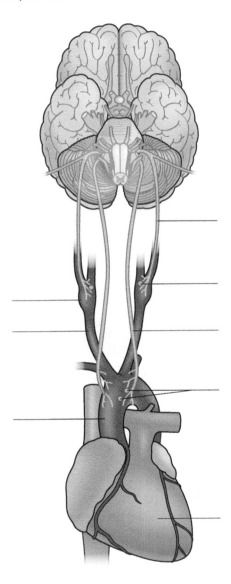

Figure 11.9 The peripheral chemoreceptors. *Source*: Peate and Nair, 2015. Reproduced with permission of John Wiley & Sons.

Gaseous exchange

Exchange of gases in the lungs takes place between alveolar air and the blood flowing through the lung capillaries. Before oxygen can enter the internal environment and before carbon dioxide can leave the internal environment they must cross the capillary and alveolar membranes. Oxygen enters the blood from the alveolar sac as the PO_2 of alveolar air is greater than the PO_2 of incoming blood. Concurrently, carbon dioxide molecules leave the blood by diffusing down the carbon dioxide pressure gradient out into the alveolar sac. The PCO_2 of venous blood is much higher than the PCO_2 of alveolar air.

Question 14

(a) Figure 11.10 demonstrates external respiration, identify the component parts of the figure. Identify the direction of blood flow through the pulmonary vein and the pulmonary artery.

(b) Colour in the vein, artery, alveolus and capillaries.

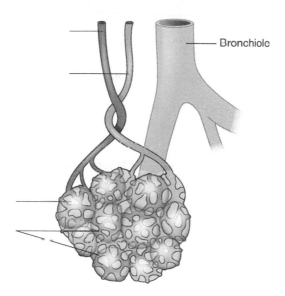

Bronchiole

Figure 11.10 External respiration. *Source*: Peate and Nair, 2015. Reproduced with permission of John Wiley & Sons.

Question 15

(a) Identify and label the features of Figure 11.11.

(b) Colour in the different components.

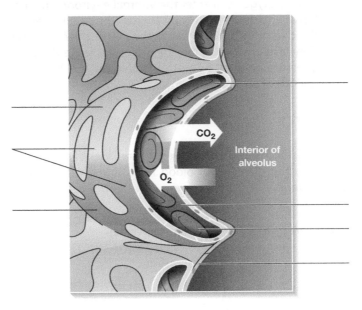

Figure 11.11   Gas exchange in the lungs. *Source*: Peate and Nair, 2015. Reproduced with permission of John Wiley & Sons.

Question 16

(a) Insert the direction of gas exchange in Figure 11.12.

(b) Colour in Figure 11.12.

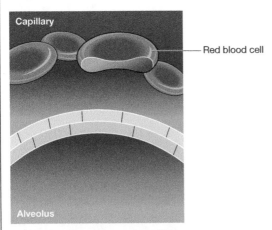

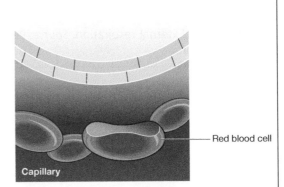

Figure 11.12   Internal respiration. *Source*: Peate and Nair, 2015. Reproduced with permission of John Wiley & Sons.

Question 17   Match the pairs.

Pulmonary ventilation concerns	how oxygen diffuses from the lungs to the bloodstream and how carbon dioxide diffuses from blood and to the lungs
External respiration concerns	how air gets in and out of the lungs
During inspiration	the respiratory centres
When intrapulmonary pressure is less than atmospheric pressure	air will naturally enter the lungs until the pressure difference no longer exists
The rate and depth of breathing are controlled by	takes place between alveolar air and the blood flowing through the lung capillaries
Exchange of gases in the lungs	the thorax expands and intrapulmonary pressure falls below atmospheric pressure

Question 18   Time yourself to unscramble these words.

Scrambled	Answer
TREPIRAISON	
LAIVENTNOTI	
SESAG	
PHISECAMORT	
VALORELA	
PROTECMECHORES	
TAXHOR	
RAMPONLYU	

Snap shot

Peak expiratory flow (PEF)

The assessment of respiratory status is important in understanding the severity of the respiratory problem a person may have, with the intention of prioritising care, ensuring safety, providing comfort and offering support.

When a person is in the acute state of a respiratory illness, for example, if they have infection or exacerbation of chronic obstructive pulmonary disease, the emphasis is placed on physiological assessment in order to detect life-threatening situations that require immediate interventions. Respiratory assessment requires observation, communication, measurement and clinical skills, and should include assessment of physiological factors, cognitive state, causative factors, symptoms, impact on the person's ability to perform the activities of living and psychosocial factors. The health care provider must aim to provide care that is effective, kind, caring, with the patient at the centre of all that is done.

A series of physiological measures that are central to assessing the needs of the person with a respiratory problem fall under an umbrella term known as lung function tests. What do you understand by peak expiratory flow (PEF) and how should this important test be carried out?

Word search

M	Z	C	F	Z	V	A	H	B	J	Y	N	I	I	R	L	M	R	T	S
E	X	I	Q	G	L	P	Y	X	I	D	N	F	Q	A	X	Z	E	R	O
M	D	X	L	U	C	N	J	N	X	U	U	G	Y	B	H	U	O	Z	H
G	Y	A	Z	O	M	E	S	E	Y	C	P	E	R	C	B	T	B	R	I
A	A	T	X	Y	U	U	U	G	P	N	T	O	P	S	P	L	L	E	K
R	Z	O	Q	K	W	S	H	Y	S	I	N	Z	P	E	E	E	U	S	S
H	E	M	D	E	B	T	K	X	U	C	E	C	C	I	P	V	N	P	T
P	Z	U	V	V	B	I	T	O	H	L	L	E	N	R	F	C	G	I	N
A	Q	E	L	Q	R	C	Q	I	O	K	R	N	O	A	B	X	U	R	P
I	F	N	U	K	R	O	O	X	V	O	V	E	I	L	B	R	Q	A	F
D	A	P	M	Z	B	L	A	K	M	C	A	Y	S	L	B	S	L	T	I
O	J	I	U	B	E	M	Y	E	Q	M	A	B	U	I	U	F	A	I	P
D	J	D	K	S	L	P	H	A	H	R	G	U	F	P	H	R	R	O	O
A	R	U	E	L	P	C	P	V	E	Y	C	B	F	A	L	D	Y	N	E
L	S	A	N	G	A	S	E	S	Z	H	Z	J	I	C	R	D	N	X	M
V	V	T	T	O	Y	C	N	Z	B	Z	C	J	D	X	T	Z	X	I	Y
Z	P	H	A	R	Y	N	X	P	J	B	T	A	I	U	L	P	H	R	W
M	Q	E	V	B	A	I	T	Z	T	N	V	L	R	D	V	T	A	C	K
D	L	V	J	U	M	D	V	E	N	T	I	L	A	T	I	O	N	T	C
H	A	B	F	O	J	I	L	O	E	V	L	A	U	K	E	D	Y	U	D

LUNG
TRACHEA
BRONCHIOLES
ALVEOLI
CAPILLARIES
PLEURA

LARYNX
PHARYNX
DIAPHRAGM
OXYGEN
DIFFUSION
GASES

VENTILATION
CHEMORECEPTORS
PNEUMOTAXIC
APNEUSTIC
RESPIRATION

Crossword

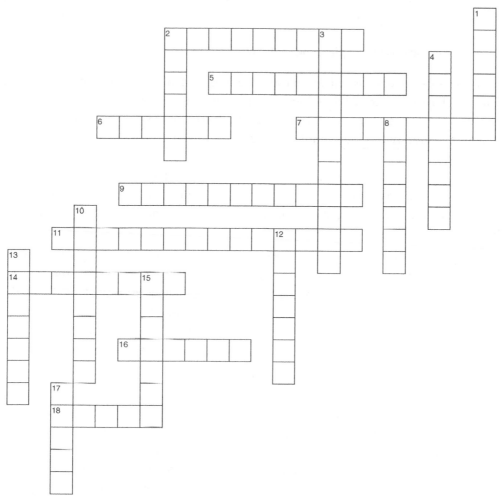

Across

2. This type of ventilation is how air gets in and out of the lungs

5. The distance between alveoli and pulmonary circulation slows the rate of what?

6. Unit peak expiratory flow is measured in what per minute?

7. This structure is said to be dome shaped

9. Type of blood cell that transports the vast majority of oxygen

11. Sensory cells which detect chemicals

14. Arterial blood pH is mainly influenced by the levels of what type of ions

16. Voice box

18. These essential organs have three lobes on the right and two on the left

Down

1. Structure which divides the nasal cavity into two equal sections

2. This space is usually filled with a small amount of fluid

3. Centres that control the rate and depth of breathing

4. The two tonsils visible when the mouth is open

8. A lack of oxygen within body tissues

10. The lungs almost fill what cavity?

12. There are 15–20 C-shaped cartilage rings found here

13. There are three regions associated with this structure

15. What the thorax does during inspiration

17. Tissue that transports oxygen from the lungs to body tissues

Fill in the blanks

Use the words in the box to complete the sentences:

air, air, air, alveolar, alveoli, alveoli, alveoli, atmosphere, breathing, bronchioles, circulatory, contraction, dioxide, gaseous, lobes, lubricating, lungs, lungs, lungs, membranes, muscles, oxygen, parietal, parietal, pleura, prevents, reduces, relaxation, respiratory, space, tension, three, tissue, tissues, two, upper, ventilation, visceral, visceral

1. The _____ system is responsible for _____ exchange between the _____ system and the _____. ___ is taken in via the _____ airways, through the lower airways and into the small _____ and _____ within the lung _____.

2. The lungs are divided into _____. There are _____ lobes in the right lung and _____ in the left. Each is surrounded by two thin protective _____: the _____ and _____ pleura. The _____ pleura lines the wall of the thorax, the _____ pleura covers the _____. The space between the two _____, the pleural _____, is minute, and contains a thin film of _____ fluid, which _____ friction between the two pleura, allowing both layers to slide over one another during _____.

3. Pulmonary _____ involves physical movement of _____ in and out of the _____. The primary function is to maintain adequate _____ ventilation. This _____ the build-up of carbon _____ in the _____ and achieves a constant supply of _____ to the _____. Air flows between the atmosphere and the _____ of the _____ as a result of pressure difference created by the _____ and _____ of the respiratory _____. The rate of _____ flow and the effort needed for breathing is influenced by the alveolar surface _____ and integrity of the lungs.

Multiple choice questions

1. Inhalation and exhalation are
   (a) Caused by chemicals changes only
   (b) Caused by contraction and relaxation of the bronchiolar smooth muscle
   (c) Referred to as ventilation
   (d) Caused by the relaxation of the diaphragm and intercostal muscles

2. The bronchi, bronchioles, and alveoli are

    (a) Concerned with the exchange of respiratory gases
    (b) Classed as part of the immune system
    (c) Referred to as the bronchial tree
    (d) All surrounded by rings of cartilage

3. What does the diameter of the bronchioles determine?

    (a) Amount of mucus secreted by the lungs
    (b) Amount of surfactant absorbed
    (c) Air flow to the alveoli
    (d) Rate of ventilation

4. Which of the following best describes the visceral and parietal pleura?

    (a) They line the diaphragm
    (b) They line the pharynx
    (c) They are serous membranes
    (d) They are surfactant-secreting membranes

5. What happens if intrapleural pressure equals or exceeds intrapulmonic pressure?

    (a) Death occurs
    (b) The lung collapses
    (c) The larynx can no longer generate sound
    (d) Pulmonary oedema develops

6. Which of the following does NOT occur on inhalation?

    (a) Air is moved into the lungs
    (b) Thoracic volume will increase
    (c) The diaphragm contracts
    (d) Pressure within the intrapleural space becomes positive

7. Boyle's law states that

    (a) When the temperature of a gas is constant, the volume is inversely proportional to its pressure
    (b) When the temperature of a gas is constant, its volume is directly proportional to its temperature
    (c) There is no relationship between intrapulmonic pressure and thoracic volume
    (d) An increase in thoracic volume causes an increase in intrapleural pressure

8. How many pieces of cartilage tissue are there in the larynx?

    (a) 3
    (b) 6
    (c) 9
    (d) 12

9. How many lobes does the right lung have?

(a) 1
(b) 2
(c) 3
(d) 4

10. What are the sensory cells that detect chemicals in the blood called?

(a) Chemoreceptors
(b) Pacini corpuscles
(c) Baroreceptors
(d) All of the above

References

Peate, I. and Nair, M. (2011) *Fundamentals of Anatomy and Physiology for Student Nurses.* Oxford: John Wiley & Sons, Ltd.

Peate, I. and Nair, M. (2015) *Anatomy and Physiology for Nurses at a Glance.* Oxford: John Wiley & Sons, Ltd.

Peate, I., Wild, K. and Nair, M. (eds) (2014) *Nursing Practice: Knowledge and Care.* Oxford: John Wiley & Sons, Ltd.

Tortora, G.J. and Derrickson, B.H. (2009) *Principles of Anatomy and Physiology*, 12th edn. Hoboken, NJ: John Wiley & Sons, Inc.

Chapter 12

The reproductive systems

In men and women the reproductive systems are the only systems that differ in terms of structure and function. In humans reproduction is sexual, meaning that children are produced as a consequence of male and female mating. The reproductive glands of the male are the testes; those in the female are the ovaries.

The key function of the reproductive system is to ensure that the human species survives by the production of offspring. The main functions of the human reproductive system are to:

1. produce egg and sperm cells
2. transport and sustain these cells
3. fertilise the egg
4. nurture the developing offspring
5. produce hormones.

Male reproductive system

The male reproductive system performs three roles:

1. produces, nourishes and transports sperm
2. deposits sperm within the female reproductive tract
3. secretes hormones.

Fundamentals of Anatomy and Physiology Workbook: A Study Guide for Nursing and Healthcare Students, First Edition. Ian Peate.
© 2017 John Wiley & Sons Ltd. Published 2017 by John Wiley & Sons Ltd.

Question 1
(a) In Figure 12.1, identify and label the structures of the male reproductive system.

(b) Colour in the various elements of the male reproductive system.

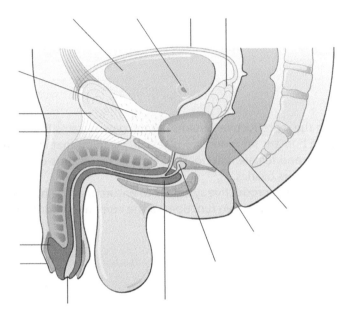

Figure 12.1   The male reproductive system. *Source*: Peate and Nair, 2015. Reproduced with permission of John Wiley & Sons.

Testes

The testes are located in the abdominal cavity of the foetus, and descend down through the inguinal canal into the scrotal sac. The testes are external to the body. There are usually two testes, each covered by three layers of serous fibrous tissue. The testes are responsible for producing testosterone and generating sperm.

Question 2
(a) In Figure 12.2, identify the component parts of the testicle.

(b) Colour the various aspects of the testicle.

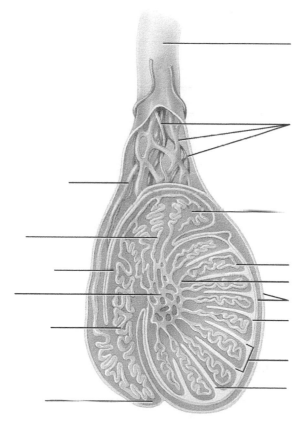

Figure 12.2 A testicle. *Source*: Tortora and Derrickson, 2009. Reproduced with permission of John Wiley & Sons.

Spermatogenesis

The production of sperm is called spermatogenesis. Sperm production occurs in the seminiferous tubules of the testes.

Question 3
(a) In Figure 12.3, identify the process of spermatogenesis.

(b) Colour in component parts.

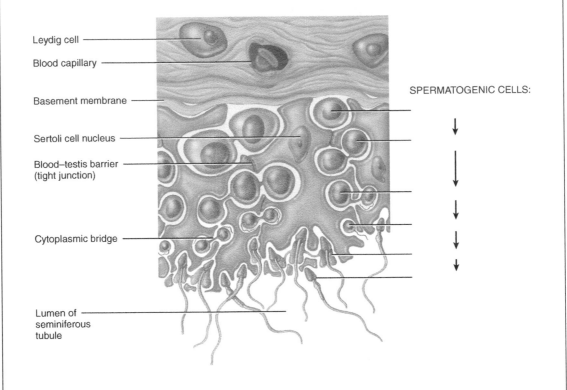

Leydig cell

Blood capillary

Basement membrane

Sertoli cell nucleus

Blood–testis barrier
(tight junction)

Cytoplasmic bridge

Lumen of
seminiferous
tubule

SPERMATOGENIC CELLS:

Figure 12.3 Stages of spermatogenesis. *Source*: Tortora and Derrickson, 2009. Reproduced with permission of John Wiley & Sons.

Question 4
(a) In Figure 12.4, label the components of a sperm.

(b) Colour in Figure 12.4.

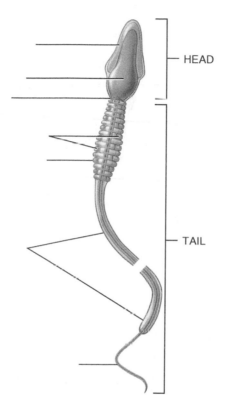

HEAD

TAIL

Figure 12.4 Components of a sperm. *Source*: Tortora and Derrickson, 2009. Reproduced with permission of John Wiley & Sons.

Testosterone

Testosterone is the primary male sex hormone, a steroid that regulates growth and development. Testosterone production increases around 18-fold during puberty. Once the man reaches approximately 40 years, testosterone production declines by about 1% per year. Testosterone functions to develop a man's primary and secondary sex characteristics.

Question 5 In Figure 12.5, identify the primary and secondary male characteristics.

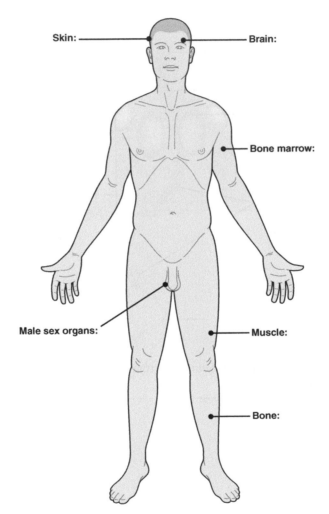

Skin:

Brain:

Bone marrow:

Male sex organs:

Muscle:

Bone:

Figure 12.5 Primary and secondary sex characteristics. *Source*: Peate and Nair, 2015. Reproduced with permission of John Wiley & Sons.

The scrotum

The scrotal sac hangs between the thighs, anterior to the anus; this is a supporting structure suspended from the root of the penis. Externally it usually appears as a single sac of skin separated into two portions by a ridge in the middle known as the raphe.

Question 6   Label the features of the scrotum in Figure 12.6.

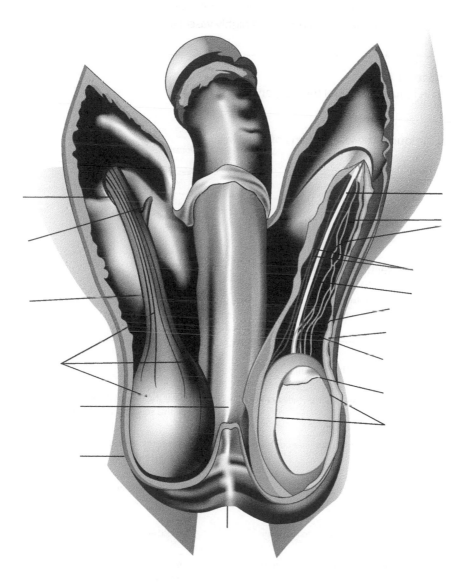

Figure 12.6   The deeper features of the scrotum. *Source*: Adapted from Edelhart Kempeneers. *Gray's Anatomy*, 20th edition. 1918.

The penis

The penis is the male organ for sexual intercourse. It has three parts:

1. the root, attached to the wall of the abdomen
2. the body or shaft
3. the glans.

In the uncircumcised male the glans is covered with a loose layer of skin, the foreskin. The urinary meatus (the opening of the urethra) is where the male passes semen and urine. The penis contains a number of sensitive nerve endings and is highly vascular.

Question 7

(a) In Figure 12.7, label the diagram.

(b) Colour in the various parts of the penis.

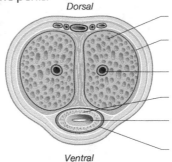

Figure 12.7 Cross-section of the penis. *Source*: Peate and Nair, 2014. Reproduced with permission of John Wiley & Sons.

Question 8   Match the pairs.

The reproductive glands of the male are the testes	near the base of the bladder, they provide sperm with a source of energy and assist with motility
Leydig cells, between the seminiferous tubules,	as sperm leaving the testes are immature, and are unable to fertilise the egg
Spermatogenesis turns each diploid spermatogonium into	which transports sperm from the epididymis to the urethra
The epididymis brings sperm to maturity	these are the male equivalent of the ovaries
The vas deferens is a long, muscular tube	manufacture and secrete testosterone and other androgens
The seminal vesicles are sac-like pouches attached to the vas deferens	four haploid sperm cells, quadrupling is accomplished through meiotic cell division

SCRAMBLE **Question 9**   Time yourself to unscramble these words.

Scrambled	Answer
LANESIM	
YIDDIMSEPI	
SNIPE	
SLANG	
PERMS	
PLIODID	
PLIODAH	
PARHE	

Prostate gland

The function of the prostate gland is not well understood. It is a single exocrine gland, approximately the size of a walnut and is doughnut shaped. It goes around the urethra under the urinary bladder and is made of 20–30 glands enclosed in smooth muscle. A thin milky fluid is secreted, adding bulk to semen. Prostatic fluid accounts for approximately one third of semen volume. Smooth muscle within the prostate gland contracts during ejaculation, helping to expel semen.

Question 10

(a) Label the diagram in Figure 12.8.

(b) Colour in the three zones.

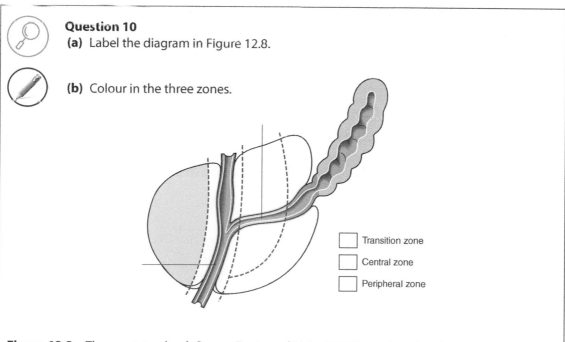

Transition zone

Central zone

Peripheral zone

Figure 12.8   The prostate gland. *Source*: Peate and Nair, 2015. Reproduced with permission of John Wiley & Sons.

Question 11   Complete Table 12.1 concerning the three zones of the prostate gland.

Table 12.1   The three zones of the prostate gland.

Zone	Description
Peripheral	
Transition	
Central	

 Question 12   Match the pairs.

The peripheral zone of the prostate gland	check for growths in or enlargement of the prostate gland
As the transition zone enlarges, it then pushes	and is farthest from the rectum
The central zone is in front of the transition zone	is the area of the prostate that is closest to the rectum
The gland cells within the prostate produce a	the peripheral zone of the prostate toward the rectum
Prostate specific antigen counteracts the clotting enzyme in the seminal vesicle fluid	thin fluid that is rich in proteins and minerals that maintain and nourish the sperm
Digital rectal examination is usually performed to	which principally glues the semen to the cervix, located next to the uterine entrance inside the vagina.

 Question 13   Time yourself to unscramble these words.

Scrambled	Answer
GIANTEN	
OPTRATSE	
REARPHILEP	
LATERNC	
TRAITSINON	
GATDILI	
ONEZ	
MUTERC	

The female reproductive system

The female reproduction system produces the female ova or oocytes, essential for reproduction, and the female sex hormones, that maintain the reproductive cycle. This system has internal and external elements.

The female internal sex organs consist of the ovaries, the fallopian tubes, the uterus and the vagina.

Question 14

(a) In Figure 12.9, identify the internal female reproductive organs.

(b) Colour in the component elements of the internal female reproductive organs.

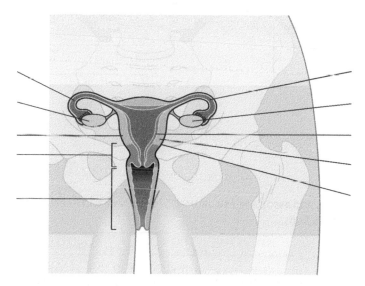

Figure 12.9 The female reproductive organs. *Source*: Peate and Nair, 2015. Reproduced with permission of John Wiley & Sons.

The uterus

The uterus is a dense, muscular, pear-shaped hollow organ and is approximately 7.5 cm long. It is situated deep in the pelvic cavity between the urinary bladder and the rectum; it also touches the sigmoid colon and the small intestine.

 Question 15
  (a) In Figure 12.10, identify the various aspects of the uterus and the associated structures.

  (b) Colour in the component elements.

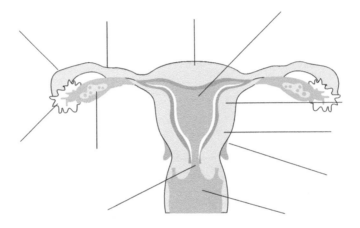

Figure 12.10   The uterus and associated structures. *Source*: Nair and Peate, 2009. Reproduced with permission of John Wiley & Sons.

   Question 16   Complete Table 12.2 regarding the layers of the uterus.

Table 12.2   The layers of the uterus.

Layers	Description
Perimetrium	
Myometrium	
Endometrium	

Ovaries and fallopian tubes

The ovaries are the primary reproductive organs; they are paired glands, flat almond-shaped structures on each side of the uterus beneath the ends of the fallopian tubes. Ligaments attach them to the uterus; they are also attached to the broad ligament. The ovaries are the site of development of the female germ cells and they also produce the female hormones, oestrogen and progesterone.

The fallopian tubes are thin cylindrical structures approximately 8–14 cm long. The lateral ends of the fallopian tubes are open, made of projections called fimbriae draped over the ovary. The fimbriae pick up the ovum after discharge from the ovary. The fallopian tubes are composed of smooth muscle lined with ciliated mucus-producing epithelial cells; muscular contractions and the actions of the cilia transport the ovum along the tubes towards the uterus.

Oogenesis

This is the development of ova from relatively undifferentiated germ cells called oogonia. The meiotic phase of development is not completed until the girl reaches puberty.

Question 17   Oogenesis is outlined in Figure 12.11. In the boxes describe the activity that takes place during development of the oogonium.

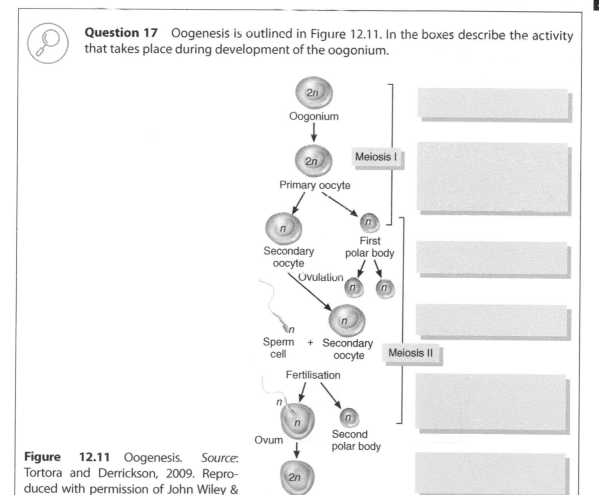

Figure   12.11   Oogenesis.   *Source*: Tortora and Derrickson, 2009. Reproduced with permission of John Wiley & Sons.

The female sex hormones and menstruation

The ovaries of a sexually mature female secrete a mixture of oestrogens. Around every 28 days, some blood and other products of the disintegration of the endometrium are discharged (menstruation); a new follicle begins to develop. After menstruation ceases, the follicle secretes an increasing amount of oestrogen which causes the endometrium to become thicker. A rising level of LH causes the developing egg to complete the first meiotic division, forming a secondary oocyte. Around 2 weeks later, a sudden surge in the production of LH occurs triggering ovulation with the release of the secondary oocyte into the fallopian tube.

Under the influence of LH, the empty follicle develops into a corpus luteum. The corpus luteum secretes progesterone stimulated by LH which continues the preparation of the endometrium for a possible pregnancy. If fertilisation does not occur, the rising level of progesterone inhibits the release of GnRH, which then inhibits further production of progesterone. As the level of progesterone drops, the corpus luteum begins to degenerate, the endometrium begins to break down, the inhibition of uterine contraction is lifted, and the bleeding and cramps of menstruation begin.

 Question 18 In Figure 12.12, the different phases of menstruation are highlighted, with the ovarian and uterine activity that take place. Identify the various phases of the menstrual cycle.

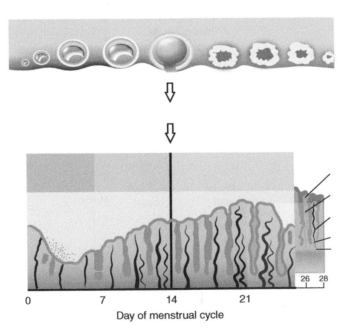

Figure 12.12 The menstrual cycle. *Source*: Rice University 2013. Reproduced with permission of Rice University.

The vagina and cervix

The vagina is tubular, fibromuscular structure approximately 8–10 cm in length. It is the receptacle for the penis during sexual intercourse, an organ of sexual response, it allows the menstrual flow to leave the body and is the passage for the birth of the child. Usually the vaginal walls are moist with a pH ranging from 3.8–4.2.

The cervix forms a pathway between the uterus and the vagina. The uterine opening of the cervix is the internal os and the vaginal opening the external os.

Question 19
(a) In Figure 12.13, label the uterus, vagina and cervix.

(b) Colour in the uterus, vagina and cervix.

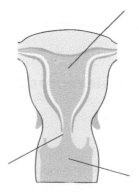

Figure 12.13 The uterus, vagina and cervix. *Source*: Nair and Peate, 2009. Reproduced with permission of John Wiley & Sons.

245

Question 20 Match the pairs.

The female reproductive system produces the ova	attached to the upper part of the uterus and serve to transport the ova from the ovaries to the uterus
The vagina is a canal that joins the	located on either side of the uterus; they produce eggs and hormones
The uterus is a hollow, pear-shaped organ divided into two parts	occurs in the fallopian tubes. The fertilised egg moves to the uterus, and implants into the lining of the uterine wall
The ovaries are small, oval-shaped glands	cervix to the outside of the body; it is also known as the birth canal
Fallopian tubes are narrow tubes	and is designed to transport the ova to the site of fertilisation
Conception is the fertilisation of an egg by a sperm; it normally	the cervix, which is the lower part that opens into the vagina, and the main body of the uterus, called the corpus

Question 21 Time yourself to unscramble these words.

Scrambled	Answer
REVIXC	
IANPOLLAF	
YAROV	
USTURE	
SPORCU	
ANIVAG	
TAUTSOMENRIN	
LICELLOF	

The external female reproductive organs

The external female genitalia are known collectively as the vulva: they include the mons pubis, the labia, the clitoris, and the vaginal and urethral openings. The external genitalia have three key functions:

- enabling sperm to enter the body
- protecting the internal genital organs from infectious organisms
- the provision of sexual pleasure

Question 22 Label Figure 12.14.

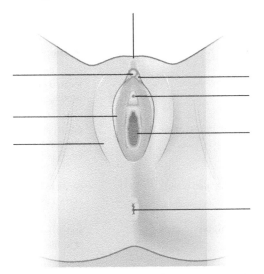

Figure 12.14 The external female genitalia. *Source*: Peate and Nair, 2015. Reproduced with permission of John Wiley & Sons.

The female breasts

The breasts (also known as the mammary glands) are dome-shaped and differ in size between individuals; they are external accessory sexual organs in the female. Located within the breast are several milk-producing glands. The hormone prolactin controls milk production.

The breasts are supported by the pectoral muscles and are provided with a rich supply of nerves, blood vessels and lymph vessels. The areola is a pigmented area situated a little below the centre of the breast containing glands, that secrete sebum, and a nipple. The nipple usually protrudes, becoming erect in response to cold and stimulation.

The breasts are made of adipose, fibrous connective and glandular tissue. There are bands of fibrous tissue supporting the breast extending from the outer breast tissue to the nipple, dividing the breast into 15 to 25 lobes. The lobes are made up of alveolar glands that are joined by ducts opening out on to the nipple.

Question 23
(a) Label Figure 12.15.

(b) Colour in the various elements.

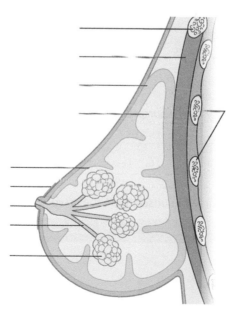

Figure 12.15 The female breast. *Source*: Peate and Nair, 2015. Reproduced with permission of John Wiley & Sons.

The breast lymph nodes and lymph

The breast lymphatic system is a network of lymph nodes and lymph ducts, axillary lymph nodes are located above the clavicle, behind the sternum as well as in other parts of the body. Breast lymph nodes include:

- supraclavicular nodes – above the clavicle
- infraclavicular (or subclavicular) nodes – below the clavicle
- axillary nodes – in the axilla
- internal mammary nodes – inside the chest around the sternum

 Question 24   Identify the breast lymphatic system and label Figure 12.16.

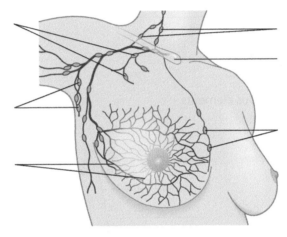

Figure 12.16   Breast lymphatic system. *Source*: Peate and Nair, 2015. Reproduced with permission of John Wiley & Sons.

 Question 25   Time yourself to unscramble these words.

Scrambled	Answer
NATALOCTI	
GRONERESTEPO	
ABIAL	
LUVVA	
SCUDT	
SONM	
RAJMAO	
RAMION	

Question 26 Match the pairs.

The labia majora are the outer lips of the vulva made of two symmetrical pads of fatty tissue	including nerves in the chest and arm, branches from the 4th, 5th and 6th thoracic nerves supply the breasts
Labia minora are thin folds of tissue within the labia majora	throughout the breast following stimulation by hormones produced after the woman has given birth
The clitoris is a small white body of oval tissue located at the top of the labia minora and the clitoral hood	providing protection for the urethral and vaginal openings
The key function of the breast is to produce, store and release milk produced in lobules located	it is composed of spongy tissue and is highly sexually sensitive
There are a number of major nerves in the breast area,	each month breast tissues are exposed to cycles of oestrogen and progesterone throughout a woman's childbearing years
Progesterone prepares the uterus for pregnancy and the breasts for producing milk for lactation,	functioning as protective structures that surround the clitoris, urinary orifice and vaginal orifice

Snap shot

Erectile dysfunction

Deniz Yayincilik is a 45-year-old gentleman with diabetes mellitus and has suffered erectile dysfunction for 2 years. The erectile dysfunction was causing disharmony with his wife. Treatment is with self-injection therapy; the injectable form of MUSE alprostadil is injected into the side of the penis.
How should Mr Yayincilik use the medication?

Word search

A	L	M	A	S	N	R	H	C	C	B	O	V	X	T	R	X	J	I	P
P	S	Y	K	K	G	A	T	E	A	E	M	Y	H	A	R	E	O	L	A
E	P	O	V	H	C	P	M	U	I	R	T	E	M	O	D	N	E	Z	U
N	E	M	J	S	F	H	J	E	D	K	M	P	L	Z	Z	L	O	H	M
I	R	E	D	Z	I	E	S	N	E	G	O	R	D	N	A	V	H	A	E
S	M	T	P	T	A	S	M	F	R	F	U	X	P	J	C	J	N	Z	E
M	O	R	P	Z	I	Y	E	W	P	E	A	I	R	B	M	I	F	W	O
U	K	I	M	Q	G	Q	W	N	U	P	A	W	Y	U	G	A	N	O	T
I	R	U	E	T	U	B	U	L	E	S	R	Q	L	A	H	W	T	E	Q
R	S	M	C	E	R	V	I	X	V	G	S	O	V	B	W	Z	S	S	V
T	I	E	B	N	N	O	B	H	D	E	O	E	S	W	U	T	M	T	U
E	Z	N	S	U	R	E	T	U	X	D	I	T	T	T	O	X	U	R	L
M	B	Q	A	N	O	Q	M	U	L	H	A	Q	A	S	A	X	O	O	V
I	K	J	C	V	L	D	E	P	G	O	K	P	T	M	E	T	E	G	A
R	P	B	Y	E	Y	B	Q	T	Q	L	W	E	J	U	R	T	E	E	R
E	T	I	P	R	O	G	E	S	T	E	R	O	N	E	N	E	F	N	F
P	E	N	E	S	V	W	H	X	P	O	Y	V	W	Z	O	H	P	S	H
X	P	S	E	I	R	A	V	O	N	S	T	A	W	K	P	Q	T	S	T
G	Z	N	K	R	O	V	L	E	M	T	B	A	Z	M	T	K	J	Z	W
T	V	L	I	P	L	I	M	U	T	O	R	C	S	C	V	X	J	D	I

VAGINA
TESTES
CERVIX
UTERUS
OVARIES
PENIS
SCROTUM
PROSTATE

SPERM
TUBULES
TESTOSTERONE
SPERMATOGENESIS
RAPHE
OVA
OESTROGENS
PROGESTERONE

ANDROGENS
ENDOMETRIUM
MYOMETRIUM
PERIMETRIUM
VULVA
FIMBRIAE
AREOLA

Crossword

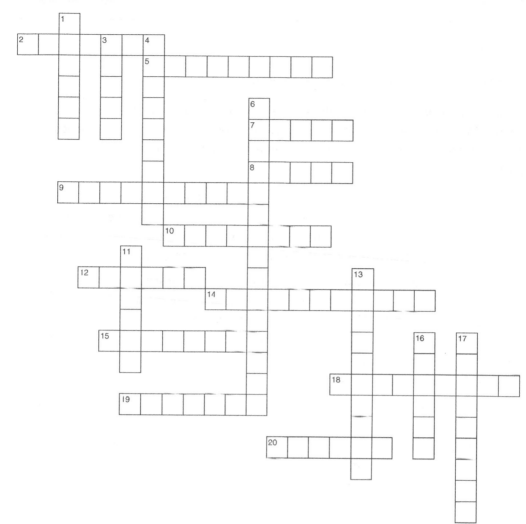

Across

2. The mammary glands
5. The male sex hormones
7. The male copulatory organ
8. Membranous folds of tissue in the vaginal wall
9. The muscular layer of the uterus
10. Gland which encircles the male urethra
12. The womb
14. A reflex occurring when the body needs to lower or raise the position of the testes
15. The fingerlike projections at the end of the fallopian tubes
18. The development of mature ova from oogonia
19. Paired flat glands on each side of the uterus
20. Part of the female reproductive system, described as tubular, fibromuscular, approximately 8–10 cm in length

Down

1. Organs suspended in the scrotal sac, hanging one on either side of the penis
3. Approximately 300 million of these mature each day
4. Fallopian tubes
6. Production of sperm
11. Structure which forms a pathway between the uterus and the vagina
13. These hormones have a key role to play in the usual structure of the skin and blood vessels
16. Term used when discussing the fallopian tubes, ovaries and supporting tissues collectively
17. A method of male surgical sterilisation

Fill in the blanks

Use the words in the box to complete the sentences:

behaviour, deliver, development, female, fertilise, gamete, genitalia, glands, hormones, hormones, infectious, internal, labia, male, mons, musculoskeletal, ova, penis, reproductive, reproductive, scrotum, sexual, sexual, sperm, sperm, spermatic, urethral, urinary, vagina, vaginal, vulva

1. The male _____ system works with other body systems, producing _____ essential for biological _____, sexual _____ and _____ performance. Other body systems involved include the neuroendocrine system and the _____ system. The male reproductive system is also central to the function of the _____ system.

2. The _____ reproductive system includes the _____, testes, _____ ducts, sex _____ and the _____. Working together these organs produce _____, the male _____, and the other components of semen. These organs also work together to _____ semen out of the body and into the _____ where it can _____ egg cells.

3. The female reproduction system produces the _____ and the _____ sex _____ that maintain the _____ cycle.

4. The external female _____ are known collectively as the _____. They include the _____ pubis, the _____, the clitoris, the _____ and _____ openings, and glands. The external _____ enable _____ to enter the body, protect the _____ genital organs from _____ organisms and provide _____ pleasure.

Multiple choice questions

1. Oestrogen and progesterone

   (a) Are gonadotropins
   (b) Are secreted by the liver
   (c) Are secreted by the ovaries
   (d) Exert their effects only on reproductive structures

2. Human chorionic gonadotropin (hCG)

   (a) Promotes the maturation of the egg
   (b) Is responsible for male characteristics
   (c) Maintains the corpus luteum
   (d) Transforms the corpus luteum into the corpus albicans

3. The luteal phase of the ovarian cycle

   (a) Is essential for menstruation
   (b) Is responsible for the uterine secretory phase
   (c) Excessively elevates plasma levels of oestrogen, progesterone and hCG
   (d) Leads the LH surge

4. Menstruation occurs in response to

   (a) Sexual activity
   (b) Diminished plasma levels of oestrogen and progesterone
   (c) Elevated plasma levels of hCG
   (d) Elevated plasma levels of FSH and LH

5. Which of the following is not true of testosterone?

   (a) Classified as androgen
   (b) Secreted by the anterior pituitary gland
   (c) Is required for the maturation of sperm
   (d) Is responsible for most of the male secondary sex characteristics

6. Which structure ejects both semen and urine?

   (a) Prostate
   (b) Epididymis
   (c) Urethra
   (d) Vas deferens

7. What are seminiferous tubules responsible for?

   (a) Producing semen
   (b) Producing the sperm cells
   (c) The sex of the child
   (d) All of the above

8. What is the ridge that separates the two sides of the scrotum?

   (a) Septum
   (b) Turbinate
   (c) Rugae
   (d) Raphe

9. What is the production of sperm called?

   (a) Semenogenesis
   (b) Spermatogenesis
   (c) Spermatogonia
   (d) Spermocyte

10. Testosterone

   (a) Increases in amount as the man ages
   (b) Is absent during puberty
   (c) Stays the same throughout the man's life
   (d) None of the above

References

Nair, M. and Peate, I. (2009) *Fundamentals of Applied Pathophysiology: An Essential Guide for Nursing Students.* Oxford: John Wiley & Sons, Ltd.

Peate, I. and Nair, M. (2015) *Anatomy and Physiology for Nurses at a Glance.* Oxford: John Wiley & Sons, Ltd.

Peate, I., Wild, K. and Nair, M. (eds) (2014) *Nursing Practice: Knowledge and Care.* Oxford: John Wiley & Sons, Ltd.

Tortora, G.J. and Derrickson, B.H. (2009) *Principles of Anatomy and Physiology*, 12th edn. Hoboken, NJ: John Wiley & Sons, Inc.

Chapter 13

The nervous system

The nervous system is a major communicating and control system within the body. It works with the endocrine system to control many body functions. The nervous system provides a rapid and short-acting response and the endocrine system provides a slower but often more sustained response. The two systems work together to maintain homeostasis. This system is large and complex.

The nervous system can be divided into two parts: the central nervous system and the peripheral nervous system. The central nervous system consists of the brain and spinal cord and is the control and integration centre for many body functions.

Question 1   In Figure 13.1, fill in the missing words.

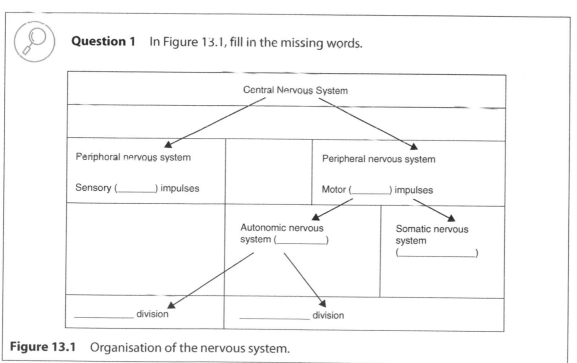

Central Nervous System

Periphoral nervous system

Sensory (_____) impulses

Peripheral nervous system

Motor (_____) impulses

Autonomic nervous system (_____)

Somatic nervous system (_____)

_____ division

_____ division

Figure 13.1   Organisation of the nervous system.

Fundamentals of Anatomy and Physiology Workbook: A Study Guide for Nursing and Healthcare Students, First Edition. Ian Peate.
© 2017 John Wiley & Sons Ltd. Published 2017 by John Wiley & Sons Ltd.

Neurones

The neurone or nerve cell is the functional unit of the nervous system, the basic building block. It has many features in common with other cells, including a nucleus and mitochondria. Neurones transmit information throughout the body. They are highly specialised nerve cells and are responsible for communicating information in chemical and electrical forms. Two characteristics of neurones are:

1. irritability, in response to a stimulus – ability to initiate a nerve impulse
2. conductivity – ability to conduct an impulse.

Neurones consist of an axon, dendrites and a cell body. Nerve impulses only travel in one direction: from the receptive area, the dendrites, to the cell body, and down the length of the axon.

Question 2
(a) Identify the key components of the nerve cell in Figure 13.2.

(b) Colour in the elements of the nerve cell.

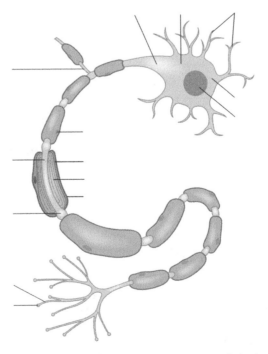

Figure 13.2 A nerve cell. *Source*: Peate and Nair, 2015. Reproduced with permission of John Wiley & Sons.

Neurotransmitters

Neurones do not come into contact with one another. Where one neurone ends and another begins, there is a space called the synapse. In order for communication to occur between neurones or between the neurone and a muscle or gland, a chemical messenger called a neurotransmitter is secreted by the neurone into the extracellular space at the synapse.

Question 3

(a) In Figure 13.3, identify the axon, synaptic vesicles, synapse, dendrites, receptor and the neurotransmitter.

(b) Colour in the component parts.

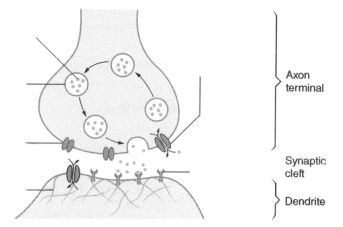

Figure 13.3   Neurotransmission. *Source*: Adapted from Thomas Splettstoesser (www.scistyle.com) 2015.

Central nervous system
The brain

The brain lies in the cranial cavity. It receives 15% of the cardiac output and has a system of autoregulation ensuring the blood supply is constant despite positional changes. The largest part of the human brain is the cerebrum; this is divided into two hemispheres. Below this lies the brain stem and behind it is the cerebellum. The outermost layer of the cerebrum is called the cerebral cortex and this comprises four lobes:

1. the frontal lobe
2. the parietal lobe
3. the temporal lobe
4. the occipital lobe.

Question 4
(a) Identify the various parts of the brain in Figure 13.4.

(b) Colour in the various parts of the brain.

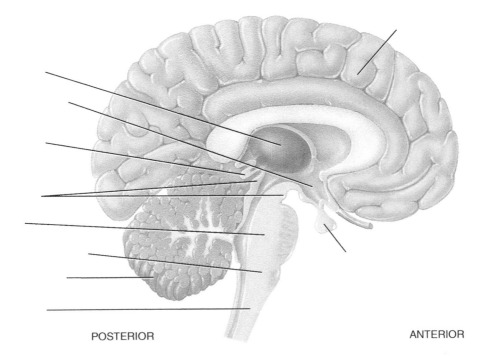

POSTERIOR   ANTERIOR

Figure 13.4 The brain. *Source*: Peate *et al.*, 2014. Reproduced with permission of John Wiley & Sons.

The spinal cord

There are two layers of the spinal cord; an outer layer of white matter and an inner layer of grey matter, surrounding a small central canal. The spinal cord is enclosed within the vertebral canal, which forms a protective ring of bone around the cord.

Question 5

(a) In Figure 13.5, identify the various aspects of the spinal cord.

(b) Colour in the various parts.

SPINAL CORD:

SPINAL
MENINGES:

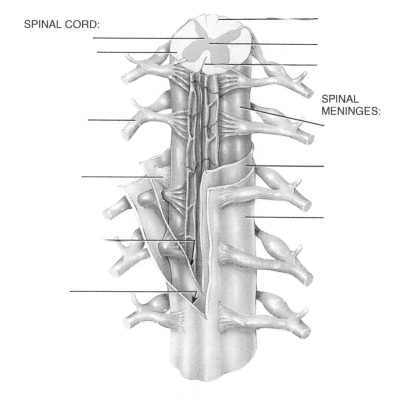

Figure 13.5 The spinal cord. *Source*: Tortora and Derrickson, 2009. Reproduced with permission of John Wiley & Sons.

Question 6
(a) In Figure 13.6, identify the bones of the spine.

(b) Colour in the cervical, thoracic, lumbar and sacral bones.

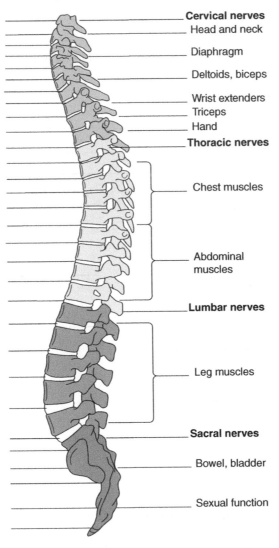

Cervical nerves
Head and neck

Diaphragm

Deltoids, biceps

Wrist extenders
Triceps
Hand
Thoracic nerves

Chest muscles

Abdominal
muscles

Lumbar nerves

Leg muscles

Sacral nerves

Bowel, bladder

Sexual function

Figure 13.6 The spinal nerves and their areas of innervation. *Source*: Peate and Nair, 2011. Reproduced with permission of John Wiley & Sons.

Cerebrospinal fluid and the ventricles of the brain

The choroid plexus in the ventricles of the brain produces cerebrospinal fluid. There are four ventricles in the brain. The paired lateral ventricles (one in each cerebral hemisphere), the third ventricle situated below this and the fourth ventricle located inferior to the third. The third and fourth ventricles communicate via the central canal and cerebrospinal fluid circulates through the central canal and into the spinal cord.

Question 7

(a) In Figure 13.7, identify the ventricles and other features of the brain.

(b) Colour in the ventricles of the brain.

POSTERIOR

ANTERIOR

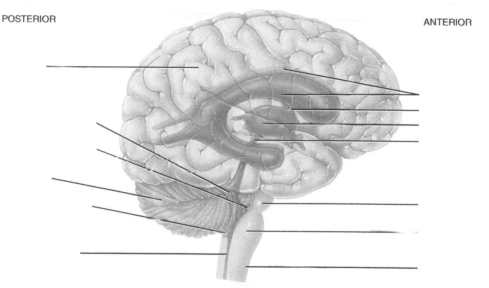

Figure 13.7 The ventricles of the brain (right lateral view). *Source:* Tortora and Derrickson, 2009. Reproduced with permission of John Wiley & Sons.

The meninges
The meninges are three layers of protective tissue:

1. dura mater
2. arachnoid mater
3. pia mater.

These three layers cover the brain and spinal cord, with a layer of cerebrospinal fluid between the arachnoid mater and the dura mater.

Question 8
(a) In Figure 13.8, identify the meninges and other features of this section of the cranium.

(b) Colour in the component parts.

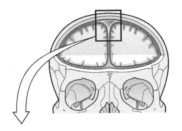
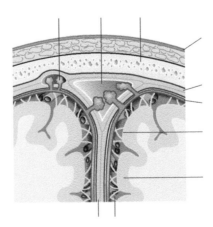

Figure 13.8 The meninges. *Source*: Peate *et al.*, 2014. Reproduced with permission of John Wiley & Sons.

Circle of Willis

The circle of Willis is an anastomotic system of arteries that sits at the base of the brain. The circle of Willis encircles the stalk of the pituitary gland and provides important communications between the blood supply of the forebrain and hindbrain. It is formed when the internal carotid artery enters the cranial cavity bilaterally and divides into the anterior cerebral artery and middle cerebral artery.

 Question 9 Identify the component parts of the circle of Willis in Figure 13.9.

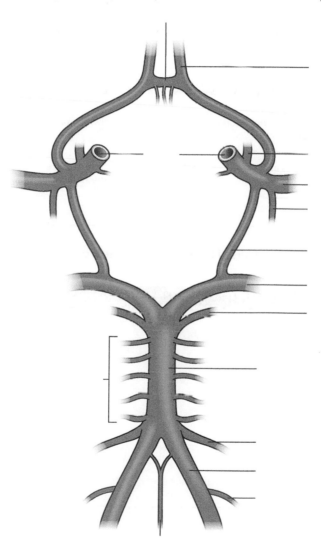

Figure 13.9 The circle of Willis. *Source*: Peate and Nair, 2015. Reproduced with permission of John Wiley & Sons.

Question 10   Match the pairs.

The nervous system can be divided into two parts:	the effector may be smooth or cardiac muscle (both involuntary muscles) or a gland
The somatic nervous system is under voluntary control	the central nervous system and the peripheral nervous system
The autonomic nervous system is responsible for involuntary motor responses	and the effector, the tissue or organ responding to instruction from the central nervous system, is skeletal muscle
The functional unit of the nervous system is	produces cerebrospinal fluid
The meninges protect the blood vessels that serve nervous tissue	the neurone or nerve cell
The choroid plexus in the ventricles of the brain	there is a layer of cerebrospinal fluid between the meninges

 Question 11   Time yourself to unscramble these words.

Scrambled	Answer
SNIGEMEN	
LIVETRENC	
SEXPLU	
BEERSLAPCROIN	
UREOSENN	
MISTRUTTEREROSNAN	
COMSATI	
MOOTNUICA	

Peripheral nervous system
Somatic nervous system

The somatic nervous system is the portion of the nervous system responsible for voluntary body movement and for sensing external stimuli. All five senses are part of this system. The somatic nervous system is a sub-part of the peripheral nervous system.

Question 12

(a) In Figure 13.10, identify the key components (the arrows indicate impulses).

(b) Colour in various aspects.

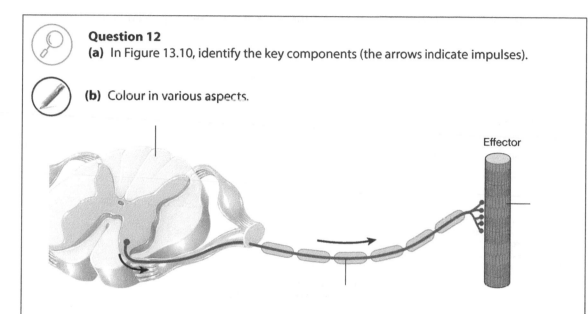

Effector

Figure 13.10 Somatic nervous system. *Source*: Peate and Nair, 2015. Reproduced with permission of John Wiley & Sons.

Motor pathway

The motor (efferent) division carries motor signals by way of efferent nerve fibres from the central nervous system to effectors (mainly glands and muscles). It can be further subdivided into the sympathetic and parasympathetic divisions.

Question 13 In Figure 13.11, draw in the reflex arc from sensory receptor to effector.

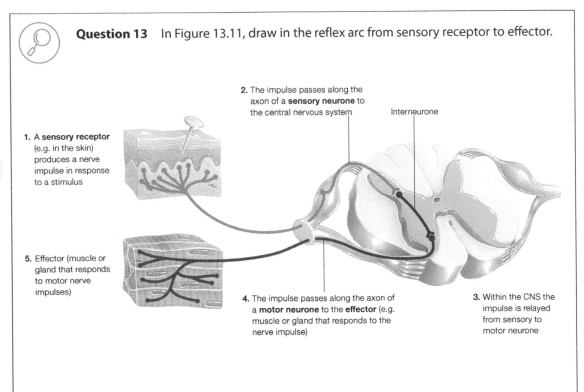

1. A **sensory receptor** (e.g. in the skin) produces a nerve impulse in response to a stimulus

2. The impulse passes along the axon of a **sensory neurone** to the central nervous system

Interneurone

3. Within the CNS the impulse is relayed from sensory to motor neurone

4. The impulse passes along the axon of a **motor neurone** to the **effector** (e.g. muscle or gland that responds to the nerve impulse)

5. Effector (muscle or gland that responds to motor nerve impulses)

Figure 13.11 Motor pathway. *Source*: Peate and Nair, 2015. Reproduced with permission of John Wiley & Sons.

Cranial nerves

There are 12 pairs of cranial nerves emerging from the brain, supplying various structures, most of which are associated with the head and neck. The 12 pairs of cranial nerves differ in their functions: some are sensory nerves, containing sensory fibres, some are motor nerves, containing only motor fibres, and some are mixed nerves, containing sensory and motor nerves.

Question 14

(a) In Figure 13.12, identify the cranial nerves.

(b) Colour in the various parts.

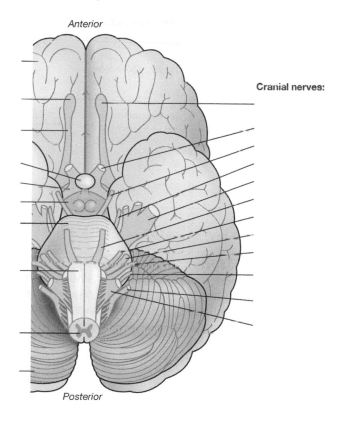

Anterior

Cranial nerves:

Posterior

Figure 13.12 The cranial nerves. *Source*: Peate *et al.*, 2014. Reproduced with permission of John Wiley & Sons.

Question 15 Complete Table 13.1 identifying the name of the nerve and the location/function.

Table 13.1 The cranial nerves.

Number	Name	Components	Location/function
I		Sensory	
II		Sensory	
III		Motor	
IV		Motor	
V		Sensory and motor	
VI		Motor	
VII		Sensory and motor	
VIII		Sensory	
IX		Sensory and motor	
X		Sensory and motor	
XI		Motor	
XII		Motor	

The autonomic nervous system

The autonomic nervous system plays a major role in the maintenance of homeostasis by regulating the body's automatic, involuntary functions, and, in common with the rest of the nervous system, consists of neurones, neuroglia and other connective tissue. Its structure is divided into two, the sympathetic division and the parasympathetic division.

Question 16 Complete Table 13.2 inserting the sympathetic and parasympathetic effects on the organs/systems listed.

Table 13.2 The effects of the sympathetic and parasympathetic divisions of the autonomic nervous system.

Organ/system	Sympathetic effects	Parasympathetic effects
Cell metabolism		
Blood vessels		
Eye		
Heart		
Lungs		
Kidneys		
Liver		
Digestive system		
Adrenal medulla		
Lacrimal glands		
Salivary glands		
Sweat glands		

Question 17 Match the pairs.

The 12 pairs of cranial nerves differ in their functions	voluntary muscle movement, balance and posture
The brain can be divided into	enclosed within the vertebral canal, which forms a protective ring of bone around the cord
The cerebrum is	the cerebrum, containing three paired structures
Diencephalon is the part of the brain surrounded by	the largest brain structure, divided into the left and right hemispheres
The cerebellum coordinates	some are sensory nerves, some are motor nerves and some are mixed nerves
The spinal cord is	four anatomical regions

Question 18 Time yourself to unscramble these words.

Scrambled	Answer
PHILDEACONNE	
CRUMBEER	
EREBELLCUM	
SWILIL	
PSYCHETMATI	
CHYMEPAPARATTSI	
AILNARC	
TOXERC	

Snap shot

Ageing and the nervous system

As we age there are a number of changes that occur throughout our body. With regard to the nervous system, these can be grouped as:

- structural changes with ageing
- cellular changes associated with ageing
- cerebrovascular changes related to ageing
- changes that have an impact on a person's function

It must be remembered that all of the areas of change will impact on each other.
Make notes on the changes related to these points above.

Word search

I	D	S	Z	J	N	E	U	R	O	M	U	S	C	U	L	A	R	X	M
E	N	E	L	N	A	H	S	C	S	H	Z	G	N	I	A	R	B	U	E
E	S	N	E	T	V	U	U	I	O	G	R	Z	W	H	M	A	A	W	P
U	Y	S	O	M	T	L	K	M	M	U	Y	Y	C	J	R	F	T	Z	A
M	M	O	A	U	I	A	E	O	A	T	Q	N	W	N	E	C	G	E	R
S	P	R	W	L	T	N	N	N	T	T	H	S	E	R	I	Z	V	S	A
H	A	Y	X	L	Z	I	I	O	I	E	T	M	P	E	V	N	Y	V	S
G	T	V	Y	E	N	P	P	T	C	E	X	J	J	C	N	N	O	T	Y
J	H	U	P	B	L	S	S	U	P	J	B	L	B	E	A	M	C	U	M
S	E	T	S	E	X	O	T	A	Y	D	R	N	S	P	R	P	E	R	P
X	T	Z	L	R	H	R	Z	S	N	E	O	S	S	T	Y	L	E	E	A
Y	I	E	Q	E	O	B	M	N	G	N	T	E	E	O	H	F	A	N	T
X	C	G	T	C	E	E	N	O	A	D	O	Z	K	R	L	E	I	O	H
N	O	X	A	R	C	R	A	P	T	R	M	J	O	E	X	D	L	R	E
N	G	A	G	U	B	E	O	K	I	I	N	T	X	K	C	S	G	U	T
R	F	K	P	P	G	C	S	F	Z	T	C	I	X	X	R	Q	O	E	I
L	A	R	E	H	P	I	R	E	P	E	E	Q	L	O	A	K	R	N	C
F	C	R	A	N	I	A	L	Y	F	S	O	R	R	E	O	P	U	J	A
J	B	Z	S	O	G	E	F	F	C	K	G	U	M	M	Y	M	E	I	F
J	P	O	L	C	K	W	E	N	C	X	Y	Z	K	Z	F	M	N	V	W

BRAIN	SENSORY	EFFECTOR
CEREBELLUM	SYMPATHETIC	RECEPTOR
PONS	PARASYMPATHETIC	RANVIER
DENDRITES	NEURONE	MYELIN
SPINE	PERIPHERAL	ARC
CRANIAL	SYNAPSE	REFLEX
AXON	NEUROMUSCULAR	CEREBROSPINAL
SOMATIC	NEUROGLIA	
MOTOR	AUTONOMIC	

Crossword

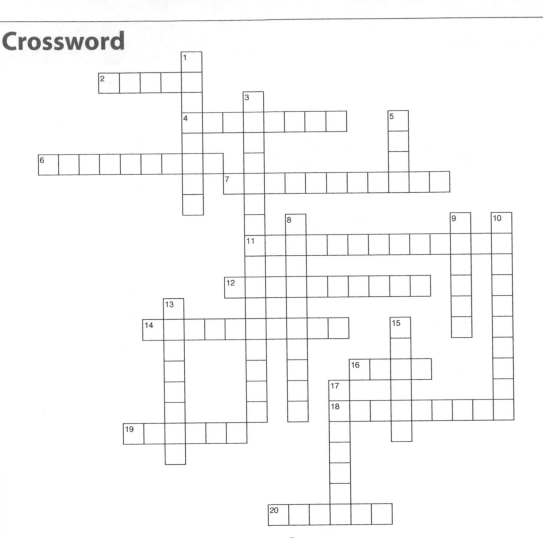

Across

2. Sense associated with the gustatory area of the brain

4. Any part of the body that produces a response to stimuli

6. Cranial nerve which has a role in the sense of smell

7. What the parasympathetic nervous system attempts to restore

11. Neurotransmitter which acts at the neuro-muscular junction

12. Star-shaped cells

14. There are four of these in the brain

16. The meningeal layer which lies closest to the bone of the skull

18. Specialised cells that are sensitive to stimuli and can turn them into electrical impulses

19. A fatty material that protects and electrically insulates the neurone

20. Clusters of cell bodies grouped together in the central nervous system

Down

1. The largest brain structure

3. A chemical messenger

5. Brain structure with a role in regulating breathing

8. The outermost part of the Schwann cell

9. The circle of _____ forms part of the blood supply to the brain

10. Photophobia is a symptom associated with which nervous system condition

13. Tissues that cover the central nervous system

15. Axons bundled together

17. Term for the nerves that emerge from the brain

Fill in the blanks

Use the words in the box to complete the sentences:

arms, axon, axons, brain, brain, chemical, chest, conscious, dendrites, electrical, information, length, lumbar, messengers, muscles, neck, nerves, nerves, nerves, nervous, neurone, neurones, neurotransmitters, organs, outside, sacral, signal, somatic, somatic, spinal, spinal, spinal, system

1. The _____ and _____ cord comprise the central nervous _____. The network of _____ connecting at different levels of the _____ cord controls _____ and unconscious activities. It is through the spinal cord that _____ flows from these _____ to the _____ and back again.

2. Neurones communicate with each other through their _____ and _____. When a _____ receives a message from another neurone, it sends an _____ signal down the _____ of its _____. At the end of the axon, the electrical _____ is converted into a _____ signal, and the axon releases chemical _____ called _____.

3. The brain sends messages via the _____ cord to peripheral _____ throughout the body that serve to control the _____ and internal _____. The _____ nervous system is made up of _____ connecting the central _____ system with the parts of the body that interact with the _____ world. _____ nerves in the cervical region are related to the _____ and _____; those in the thoracic region serve the _____; and those in the _____ and _____ regions interact with the legs.

Multiple choice questions

1. The precentral gyrus is

(a) Situated in the parietal lobe
(b) The primary motor cortex
(c) The primary visual cortex
(d) A part of the brain stem

2. Which of the following is true?

(a) The medulla oblongata is a cerebral structure
(b) The hypothalamus is a brain stem structure
(c) The medulla oblongata descends as the spinal cord
(d) The midbrain, pons and medulla oblongata are supratentorial structures

3. The postcentral gyrus

(a) Is found in the parietal lobe
(b) Regulates all voluntary motor activity
(c) Is where Broca's area can be found
(d) Contains the primary visual cortex

4. Cerebrospinal fluid

(a) Drains out of the subarachnoid space into the choroid plexus
(b) Circulates within the subarachnoid space
(c) Is also known as mucus
(d) Flows up the central canal into the fourth, third and lateral ventricles

5. Which is accurate?

(a) Temporal lobe: vision
(b) Frontal lobe: somatosensory (touch, pressure, pain)
(c) Occipital lobe: vision
(d) Parietal lobe: hearing

6. Neuroglia

(a) Are categorised as sensory and motor
(b) Include astrocytes, oligodendrocytes, Schwann cells and ependymal cells
(c) When stimulated fire action potentials
(d) Contain CSF, dendrites and axons

7. Activation of the emetic centre

(a) Descrases blood pressure
(b) Increases body temperature
(c) Stops diaphoresis
(d) Causes vomiting

8. The hypothalamus

(a) Is within the diencephalon
(b) Synthesises antidiuretic hormone and oxytocin
(c) Regulates pituitary gland activity
(d) All of the above are true

9. The meninges consist of how many connective tissue layers?

(a) 1
(b) 2
(c) 3
(d) 4

10. What is the name of cranial nerve IV?

(a) Trochlear
(b) Optic
(c) Trigeminal
(d) Vagus

References

Peate, I. and Nair, M. (2011) *Fundamentals of Anatomy and Physiology for Student Nurses*. Oxford: John Wiley & Sons, Ltd.

Peate, I. and Nair, M. (2015) *Anatomy and Physiology for Nurses at a Glance*. Oxford: John Wiley & Sons, Ltd.

Peate, I., Wild, K. and Nair, M. (eds) (2014) *Nursing Practice: Knowledge and Care*. Oxford: John Wiley & Sons, Ltd.

Tortora, G.J. and Derrickson, B.H. (2009) *Principles of Anatomy and Physiology*, 12th edn. Hoboken, NJ: John Wiley & Sons, Inc.

Chapter 14

The senses

There is no agreement as to how many special senses there are. The special senses here are referred to as:

- smell
- taste
- vision
- hearing

They are known as the special senses because their sensory receptors are located within relatively large sensory organs located in the head: the nose, tongue, eyes and ears.

 Question 1 Complete Table 14.1 by providing examples of the various types of sensory receptors.

Table 14.1 Sensory receptors.

Receptor	Stimulus	Example
Chemoreceptors	Alterations in concentrations of chemical substances	
Nociceptors (pain receptors)	Damage to tissues	
Thermoreceptors	Heat changes	
Sensory receptor (mechanoreceptors)	Changes in pressures (can also include change in the movement of fluids)	
Photoreceptors	Light energy	

Olfaction

Olfaction, the sense of smell, is (along with taste) a chemical sense. The sensations come from the interaction of molecules with smell receptors. Some smells can evoke strong emotional responses as the impulse for smell spreads to the limbic system.

Fundamentals of Anatomy and Physiology Workbook: A Study Guide for Nursing and Healthcare Students, First Edition. Ian Peate.
© 2017 John Wiley & Sons Ltd. Published 2017 by John Wiley & Sons Ltd.

Question 2   In Figure 14.1, fill in the missing word in each of the boxes related to the pathway of smell.

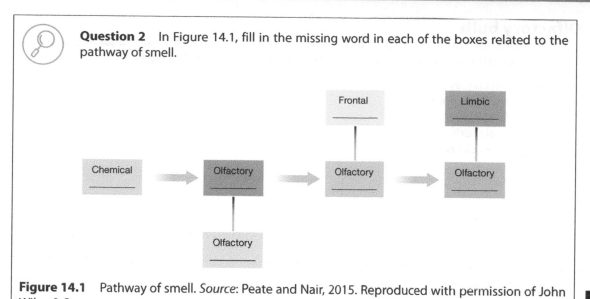

Figure 14.1   Pathway of smell. *Source*: Peate and Nair, 2015. Reproduced with permission of John Wiley & Sons.

The nose contains between 10 and 100 million olfactory receptor neurones. They form part of the olfactory epithelium that lines the nasal mucosa in the nasal cavity and are able to detect odours.

Question 3   In Figure 14.2, identify the various aspects related to olfaction.

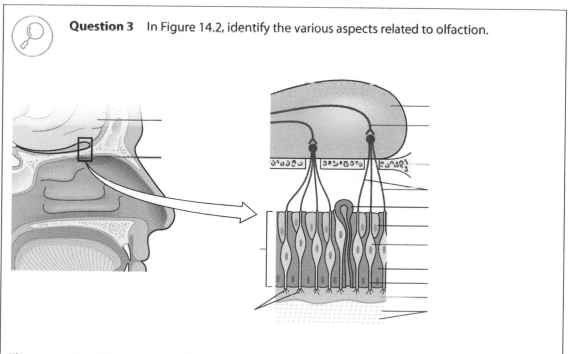

Figure 14.2   Olfactory epithelium and olfactory receptor cells. *Source*: Peate and Nair, 2015. Reproduced with permission of John Wiley & Sons.

Olfactory bulb

The olfactory bulb lies inferior to the basal frontal lobe and is a highly organised structure composed of several distinct layers and synaptic specialisations. The layers are:

- glomerular layer
- external plexiform layer
- mitral cell layer
- internal plexiform layer
- granule cell layer

Question 4
(a) In Figure 14.3, identify the various components associated with the olfactory bulb.

(b) Colour in the component parts.

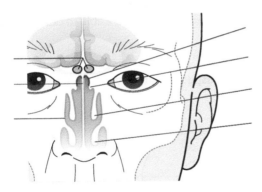
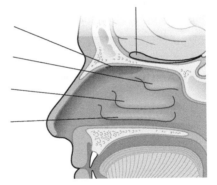

Figure 14.3   The olfactory bulb (nerve). *Source*: Peate and Nair, 2015. Reproduced with permission of John Wiley & Sons.

Question 5 Match the pairs.

The sense of smell is useful for	in the nasal cavity there are paired olfactory organs made up of two layers.
Olfaction is dependent on	the identification of food that is safe to eat and that which has gone rotten
On either side of the nasal septum	receptors that respond to airborne particles
When air is inhaled through the nasal cavity	highly modified neurones contained within the olfactory epithelium
The olfactory receptors are	that respond to certain irritants such as ammonia, chillies and menthol
The nasal cavity contains pain receptors	it is subject to turbulent flow ensuring that airborne smell particles are brought to the olfactory organs

Question 6 Time yourself to unscramble these words.

Scrambled	Answer
TAYFORCLO	
CREEPROST	
LUBB	
BLICIM	
IMCHELAC	
LLEMS	
IRCIMBFOR	
DRATOON	

Gustation

Gustation is the formal term for the sense of taste. In order to create the sensation of taste, a substance has to be in a solution of saliva so that that substance can enter the taste pores. Taste drives the appetite and also protects us from poison. Mostly when we taste bitter or sour this causes dislike; most poisons are bitter, while foods that have gone off taste acidic.

The tongue

This is a muscular organ in the mouth and is covered with moist, pink tissue called mucosa. Like the sense of smell, the sense of taste helps to protect us from poisons but also drives our appetite. There are five basic tastes:

1. sweet
2. sour
3. bitter
4. salt
5. umami.

Taste is associated with the taste buds, the sensory receptor found primarily in the oral cavity. Most of the taste buds are found in peg-like projections of the tongue's mucosa known as papillae, which give the tongue its slightly rough feel.

Question 7
(a) In Figure 14.4, identify the sites of the various papillae and the associated structures.

(b) Colour in the tongue.

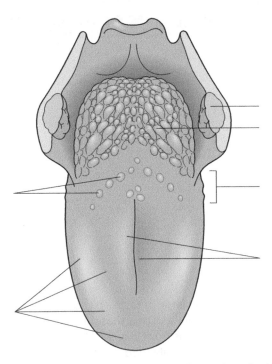

Figure 14.4 The tongue. *Source*: Peate and Nair, 2015. Reproduced with permission of John Wiley & Sons.

Taste buds

Each taste bud is globular in structure and consists of 40–60 epithelial cells of three major types:

1. supporting cells, form the greatest part of the taste bud
2. gustatory (or taste) cells, the chemoreceptors responsible for sensing taste
3. basal cells, stem cells that mature into new receptor cells replacing those that die.

Question 8

(a) In Figure 14.5, identify the parts of the tongue and the various components of the taste bud.

(b) Colour in the component parts.

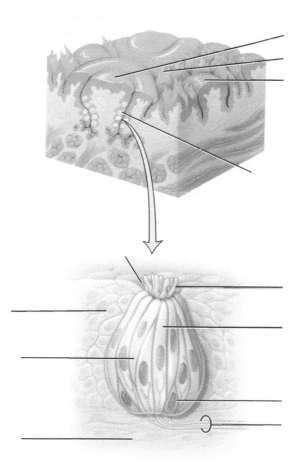

Figure 14.5 Cross-section of part of the tongue with a microscopic view of a taste bud. *Source:* Tortora and Derrickson, 2009. Reproduced with permission of John Wiley & Sons.

Question 9   Match the pairs.

Mostly when we taste bitter or sour this causes dislike because most	in conjunction with the needs of the body
The tongue is a muscular structure	with squamous epithelium
The papillae are projections of a connective tissue core covered	through this pore extend microvilli from the taste cells
The taste cells within a bud are arranged so that their tips form a small taste pore	poisons are bitter, while foods that have gone off taste acidic
When the taste signals are transmitted to the brain,	a number of efferent neural pathways are activated, these are important to digestive function
Taste preferences often change	papillae give the tongue its rough texture with thousands of taste buds covering the surfaces of the papillae

Question 10   Time yourself to unscramble these words.

Scrambled	Answer
DUBS	
TOSINGUTA	
ORCHERTECEMPO	
IMAMU	
ALPEALIP	
UNGOTE	
SIPONO	

Vision

The eye permits us to see and understand shapes, colours and dimensions of objects by processing the light reflected or emitted. The eye consists of the cornea, iris, pupil, lens and retina (housing light-sensitive photoreceptors).

Accessory structures of the eye

The accessory structures of the eye help to protect the eye and preserve vision. Table 14.2 outlines the structure and function of the accessory structures of the eye.

Question 11   Complete Table 14.2 with notes on the various functions of the accessory structures of the eye.

Table 14.2   The structure and function of the accessory structures of the eye.

Structure	Function
Eyelids (palpebrae)	
Eyelashes	
Lacrimal caruncle	
Commissure	
Conjunctiva	
Eyebrows	

Question 12   In Figure 14.6, identify the accessory structures of the eye.

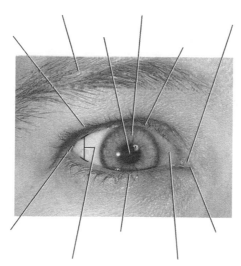

Figure 14.6   The accessory structures of the eye. *Source*: Tortora and Derrickson, 2009. Reproduced with permission of John Wiley & Sons.

The lacrimal apparatus

A constant flow of tears washes over the eyes keeping the conjunctiva moist and clean. Tears have several functions. The lacrimal apparatus produces, distributes and removes tears. It consists of:

- a lacrimal gland
- lacrimal canaliculi
- lacrimal sac
- nasolacrimal duct

Question 13
(a) In Figure 14.7, identify the component parts of the lacrimal apparatus.

(b) Colour in the component parts.

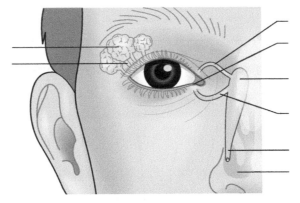

Figure 14.7 The lacrimal apparatus. *Source*: Peate *et al.*, 2014. Reproduced with permission of John Wiley & Sons.

Question 14 Complete Figure 14.8, giving the route of the flow of tears from the lacrimal gland to the nasal cavity.

Flow of tears: Lacrimal gland → → → → → Nasal cavity

Figure 14.8 The flow of tears from the lacrimal gland to the nasal cavity.

Question 15 Match the pairs.

Continual blinking keeps the surface of the eye	the tarsal glands which produce a lipid-rich secretion that helps to prevent the eyelids from sticking together
Eyelashes are robust hairs that help to keep foreign matter out of the eyes associated with	occupied by adipose tissue
Conjunctiva is	arched protecting the eyeball from foreign bodies, dust and sweat
The eyebrows are	the optic nerve (cranial nerve II)
The organ of sight is the eye which is supplied by	the epithelial cell layer that lines the inside of the eyelids and the outer surface of the eye
The space between the eye and the orbital cavity is	lubricated and removes dirt. The gap between the eyelids is known as the palpebral fissure

Question 16 Time yourself to unscramble these words.

Scrambled	Answer
TAILORB	
POISEDA	
PREPABALL	
IFSURES	
RATSAL	
VACUNJONTIC	
BREWSYEO	
SPHEROPROTECTO	

The eye

Question 17
(a) In Figure 14.9, identify the parts of the eye.

(b) Colour in the component parts of the eye.

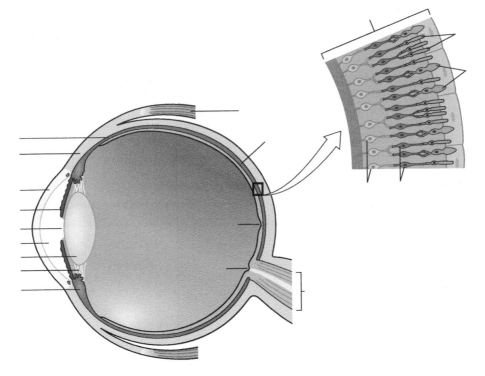

Figure 14.9 The eye. *Source*: Peate and Nair, 2015. Reproduced with permission of John Wiley & Sons.

The retina

The retina is a transparent thin tissue designed to capture photons of light and initiate processing of the image by the brain. There are two types of receptors, rods and cones. The outer segment contains light-sensitive visual pigment molecules – opsins – in stacked discs (rods) or invaginations (cones).

Question 18 Identify the various components of the rods and cones of the retina in Figure 14.10.

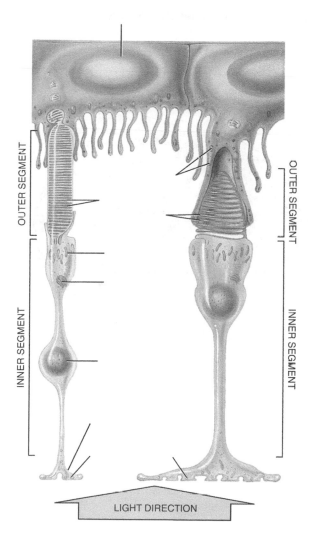

Figure 14.10 Cross-section of the retina. *Source*: Tortora and Derrickson, 2009. Reproduced with permission of John Wiley & Sons.

The muscles of the eye

The two groups of muscles associated with the eyes are the extrinsic and intrinsic eye muscles. The extrinsic eye muscles move the eyeball in the bony orbit; the intrinsic muscles move those structures within the eyeball.

Question 19

(a) Identify the extrinsic muscles of the eye in Figure 14.11.

(b) Colour in the muscles and other components.

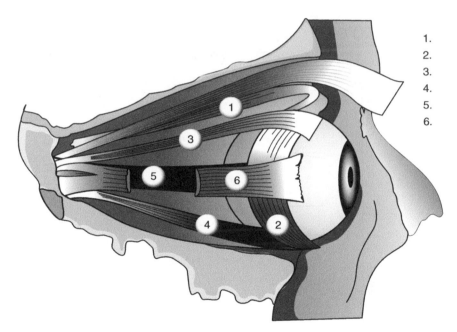

1.
2.
3.
4.
5.
6.

Figure 14.11   The extrinsic muscles of the eye. *Source*: Adapted from Edelhart Kempeneers. *Gray's Anatomy*, 20th edition. 1918.

The visual system pathways to the brain

The optic nerves meet at the optic chiasma, here axons from the medial half of each retina cross to the opposite side, forming pairs of axons from each eye – the left and right optic tracts. The crossing of the axons results in each optic tract carrying information from both eyes: the left carries visual information from the lateral half of the retina of the left eye and the medial half of the retina of the right eye; the right one carries visual information from the lateral half of the retina of the right eye and the medial half of the retina of the left eye.

Question 20

(a) Identify the various components associated with the visual pathway in Figure 14.12.

(b) Colour in the features.

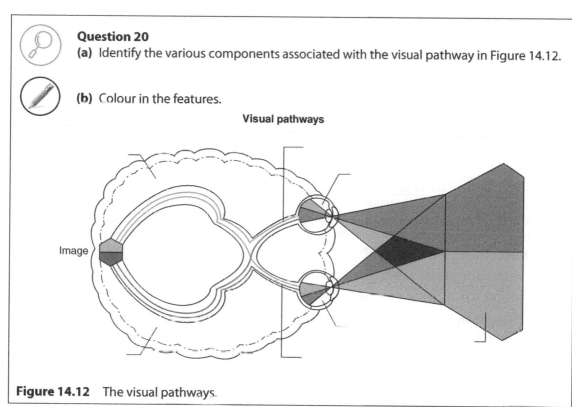

Figure 14.12 The visual pathways.

Question 21 Match the pairs.

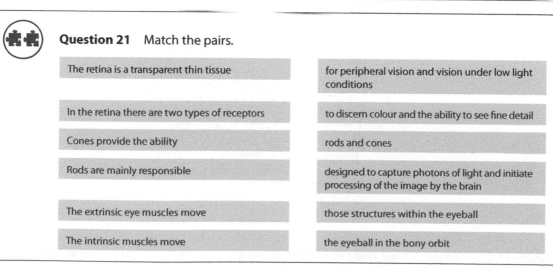

The retina is a transparent thin tissue	for peripheral vision and vision under low light conditions
In the retina there are two types of receptors	to discern colour and the ability to see fine detail
Cones provide the ability	rods and cones
Rods are mainly responsible	designed to capture photons of light and initiate processing of the image by the brain
The extrinsic eye muscles move	those structures within the eyeball
The intrinsic muscles move	the eyeball in the bony orbit

Question 22   Time yourself to unscramble these words.

Scrambled	Answer
SCONE	
RIPERSUO	
QUILBEO	
TRIBO	
ATERIN	
SHOOTNP	
LAPERHIREP	
ISNOVI	

290

Hearing and equilibrium

Sound represents a combination of waves, generated by a vibrating sound source(s), propagated through the air until they reach the ear. Wave frequency corresponds to what is perceived as pitch; amplitude corresponds to the loudness or intensity of sound. The ear has two key functions: to assist equilibrium and to allow us to hear the sounds around us. The ear is composed of three sections:

1. external   **2.** middle   **3.** inner

Question 23   Identify the component parts that make up the external, middle and inner ear in Figure 14.13.

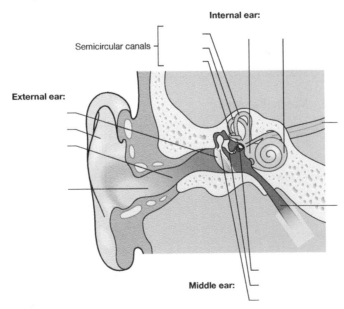

Figure 14.13   The ear. *Source*: Peate *et al.*, 2014. Reproduced with permission of John Wiley & Sons.

The external ear

This aspect of the ear assists with functions of the middle ear although it is not an anatomical part of it. The auricle and external acoustic meatus compose the external ear. It functions to collect and amplify sound, which is transmitted to the middle ear. The asymmetric shape introduces delays in the path of sound, assisting in sound localisation.

Question 24
(a) In Figure 14.14, identify the component parts of the external ear.

(b) Colour in the various parts.

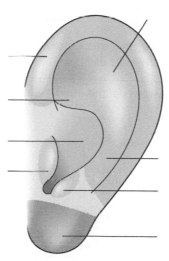

Figure 14.14   The external ear. *Source*: Peate *et al.*, 2014. Reproduced with permission of John Wiley & Sons.

The middle ear

The key function of the middle ear (tympanic cavity) is that of bony conduction of sound from the tympanic membrane to the fluid of the inner ear. It sits in the petrous portion of the temporal bone and is filled with air as it communicates with the nasopharynx via the eustachian tube.

Tympanic membrane and ossicles

The tympanic membrane is an oval, thin, semi-transparent membrane separating the external and middle ear. Air vibrations collected by the auricle are transferred to the mobile tympanic membrane, which transmits the sound to the ossicles. The ossicles (the malleus, incus and stapes) are a chain of movable bones between the deep surface of the tympanic membrane and the oval window. They transmit and amplify sound waves from the air to the perilymph of the internal ear.

Question 25

(a) In Figure 14.15, identify the three bones, the tympanic membrane and other component parts of the middle ear.

(b) Colour in the various aspects of the middle ear.

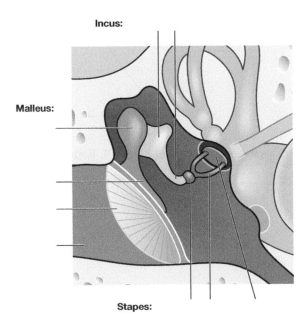

Figure 14.15 The middle ear. *Source:* Peate *et al.*, 2014. Reproduced with permission of John Wiley & Sons.

The inner ear

The inner ear consists of a membranous 'labyrinth' encased in an osseous labyrinth. The vestibule and semicircular canals are associated with vestibular function (balance). The cochlea is concerned with hearing. A layer of dense bone creates the surface outline of the inner ear. The inner aspects of the bony labyrinth closely follow the contours of the membranous labyrinth, a delicate, interconnected network of fluid-filled tubes where the receptors are found. Perilymph flows between the bony and membranous labyrinths. Endolymph is contained in the membranous labyrinth. These fluids are in separate compartments. The bony labyrinth can be subdivided into the vestibule, three semicircular canals and the cochlea.

Question 26

(a) In Figure 14.16, identify the component parts of the inner ear.

(b) Colour the various aspects of the inner ear.

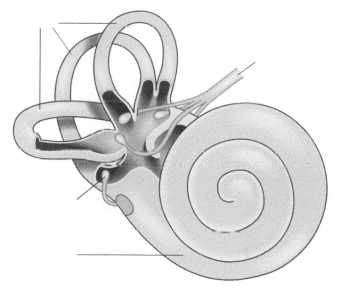

Figure 14.16   The inner ear. *Source:* Peate *et al.*, 2014. Reproduced with permission of John Wiley & Sons.

Equilibrium

The sense of equilibrium is part of the sense of balance controlled by receptors in the semicircular ducts, the utricle and the saccule of the inner ear. Sensory receptors in the semicircular ducts are active during movement but inactive when the body is motionless. The sensory receptors in the ducts respond to rotational movements of the head. There are three of these ducts:

1. lateral
2. posterior
3. anterior.

Question 27 In Figure 14.17, identify the position of the macula with the head upright and tilted forward and identify the component parts.

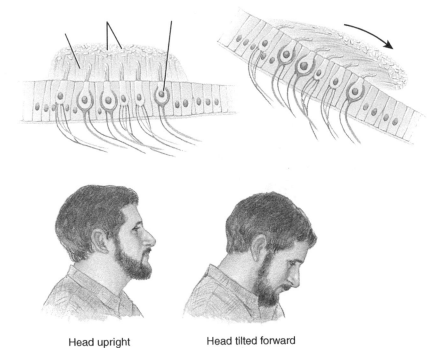

Head upright   Head tilted forward

Position of macula with head upright (left) and tilted forward (right)

Figure 14.17 The action of gravity on the otolith. *Source:* Tortora and Derrickson, 2009. Reproduced with permission of John Wiley & Sons.

The cochlea

The cochlea is a bony, spiral-shaped chamber, containing the cochlear duct of the membranous labyrinth. The sense of hearing is provided by receptors within the cochlear duct. Two perilymph-filled chambers are on either side of the duct.

Question 28
(a) Identify the various aspects of the cochlea depicted in Figure 14.18.

(b) Colour in the various components.

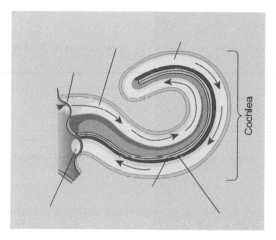

Figure 14.18 The cochlea showing the continuous nature of the vestibular and lymphatic ducts.
Source: Peate and Nair, 2011. Reproduced with permission of John Wiley & Sons.

Question 29   Match the pairs.

The cochlea is a bony, spiral-shaped chamber	kill bacteria and, in conjunction with the hairs, keep the canal free of debris
The purpose of the oils and the cerumen is to lubricate the ear canal	containing the cochlear duct of the membranous labyrinth
The tympanic cavity is a small, air-filled cavity	and is controlled by receptors in the semicircular ducts, the utricle and the saccule of the inner ear
The inner ear is also known as the labyrinth due to the complicated series of canals it contains	lined with mucosa and contained within the temporal bone
The sense of equilibrium is part of the sense of balance	they are hair cells similar to those of the semicircular canals and vestibule
The sense of hearing is provided by receptors in the cochlear duct,	it is composed of two main fluid-filled parts

Question 30 Time yourself to unscramble these words.

Scrambled	Answer
LEACHOC	
IRUBIQMILEU	
TOTHLIO	
SMALLUE	
SUCIN	
PASTES	
THYINLABR	
CAMPYTIN	

Snap shot

Visual acuity

The term 20/20 vision is used to express normal visual acuity; this is the clarity or sharpness of vision. 20/20 vision is cited when the imperial system is used, with the metric system normal visual acuity quoted as being 6/6.

What does 6/6 vision mean?

Word search

A	H	O	C	J	M	M	D	L	E	Q	Q	R	E	L	T	H	G	I	S
S	R	E	T	I	N	A	S	U	C	N	I	E	C	G	K	S	Y	W	A
M	T	R	A	D	X	O	U	C	V	F	D	Q	I	V	F	V	F	I	Z
E	H	A	W	R	O	T	P	E	C	E	R	O	M	E	H	C	M	I	Z
L	J	A	P	W	L	A	C	R	I	M	A	L	O	S	N	S	I	U	Y
L	J	J	L	E	N	O	I	T	A	T	S	U	G	C	O	S	J	G	E
N	J	Q	Q	S	S	C	G	V	P	X	W	G	Y	N	U	U	W	V	A
G	N	C	K	P	I	U	G	K	Q	H	N	M	A	Q	A	L	R	D	C
G	A	O	Q	H	Q	R	M	P	H	N	A	V	M	X	J	I	A	C	C
J	E	H	I	E	J	C	I	A	A	L	R	A	E	L	H	C	O	C	E
E	S	D	T	T	I	E	C	B	L	K	U	T	D	O	N	R	P	H	R
E	C	Y	Y	B	C	W	F	E	O	A	V	Q	L	W	T	T	B	X	U
O	N	U	M	Y	B	A	U	U	O	L	H	X	E	I	E	R	Z	V	M
G	Z	I	P	Z	K	S	F	T	C	O	G	T	R	R	I	D	O	U	E
N	L	P	A	X	W	X	F	L	E	H	A	Q	O	L	C	S	F	J	N
I	Z	U	N	D	Z	Z	A	U	O	E	P	A	L	P	E	B	R	A	E
R	G	G	I	O	B	U	M	A	M	I	W	S	V	C	Y	H	M	P	U
A	U	H	C	C	R	A	N	I	A	L	C	S	K	J	C	H	U	F	T
E	K	G	Y	D	G	A	U	I	A	I	S	U	E	G	A	R	E	B	E
H	H	Q	I	V	E	N	R	P	C	O	G	M	Z	X	N	M	I	H	N

RETINA   HYPOTHALAMUS   INCUS
HEARING   ANOSMIA   STAPES
SIGHT   UMAMI   COCHLEAR
GUSTATION   SWEET   CORTI
OLFACTION   SOUR   PALPEBRAE
CHEMORECEPTOR   AGEUSIA   LACRIMAL
SMELL   TYMPANIC   IRIS
CRANIAL   CERUMEN
LIMBIC   MALLEUS

Crossword

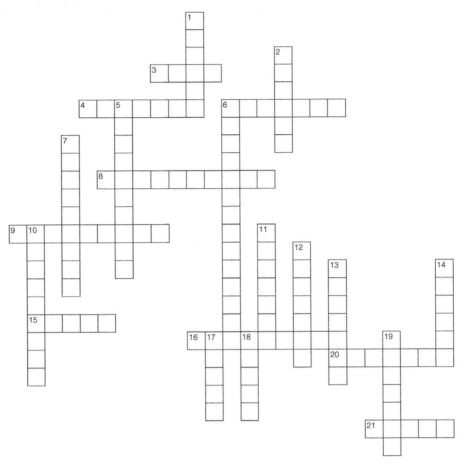

Across

3. The central, coloured portion of the eye
4. Complete loss of sense of taste
6. Ear wax
8. Anosmia is an early indicator of what disease?
9. The sense of smell
15. Bone which attaches the malleus to the stapes
16. Taste
20. Perilymph is found in here
21. Dissolved chemicals interact with odorant-binding proteins on the surface of what?

Down

1. The innermost layer of the eye
2. When the head is in a neutral position what does the statoconia sit on top of?
5. Tube which connects the middle ear to the nasopharynx
6. What do the chemical senses (smell and taste) rely on?
7. The nasal cavity contains pain receptors that respond to what?
10. The inner ear
11. Singular of papillae
12. Loss of the sense of smell
13. Equilibrium
14. Tissue that covers most of the ocular surface
17. Basic taste associated with the proteins found in meat and fish
18. Number of bones in the middle ear
19. The vascular layer that separates the fibrous and neural tunics

Fill in the blanks

Use the words in the box to complete the sentences:

acidic, airborne, appetite, bitter, bitter, blind, cavity, cells, chemicals, cornea, dangers, dimensions, dislike, ear, emitted, equilibrium, external, eye, flowers, frequency, gustation, hear, identification, inner, insensitive, layers, light, light, loudness, optic, organs, paired, perfume, poison, pupil, receptors, retina, rods, rotten, safe, saliva, see, shapes, smell, solution, sound, source(s), taste, three, two, vibrating, waves

1. The sense of _____ is one of the oldest senses. The sense of smell is useful to us for the _____ of food that is _____ to eat and that which has gone _____; it helps us to identify _____, such as dangerous _____, and gives us pleasure through the smell of _____ and _____. Olfaction is dependent on _____ that respond to _____ particles. In the nasal _____, either side of the nasal septum, there are _____ olfactory _____ made up of two _____.

2. _____ is the formal term for the sense of taste. In order to create the sensation of _____, a substance has to be in _____ of _____ so that it can enter the taste pores. Taste drives the _____ and also protects us from _____. Mostly when we taste _____ or sour this causes _____, most poisons are _____, while foods that have gone off taste _____.

3. The eye permits us to _____ and understand _____, colours and _____ of objects by processing the _____ reflected or _____. The eye consists of the _____, iris, _____, lens and retina. The lens focuses _____ on the retina. The retina is covered with _____ basic types of light-sensitive _____ – _____ and cones. The _____ is connected to the brain through the _____ nerve. The point of this connection is called the "_____ spot" because it is _____ to light.

4. Sound represents a combination of _____ generated by a _____ sound _____, propagated through the air until they reach the _____. Wave _____ corresponds to what is perceived as pitch, amplitude corresponds to the _____ or intensity of _____. The ear has two key functions: to assist _____ and to allow us to _____ the sounds around us. The ear is composed of _____ sections: the _____, middle and _____ ear.

Multiple choice questions

1. The retina

   (a) Is easily infected
   (b) Contains rods and cones
   (c) Covers the eye lid
   (d) Secretes vitreous humour

2. The consequence of diminished blood flow to the choroid can result in

   (a) Aqueous humour cannot be formed and the intraocular pressure increases
   (b) Light cannot be refracted
   (c) The retina dies
   (d) The pupil constricts

3. A drug that is described as mydriatic

   (a) Increases intraocular pressure
   (b) Dilates the pupil
   (c) Decreases the secretion of aqueous humour
   (d) Increases the numbers of rods

4. Which of the following does not describe the middle ear?

   (a) It contains the malleus, incus and stapes
   (b) It connects with the pharynx by the eustachian tube
   (c) It is the location of the organ of Corti
   (d) It is concerned with bony conduction of sound

5. The organ of Corti

   (a) Is the receptor for hearing
   (b) Refers to the bones within the middle ear
   (c) Is easily identified with a ophthalmoscope
   (d) Deactivates CN II

6. Touch, pressure, pain, and temperature are

   (a) Mediated through mechanoreceptors
   (b) Classified as general senses
   (c) Translated in the precentral gyrus
   (d) General senses that are interpreted in the occipital lobe

7. Cranial nerves III, IV and VI

   (a) Carry sensory information from the iris to the occipital lobe
   (b) Carry sensory information from the organ of Corti to the primary auditory cortex
   (c) Innervate the extrinsic eye muscles
   (d) Are the motor nerves involved in tear production

8. Which of the following is not a sense?

    (a) Gustation
    (b) Lacrimation
    (c) Olfaction
    (d) Proprioception

9. What are these structures: superior oblique, inferior oblique, superior rectus, inferior rectus, medial rectus and lateral rectus?

    (a) Cranial nerves that stimulate the extrinsic eye muscles
    (b) Muscles that form the iris
    (c) Structures of the middle ear
    (d) Extrinsic eye muscles

10. What does ptosis refer to?

    (a) Drooping of the upper eyelid
    (b) A cranial nerve
    (c) Another name for earache
    (d) None of the above

References

Peate, I. and Nair, M. (2011) *Fundamentals of Anatomy and Physiology for Student Nurses*. Oxford: John Wiley & Sons, Ltd.

Peate, I. and Nair, M. (2015) *Anatomy and Physiology for Nurses at a Glance*. Oxford: John Wiley & Sons, Ltd.

Peate, I., Wild, K. and Nair, M. (eds) (2014) *Nursing Practice: Knowledge and Care*. Oxford: John Wiley & Sons, Ltd.

Tortora, G.J. and Derrickson, B.H. (2009) *Principles of Anatomy and Physiology*, 12th edn. Hoboken, NJ: John Wiley & Sons, Inc.

Chapter 15

The endocrine system

There are two major systems in the body for maintaining homeostasis: the nervous system and the endocrine system. The nervous system reacts rapidly to stimuli and effects its changes over a period of seconds or minutes; it is involved in the immediate and short-term maintenance of homeostasis. The endocrine system is often responsible for the regulation of longer-term processes.

The endocrine system is made up of a collection of small organs scattered throughout the body, each of which releases hormones into the bloodstream.

Question 1 Complete Table 15.1 in relation to the two systems.

Table 15.1 Nervous system versus endocrine system.

	Nervous system	Endocrine system
Speed of action		
Duration of action		
Method of transmitting messages		
Transport method		

Fundamentals of Anatomy and Physiology Workbook: A Study Guide for Nursing and Healthcare Students, First Edition. Ian Peate.
© 2017 John Wiley & Sons Ltd. Published 2017 by John Wiley & Sons Ltd.

The endocrine organs

Each of these organs typically has a rich blood supply delivered by numerous blood vessels. The hormone-producing cells within the organ are arranged into branching networks around this supply, which ensures that hormones enter into the bloodstream rapidly and are then transported throughout the body to the target cells.

Question 2   In Figure 15.1, identify the major endocrine glands.

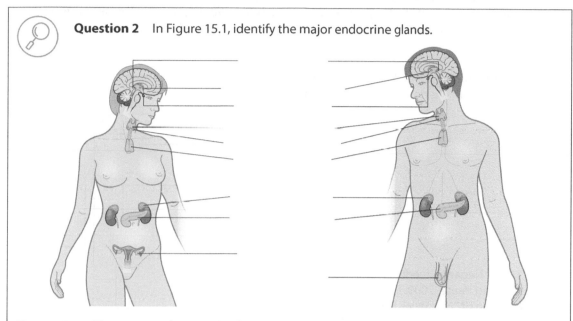

Figure 15.1   The major endocrine glands. *Source*: Peate and Nair, 2015. Reproduced with permission of John Wiley & Sons.

Question 3   Provide definitions for the words in Table 15.2.

Table 15.2   Endocrine, paracrine, autocrine and exocrine.

	Definition
Endocrine	
Paracrine	
Autocrine	
Exocrine	

Hormones

Hormones are chemical messengers secreted into the blood or the extracellular fluid by one cell and have an effect on the functioning of other cells. As hormones circulate in the blood they come into contact with virtually every cell in the body but only exert their specific effect on the target cells. Like a lock and key mechanism, only the right hormone can unlock a particular receptor.

The creation and release of most hormones are preceded by a stimulus, internal or external; for instance, a rise in blood glucose levels or a cold environment. The further synthesis and release of hormones is then usually controlled by a negative feedback system.

Question 4   Complete the diagram in Figure 15.2, filling in the boxes and using arrows to explain the negative feedback system.

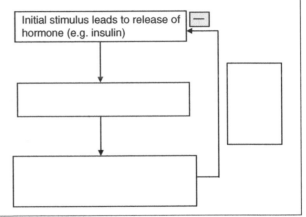

Figure 15.2   Negative feedback system.
Source: Nair and Peate, 2009. Reproduced with permission of John Wiley & Sons.

Question 5   Match the pairs.

Homeostasis refers to	a collection of small organs scattered throughout the body, each of which releases hormones into the blood supply
The endocrine system is made up of	hormones that act locally and diffuse to the cells in the immediate neighbourhood to produce their action
Paracrine refers to	the maintenance of normal physiological balance and functioning within the body
Hormones are chemical	as up-regulation and down-regulation
Changes in the number of receptors are known	messengers that are secreted into the blood or the extracellular fluid by one cell and have an effect on the functioning of other cells
Most hormones are inactivated by enzyme systems in the liver and kidneys	and excreted mostly in the urine, some are excreted in the faeces

Question 6   Time yourself to unscramble these words.

Scrambled	Answer
SHOREMON	
CREEDINON	
CROXEINE	
RATGET	
BEEFCAKD	
USMUTLIS	
PORCESTER	
RINCETOAU	

The pituitary gland and the hypothalamus

The hypothalamus has a number of functions. The pituitary gland is the size of a pea and is cone shaped. It rests in the hypophyseal fossa and is connected to the hypothalamus by the infundibulum. The pituitary gland and the hypothalamus act as a unit, controlling other endocrine glands. There are two distinct areas: the anterior lobe and the posterior lobe.

Question 7
(a) Identify the pituitary gland (posterior and anterior aspects) and the surrounding structures in Figure 15.3.

(b) Colour in the pituitary gland and the surrounding structures.

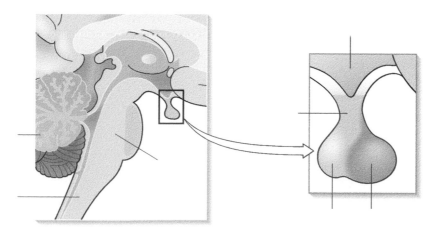

Figure 15.3   The pituitary gland and surrounding structures. *Source*: Peate and Nair, 2015. Reproduced with permission of John Wiley & Sons.

Hormones released by the anterior pituitary gland

 Question 8   Table 15.3 shows hormones released by the hypothalamus and the anterior pituitary gland. Complete this table by adding the name of the hormones that are released by the anterior pituitary gland and the target organ or tissues.

Table 15.3   Hormones released by the hypothalamus and the anterior pituitary gland.

Hypothalamus	Anterior pituitary gland	Target organ or tissues	Action
Growth hormone releasing factor			Stimulates growth of body cells
Growth hormone release inhibiting factor			–
Thyroid releasing hormone (TRH)			Stimulates thyroid hormone release
Corticotropin releasing hormone (CRH)			Stimulates corticosteroid release
Prolactin releasing hormone			Stimulates milk production
Prolactin inhibiting hormone			–
Gonadotropin releasing hormone			Various reproductive functions

The thyroid gland

The thyroid gland is located in the front of the neck on the trachea, just below the larynx. It is made up of two lobes joined by an isthmus. The upper extremities of the lobes are known as the upper poles and the lower extremities the lower poles.

Question 9
(a) Label the diagram in Figure 15.4.

(b) Colour in the various components.

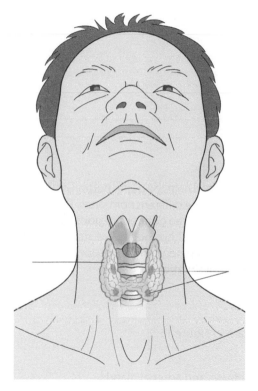

Figure 15.4 The thyroid and parathyroid glands. *Source*: Peate 2015. Reproduced with permission of John Wiley & Sons.

Thyroid hormones are required for normal growth and development. The thyroid releases two types of thyroid hormone, thyroxine (T_4) and triiodothyronine (T_3).

Question 10 Table 15.4 provides a list of outcomes that can occur when there is an increased secretion of T_3 and T_4 (hyperthyroidism). Complete the list in relation to decreased secretion of T_3 and T_4 (hypothyroidism).

Table 15.4 Some effects associated with an abnormal secretion of thyroid hormones.

Increased secretion of T_3 and T_4 (hyperthyroidism)	Decreased secretion of T_3 and T_4 (hypothyroidism)
Increased basal metabolic rate	
Weight loss (despite good/increased appetite)	
Tachycardia, palpitations, arrhythmia	
Excitability, nervousness, irritability	
Tremor	
Hair loss	
Changes in menstruation patterns	
Goitre	
Diarrhoea	
Exophthalmos	

The adrenal glands

The two adrenal glands are located near the upper portion of the kidneys. They have an outer cortex and an inner medulla, which secrete different hormones. The adrenal cortex is essential to life.

The adrenal cortex consists of three different regions; each region produces a different group or type of hormone. All the cortical hormones are steroids. The adrenal medulla secretes two hormones, epinephrine and norepinephrine, in response to stimulation by sympathetic nerves, predominantly during stressful situations.

Question 11
(a) Label the diagram in Figure 15.5.

(b) Colour in the kidneys and adrenal glands.

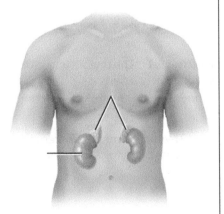

Figure 15.5 The position of the adrenal glands.
Source: Tortora and Derrickson, 2009. Reproduced with permission of John Wiley & Sons.

Question 12

(a) In Figure 15.6, identify the cortex, medulla and capsule of the adrenal gland.

(b) Colour in the cortex, medulla and capsule.

Transverse section

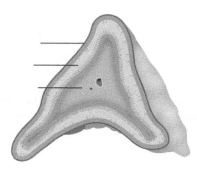

Figure 15.6 Cross-section of an adrenal gland. *Source*: Nair and Peate, 2009. Reproduced with permission of John Wiley & Sons.

Question 13

(a) In Figure 15.7, identify the capsule, medulla and three zones of the cortex.

(b) Colour in the capsule, medulla and three zones.

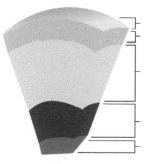

Figure 15.7 Cross-section of the adrenal cortex. *Source*: Nair and Peate, 2009. Reproduced with permission of John Wiley & Sons.

Question 14 Match the pairs.

The thyroid is made up of two lobes	made up of three distinct functional layers
One unique factor of the thyroid gland is	the top of each of the two kidneys
The parathyroid glands are small glands located on	its ability to create and store large amounts of hormone
The two adrenal glands are found on	the posterior of the thyroid gland
The outer part of each adrenal gland is	the regulation of the concentration of electrolytes in the blood
Mineralocorticoids are the group of hormones whose main function is	joined by an isthmus

 Question 15 Time yourself to unscramble these words.

Scrambled	Answer
IDRYTHO	
RECXOT	
ANDRIOILOCOMETCRI	
SMUTHSI	
SUGERMOLAOL	
NOIDEI	
DALELUM	
ASLUPEC	

Pancreas

The pancreas is composed of two different types of tissues, the majority of which is exocrine tissue and the associated ducts producing and secreting a fluid rich with digestive enzymes into the small intestine. Scattered throughout the exocrine tissue are the islets of Langerhans, the site of the endocrine cells of the pancreas. Each islet has three major cell types producing a different hormone:

1. alpha cells, which secrete glucagon
2. beta cells, the most abundant of the three cell types and which secrete insulin
3. delta cells, which secrete somatostatin.

Question 16

(a) Identify the various aspects of the pancreas and associated structures in Figure 15.8.

(b) Colour in the component parts.

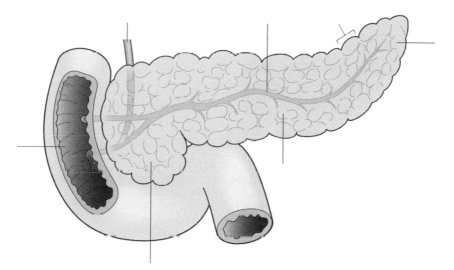

Figure 15.8 The pancreas. *Source*: Peate and Nair, 2015. Reproduced with permission of John Wiley & Sons.

The gonads and other endocrine glands

The gonads are the primary reproductive organs: the testes in the male and the ovaries in the female. These organs are responsible for producing the sperm and ova and they also secrete hormones, so are considered endocrine glands.

As well as the major endocrine glands discussed in this chapter, other organs have some hormonal activity as part of their function. These include the thymus, stomach, small intestines, heart and placenta.

Question 17 In Table 15.5 provide a description of the endocrine function of the endocrine glands listed.

Table 15.5 Other endocrine glands.

Organ	Description
Thymus gland	
Stomach	
Small intestine	
Heart	
Placenta	

Question 18 Match the pairs.

The gonads are the primary reproductive organs:	the gastric mucosa produces gastrin
The pancreas is an elongated organ and	exocrine tissue and the associated ducts
The pancreas is innervated	is found next to the first part of the small intestine
Special cells in the wall of the atria produce	the testes in the male and the ovaries in the female
The majority of the pancreas is made up of	by the parasympathetic and sympathetic nervous systems
when food is present in the stomach	atrial natriuretic hormone

Question 19   Time yourself to unscramble these words.

Scrambled	Answer
REANCAPS	
STEETS	
VARSIEO	
MOYSTHIN	
TAPACELN	
ANALSHERGN	
PALAH	
TEDAL	

Snap shot

Polydipsia and polyuria

John James, a 46-year-old, has been referred to and has been admitted to a specialist center by his GP. He has been complaining of intense thirst that is not relieved by drinking copious amounts of fluid (polydipsia) (he has preference for ice cold water). John is passing large amounts of very pale diluted urine (polyuria). Today he has passed over 7 L, he has been experiencing nocturia and has wet his bed on two occasions.

What might the diagnosis and treatment be?

Word search

J	M	L	H	J	H	Y	P	O	T	H	A	L	A	M	U	S	O	G	S
D	I	Q	A	D	R	E	N	A	L	I	N	E	V	P	W	K	R	Y	T
J	K	B	L	I	N	F	U	N	D	I	B	U	L	U	M	Q	S	F	I
G	W	N	P	I	T	U	I	T	A	R	Y	Y	H	L	L	A	Q	S	S
U	H	U	H	O	J	C	D	T	S	A	E	R	C	N	A	P	Y	T	T
L	A	R	O	T	H	Y	R	O	X	I	N	E	E	K	V	D	Y	E	H
N	M	D	M	Z	T	T	F	B	Y	L	Q	T	Q	I	W	H	T	R	M
O	H	S	E	N	I	M	A	L	O	H	C	E	T	A	C	E	D	O	U
R	Y	D	O	N	N	E	U	R	O	H	Y	P	O	P	H	Y	S	I	S
A	T	N	S	F	O	T	D	I	O	R	Y	H	T	A	R	A	P	D	U
D	E	A	T	P	S	H	E	N	I	R	C	O	D	N	E	R	J	Y	A
R	N	L	A	P	G	H	Y	P	O	T	H	Y	R	O	I	D	I	S	M
E	I	G	S	K	P	B	P	P	M	V	B	E	T	T	B	S	Q	G	M
N	R	D	I	H	H	O	R	M	O	N	E	S	E	V	P	N	E	I	H
A	C	P	S	Q	G	Y	D	Y	F	P	B	U	L	S	I	J	N	K	N
L	O	C	M	U	K	R	T	B	P	B	H	I	T	M	O	S	N	X	W
I	T	N	C	L	A	N	E	R	D	A	Y	Y	E	R	U	C	Z	S	O
N	U	X	D	H	C	R	J	L	I	W	D	A	S	L	I	F	U	A	O
E	A	J	B	L	T	H	Y	R	O	I	D	Q	I	I	S	S	A	L	A
M	G	L	T	B	A	R	E	E	L	T	M	N	N	F	S	T	D	C	G

HORMONES	HYPOTHALAMUS	INFUNDIBULUM
HOMEOSTASIS	PANCREAS	NEUROHYPOPHYSIS
ENDOCRINE	ISTHMUS	ADENOHYPOPHYSIS
GLAND	AUTOCRINE	HYPOTHYROIDISM
PITUITARY	STEROID	CATECHOLAMINES
THYROID	GLUCOSE	ADRENALINE
PARATHYROID	INSULIN	NORADRENALINE
ADRENAL	THYROXINE	

Crossword

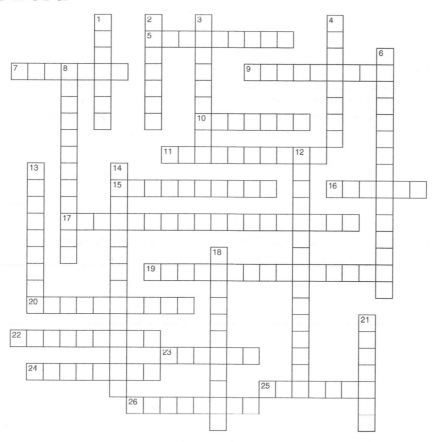

Across

5. T4

7. A narrow strip

9. Gland the size of a pea

10. Butterfly-shaped gland located in the front of the neck

11. Islets of endocrine tissue in the pancreas

15. Hormone that frequently evokes anxiety and fear

16. The stimulus for the release of a hormone due to direct nervous stimulation

17. The group of hormones whose main function is the regulation of the concentration of the electrolytes in the blood

19. The anterior lobe lobe of the pituitary gland

20. A normal blood volume

22. Hormones which diffuse to cells in the immediate neighbourhood to produce their action

23. The outer part of the adrenal gland

24. An elongated organ found next to the duodenum

25. Hormone which reduces blood glucose levels

26. Glands/organs that secrete substances into ducts that eventually lead outside the body

Down

1. The inner part of the adrenal gland

2. Type of hormone that can cross the cell membrane

3. Hormone that stimulates the secretion of milk

4. Hormone that has an effect on uterine contraction in childbirth

6. An overactive thyroid gland

8. Part of the brain

12. The posterior lobe of the pituitary gland

13. Hormones secreted into the blood and have an effect on distant cells

14. Secreted by the adrenal medulla

18. The process of maintaining a stable internal environment

21. Glands found on the top of the kidneys

Fill in the blanks

Use the words in the box to complete the sentences:

adenohypophysis, adrenal, butterfly, development, digestion, ducts, duodenum, endocrine, endocrine, endocrine, exocrine, function, functions, glandular, glucagon, hormones, hormones, hormones, hypothalamus, infundibulum, insulin, islands, isthmus, Langerhans, larynx, levels, lobes, main, metabolism, neck, nervous, neurohypophysis, ovaries, pancreas, pituitary released, reproduction, rings, T4, thyroid, thyroxine, trachea

1. The _____ system is the collection of glands producing _____ that regulate
    _____, growth and _____, tissue _____, sexual function, _____,
    sleep and mood, and other things. The endocrine system is made up of the _____
    gland, thyroid gland, parathyroid glands, _____ glands, pancreas, _____ and
    testes.

2. The pituitary gland is connected to the _____ by the _____. The pituitary gland
    and the hypothalamus act as a unit, controlling most of the other _____ glands.
    Within the pituitary there are two distinct areas: the _____, composed of _____
    epithelium, and the _____ made of a down-growth of _____ tissue from the
    brain.

3. The thyroid gland is located in the _____, anterior to the _____ and the
    trachea. This is a _____-shaped gland with two _____ on either side of the
    _____ cartilage and the upper incomplete cartilaginous _____ of the
    _____. Lying in front of the trachea is the narrow _____ joining the left and
    right lobes. The thyroid gland secretes several hormones, collectively called thyroid
    _____. The main hormone is _____, also called _____.

4. The _____ has both _____ and exocrine _____. The bulk of the pancreas
    is composed of _____ cells producing enzymes to help with the _____ of food.
    These release their enzymes into a series of progressively larger _____ that
    eventually join together to form the _____ pancreatic duct, this runs the length of
    the pancreas and drains into the _____. The second functional component of the
    pancreas is the endocrine pancreas, composed of small _____ of cells, the islets of
    _____. Hormones, such as _____ and _____, are _____ into the
    bloodstream. These _____ help control glucose _____.

Multiple choice questions

1. Which of the following is true of cortisol?

   (a) It is an enzyme
   (b) It is secreted by the adrenal cortex in response to ACTH
   (c) It stimulates the secretion of ATP
   (d) It is released by the adrenal medulla

2. Aldosterone is

   (a) A mineralocorticoid
   (b) A glucocorticoid
   (c) An enzyme
   (d) A carbohydrate

3. The pancreas

   (a) Secretes only steroids
   (b) Is controlled by a hormone secreted by the ovaries
   (c) Secretes both insulin and glucagon
   (d) Secretes hormones that only lower blood glucose levels

4. What is the best way to describe the function of insulin?

   (a) Regulates blood viscosity
   (b) It is only concerned with gluconeogenesis
   (c) Causes ketone body formation
   (d) Lowers blood glucose

5. As calcium decreases in the blood

   (a) Insulin ceases to be secreted
   (b) The parathyroid glands secrete calcitonin
   (c) The kidneys excrete calcium and phosphate
   (d) PTH is secreted, thereby stimulating osteoclastic activity

6. Hypocalcaemic tetany is

   (a) Due to a deficiency of PTH
   (b) A key cause of death
   (c) A consequence of osteoclastic inactivity
   (d) A natural phenomenon when a person is obese

7. Autocrine

   (a) Refers to hormones that act on the cells that produce it
   (b) Refers to hormones that act locally and diffuse to the cells in the immediate neighbourhood to produce their action
   (c) Refers to an immune disorder
   (d) All of the above

8. Hyperglycaemia, polyuria, polydipsia and ketoacidosis may indicate a deficiency of

   (a) Thyroxine
   (b) Insulin
   (c) Epinephrine
   (d) Oestrogen

9. Which of the following is not a steroid?

   (a) Adrenal cortical hormones
   (b) ACTH
   (c) Oestrogen
   (d) Androgens

10. The pituitary gland is said to be

   (a) Located close to the retina
   (b) Enlarged during the menstrual cycle
   (c) The size of a pea and is cone shaped
   (d) The size of a walnut and doughnut shaped

References

Nair, M. and Peate, I. (2009) *Fundamentals of Applied Pathophysiology: An Essential Guide for Nursing Students*. Oxford: John Wiley & Sons, Ltd.

Peate, I. and Nair, M. (2015) *Anatomy and Physiology for Nurses at a Glance*. Oxford: John Wiley & Sons, Ltd.

Tortora, G.J. and Derrickson, B.H. (2009) *Principles of Anatomy and Physiology*, 12th edn. Hoboken, NJ: John Wiley & Sons, Inc.

Chapter 16

The immune system

The immune system is an intricate system of cells, enzymes and proteins providing protection and rendering us resistant or immune to infections caused by various microorganisms, for example, bacteria, viruses and fungi. The immune system is capable of doing more than fighting infection and protecting from infectious diseases; other functions include the removal and destruction of damaged or dead cells and the identification and destruction of malignant cells.

Question 1

(a) Figure 16.1, provides an overview of the cells of the immune system with some cells identified. Complete the image, identifying the various cells.

(b) Colour in the cells.

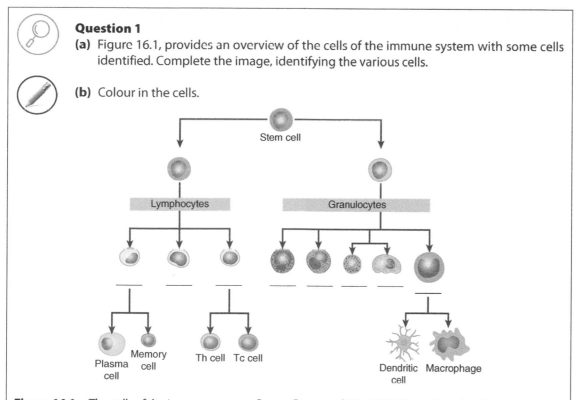

Figure 16.1 The cells of the immune system. *Source*: Peate and Nair, 2015. Reproduced with permission of John Wiley & Sons.

Fundamentals of Anatomy and Physiology Workbook: A Study Guide for Nursing and Healthcare Students, First Edition. Ian Peate.
© 2017 John Wiley & Sons Ltd. Published 2017 by John Wiley & Sons Ltd.

Question 2 In Table 16.1 describe the various elements associated with the immune system.

Table 16.1 The immune system.

Component of the immune system	Description
B-lymphocytes	
Bone marrow	
Immunoglobulins	
Monocytes	
Plasma cells	
Polymorphonuclear leucocytes	
Stem cells	
Thymus	
T-effector lymphocytes	
T-helper lymphocytes	
T-lymphocytes	

Types of immunity

Active immunity is protection that is produced by the person's own immune system. This type of immunity is usually permanent.

Passive immunity is protection by products produced by an animal or human, and transferred to another human, usually by injection. Passive immunity often provides effective protection, but this protection wanes with time, usually a few weeks or months.

Question 3

(a) Identify the types of acquired immunity by filling in the blank boxes in Figure 16.2.

(b) Colour in the boxes.

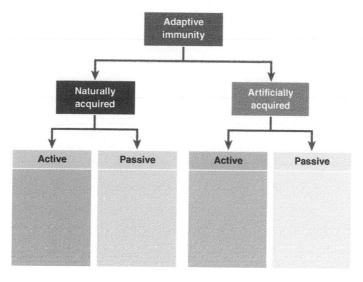

Figure 16.2 Types of acquired immunity. *Source*: Peate and Nair, 2015. Reproduced with permission of John Wiley & Sons.

Question 4 There are five types of antibody. The types of antibody are listed in Table 16.2; complete the table with the functions of the antibodies.

Table 16.2 Types of antibodies.

Type of antibody	Functions
IgA	
IgD	
IgE	
IgG	
IgM	

Question 5 Match the pairs.

Innate immunity is acquired at birth	been met and overcome known as immunological memory
A central role of the innate immune responses is to prevent or restrict	the foetus acquires some immunity via the placenta, this is called passive immunity
Acquired immunity has the ability to remember when a particular immunological threat has	associated with activation of the T-lymphocyte system that stimulates B-lymphocyte separation
The primary response generates a slow and delayed rise in antibody levels	the entrance of microorganisms into the body, so that tissue damage is limited
The secondary response occurs on subsequent exposure to the same antigen	this is relatively short acting as the antibodies eventually break down
Passive immunity occurs when the person has been given antibodies	the response is much faster as the memory B-lymphocytes generated after the first infection divide and separate a faster rate

Question 6 Time yourself to unscramble these words.

Scrambled	Answer
VESPASI	
TABIESDINO	
TENAGIN	
QUACREDI	
TUMMYINI	
CHYMESYPOTL	
GRAPHSOMEAC	
SYMHUT	

Organs of the immune system

The key organs of the immune system are all part of the lymphatic system and consist of:

- thymus
- spleen
- bone marrow
- lymph nodes
- lymphoid tissues scattered throughout the gastrointestinal, respiratory and urinary tracts

Question 7

(a) In Figure 16.3, identify the various aspects of the immune system.

(b) Colour in the various organs.

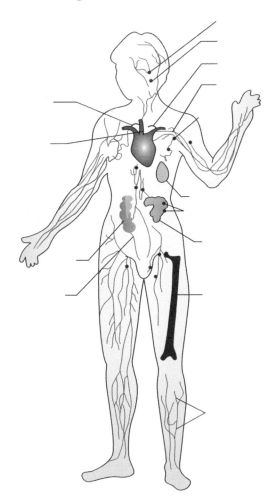

Figure 16.3 Organs of the immune system.

The thymus

The thymus is situated in the chest.

Question 8

(a) In Figure 16.4, identify the position of the thymus gland and associated structures.

(b) Colour in the thymus and the associated structures.

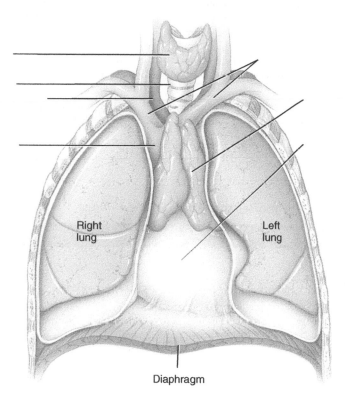

Figure 16.4 The position of the thymus in an adolescent. *Source*: Tortora and Derrickson, 2009. Reproduced with permission of John Wiley & Sons.

Question 9 Match the pairs.

The key primary lymphoid organs of the immune system include	by the early teens, the thymus begins to atrophy
The secondary lymphatic tissues include	is a key element of the lymphatic system, being one of the primary lymphoid organs that generates lymphocytes
The thymus is largest and most active during the neonatal and pre-adolescent periods of development	the thymus and bone marrow, they are involved in the production and early selection of lymphocytes
Bone marrow is the flexible tissue found in the interior of bones, the red bone marrow	conduits called lymphatic vessels that carry a clear fluid, called lymph towards the heart
The lymphatic system is a part of the circulatory system, comprising a network of	spleen, tonsils, lymph vessels, lymph nodes, adenoids, skin and liver

Question 10 Time yourself to unscramble these words.

Scrambled	Answer
SLEEPN	
RAWMOR	
PLYMH	
REYSEP	
HLYOPMID	
ORAPHYT	
DIEDANSO	
NOSLITS	

The lymphatic system

The lymphatic system is a network of tissues and organs primarily consisting of lymph vessels, lymph nodes and lymph. There are 600 to 700 lymph nodes in the body that filter the lymph before it returns to the circulatory system.

Question 11

(a) In Figure 16.5, identify the various components of the lymphatic system.

(b) Colour in the structures.

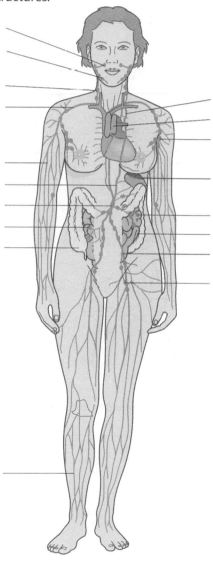

Figure 16.5   The lymphatic system. *Source*: Peate *et al.*, 2014. Reproduced with permission of John Wiley & Sons.

Lymphatic capillaries

Lymphatic capillaries differ from blood capillaries. They originate as pockets rather than forming continuous vessels, have larger diameters, thinner walls and have an irregular outline.

Lymph nodes

Lymph nodes are bean-shaped organs scattered along the lymphatic vessels.

Question 12   In Figure 16.6, identify the component parts.

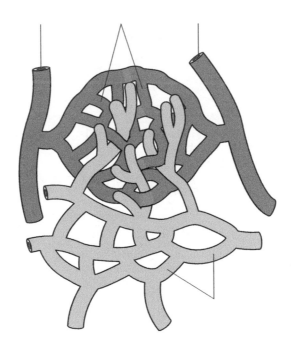

Figure 16.6   Lymphatic capillaries. *Source*: Peate, 2015. Reproduced with permission of John Wiley & Sons.

Question 13
(a) In Figure 16.7, identify the various components of the lymph node.

(b) Colour in the parts of the lymph node.

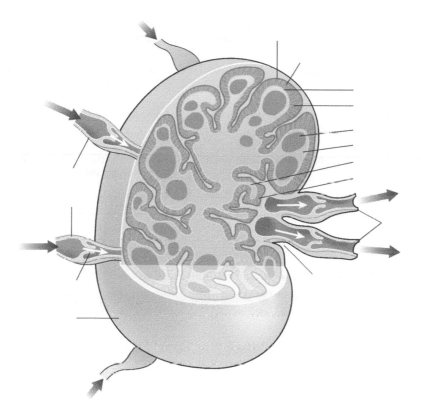

Figure 16.7 A lymph node. *Source:* Peate *et al.*, 2014. Reproduced with permission of John Wiley & Sons.

Question 14   Match the pairs.

The lymphatic system is a specialised system	but it does not have a pump like the heart
The lymphatic vessels are drainage vessels that	of lymph vessels and lymph nodes
The lymphatic system can be thought of as a parallel system to the blood circulatory system	in that their walls consist of a layer of endothelial cells
The lymph vessels and capillaries form a network throughout the body	collect the excess interstitial fluid and return it to the bloodstream
Lymphatic capillaries have some anatomical similarities to blood capillaries	the right lymphatic duct and the thoracic duct
The lymph eventually flows into two large lymph ducts,	and connect the tissues of the body to the lymphoid organs,

Question 15   Time yourself to unscramble these words.

Scrambled	Answer
TUCD	
LILIESCRAPA	
BALACUTREE	
SOFILLECL	
TICYCOGAHP	
FRETEEFN	
RIFTEL	
SLANGD	

Inflammation

Inflammation is an innate response to tissue damage. When tissue damage occurs this triggers a number of proteins to act as the catalysts for the immune response. This response is non-specific and attacks any and all foreign invaders, attempting to rid the body of microbes, toxins or other foreign matter, and to prevent their spread to other tissues. There are four signs related to the inflammatory response:

1. redness
2. swelling
3. heat
4. pain.

 Question 16   Complete Figure 16.8, identifying causes of the inflammatory response.

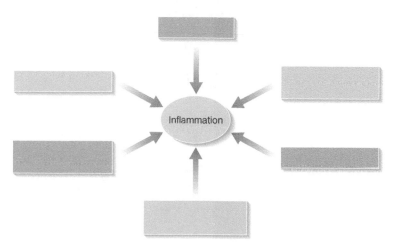

Figure 16.8 Causes of the inflammatory response. *Source*: Peate and Glencross, 2015. Reproduced with permission of John Wiley & Sons.

Question 17

(a) In Figure 16.9, identify the various aspects that are associated with the steps of inflammatory response.

(b) Colour in Figure 16.9.

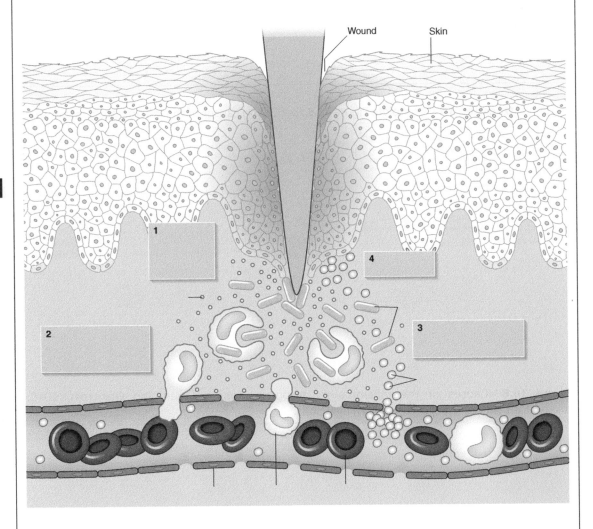

Figure 16.9 The steps of the inflammatory response. *Source*: Peate and Glencross, 2015. Reproduced with permission of John Wiley & Sons.

Question 18   Match the pairs.

Inflammation is	three processes occur at the same time
The inflammatory process involves the movement of	and immunoglobulins help in the destruction of bacteria
Following injury or other damage to the body	the body's immediate reaction to tissue injury or damage
The complement system activates and assists the inflammatory and immune processes	are cytokines which promote inflammation, attracting white blood cells to the affected area
The kinin system helps to control vascular permeability	playing a major role in the destruction of bacteria
Other factors involved in vascular permeability	white cells, complement and other plasma proteins

Question 19   Time yourself to unscramble these words.

Scrambled	Answer
SINKIN	
SINKTOECY	
LACRO	
PELEMMCONT	
THINEISAM	
LARGENATIONDU	
STAM	
POETSHANG	

Snap shot

Immunisations

Immunisation protects people against harmful infections before they come into contact with them in the community. Immunisation is the most important way of protecting people from vaccine-preventable diseases.

All health professionals who become involved in immunisation in any context, administering or advising, should have an understanding of the key issues associated with immunisation.

Throughout their life span people are recommended to have a number of vaccines. Give details of the UK vaccine programme.

Word search

O	W	S	Q	U	K	L	U	F	M	A	R	T	L	A	I	O	X	N	J
N	I	G	E	D	L	M	P	A	S	S	I	V	E	V	I	T	C	A	E
L	M	E	V	T	R	H	W	V	H	B	L	A	P	S	F	A	G	B	L
W	M	G	Z	U	Y	G	Y	T	I	N	U	M	M	I	B	E	G	M	G
Z	U	A	C	J	Y	C	O	Z	H	X	Z	U	S	O	S	H	R	Q	I
O	N	H	Y	Z	A	U	O	Z	O	T	U	F	H	N	Z	J	T	V	S
Z	O	P	T	F	N	Y	P	G	K	S	C	T	I	K	S	A	H	I	P
W	L	O	O	B	T	U	R	I	A	A	P	L	U	C	E	M	Y	I	L
R	O	R	T	G	I	R	O	J	S	H	U	K	S	E	T	E	M	J	E
S	G	C	O	J	G	M	S	U	C	B	P	R	A	S	Y	D	U	H	E
E	Y	A	X	E	E	Y	T	S	O	D	W	J	G	D	C	E	S	G	N
I	X	M	I	A	N	B	A	L	F	P	G	A	T	V	O	O	I	V	X
D	L	T	C	Q	S	E	G	O	J	A	Y	C	J	W	N	L	V	F	J
O	L	J	P	Z	V	O	L	N	K	Q	R	C	P	I	O	Y	K	O	K
B	R	Z	O	F	N	C	A	I	S	B	E	D	P	U	M	G	N	M	R
I	J	Z	H	U	S	D	N	X	N	S	E	N	I	K	O	T	Y	C	O
T	N	C	M	Y	L	I	D	P	C	E	Z	H	P	M	Y	L	Z	E	N
N	U	M	Z	X	N	Q	I	P	C	F	T	Y	E	N	J	T	G	U	O
A	I	H	Y	S	S	A	N	M	V	A	L	C	Q	L	P	B	L	S	D
O	N	Z	W	B	D	M	S	L	T	I	W	S	S	N	X	G	S	I	E

IMMUNOGLOBULINS
MONOCYTES
THYMUS
SPLEEN
ACTIVE
PASSIVE
PHAGOCYTES

ANTIBODIES
ANTIGENS
CYTOKINES
CYTOTOXIC
IMMUNOLOGY
IMMUNITY
KININS

LYMPH
NODE
OEDEMA
MACROPHAGE
PROSTAGLANDINS

Crossword

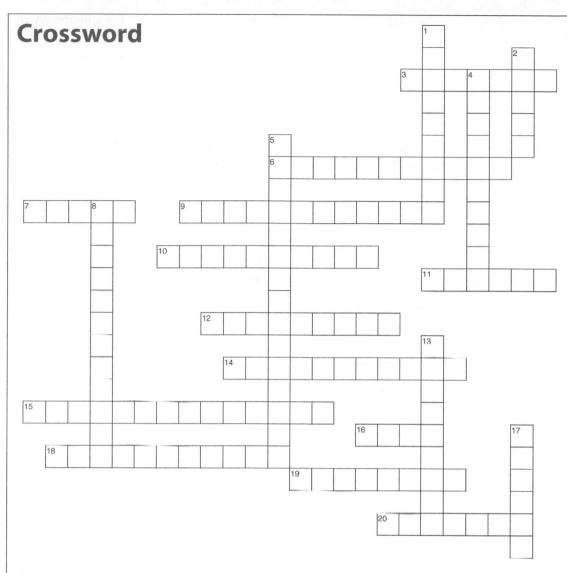

Across

3. Anything that provokes an antibody response
6. Type of stem cell
7. Fluid within lymphatic vessels
9. Neutrophils, eosinophils and basophils
10. A type of white blood cell
11. An immune organ located in the chest
12. Related to damage to or death of cells
14. 60% of the leucocytes in the body
15. Fatty acids functioning as part of the inflammatory process
16. Number of classes of immunoglobulin
18. 1% of leucocytes
19. One of the major types of immunity
20. Type of immunisation in which the individual is injected with antibodies

Down

1. Phagocytic white blood cells
2. Fluids from the eyes that act as a mechanical barrier
4. The study of the immune system
5. Antibodies
8. Destruction of infectious organisms/non-self matter by specialised cells
13. Blood cells with an important role in blood clotting
17. An encapsulated organ associated with the immune system

Fill in the blanks

Use the words in the box to complete the sentences:

antibodies, body, breastbone, cells, chest, disease, enlarged, entry, environment, fat, fight, fungi, health, immune, infants, infection, infection, limits, lymph, lymphatic, nodes, parasites, produce, protect, puberty, shrink, system, T-cells, thymus, thymus, trigger, viruses

1. The immune _____ is a network of _____, tissues and organs working together to _____ the body from _____. The body provides an ideal _____ for many microbes, such as _____, bacteria, _____ and _____, and the _____ system prevents and _____ their _____ and growth to maintain optimal _____.

2. Lymph _____ are small bean-shaped structures that _____ and store cells that _____ infection and _____, and are part of the _____ system. _____ is a clear fluid that carries those cells of the immune system to different parts of the _____. When the body is fighting _____, lymph nodes can become _____.

3. The _____ is a small organ and is where _____ mature. It is situated in the _____ beneath the _____. It can _____ or maintain the production of _____. The _____ is somewhat large in _____, grows until _____, then starts to slowly _____ and become replaced by _____ with age.

Multiple choice questions

1. What are complement and interferons?

   (a) Considered to be specific immunity
   (b) Protective proteins engaged in non-specific immunity
   (c) Secreted by B-cells and T-cells
   (d) Hormones

2. What are T- and B-cells?

   (a) Types of red blood cells
   (b) Platelets
   (c) Viruses
   (d) Lymphocytes that are responsible for specific immunity

3. Active immunity is protection that is

   (a) Produced by the person's own immune system
   (b) Only activated when the person becomes seriously ill
   (c) Is only activated during times of stress
   (d) None of the above

4. B-cells

   (a) Can only connect to virus antigens on the outside of infected cells
   (b) Are types of red blood cells
   (c) All of the above
   (d) None of the above

5. Pyrexia, pyrogens and febrile seizures are most related to which non-specific form of immunity?

   (a) Hypotension
   (b) Fever
   (c) Anaphylaxis
   (d) Hypertension

6. Plasma cells

   (a) Are also called T-cells
   (b) Are known as NK cells
   (c) Secrete antibodies
   (d) Secrete viruses

7. With which of the following is anaphylaxis most associated?

   (a) Interferons
   (b) Phagocytosis
   (c) IgE
   (d) Only with nut allergy

8. What is the primary concern concerning the care of a patient experiencing anaphylaxis?

   (a) Development of rash
   (b) Inability to breathe
   (c) Development of seizure
   (d) Inability to communicate

9. Where is the thymus located?

(a) Abdomen
(b) Brain
(c) Thorax
(d) Small intestine

10. Inflammation is

(a) Related to anxiety
(b) Characterised by redness, heat, swelling and pain
(c) Called cell-mediated immunity
(d) The same as infection

References

Peate, I. and Glencross, W. (2015) *Wound Care at a Glance*. Oxford: John Wiley & Sons, Ltd.
Peate, I. and Nair, M. (2015) *Anatomy and Physiology for Nurses at a Glance*. Oxford: John Wiley & Sons, Ltd.
Peate, I., Wild, K. and Nair, M. (eds) (2014) *Nursing Practice: Knowledge and Care*. Oxford: John Wiley & Sons, Ltd.
Tortora, G.J. and Derrickson, B.H. (2009) *Principles of Anatomy and Physiology*, 12th edn. Hoboken, NJ: John Wiley & Sons, Inc.

Chapter 17

The skin

The skin (also called the integumentary system) is the largest organ of the body, accounting for around 15% of an adult's body weight. It is composed of specialised cells and structures. The skin carries out a number of vital functions, including protecting the person against external physical, chemical, and biological attack, preventing the loss of excess water from the body and playing a central role in thermoregulation.

The skin structure

The skin has two regions the epidermis and the dermis; the subcutaneous layer lies below the skin. The skin covers the entire surface of the body and is continuous with the mucous membranes of the mouth, eyes, ears, nose vagina and rectum.

Question 1

(a) Identify the various aspects of the cross-section of the skin in Figure 17.1.

(b) Colour in the three layers of the skin.

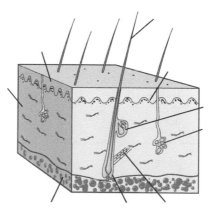

Figure 17.1 The skin. *Source*: Nair and Peate, 2009. Reproduced with permission of John Wiley & Sons.

Question 2   Match the pairs.

The skin is sometimes referred to as this	Nearly one third of all blood that flows thorough the body
The thinnest part of the skin is	The brain
The skin is composed of two distinct regions	The epidermis
The skin is twice as heavy as	The dermis and epidermis
The appendages are	Manifestations of the skin
The skin receives	The integummary system

Question 3   Time yourself to unscramble these words.

Scrambled	Answer
DRMIES	
ENCOUTASSUBU	
SNLAGD	
OSCUMU	
SPIDEREMI	
PAILLEAP	
SIREGD	
ROPE	

Question 4
(a) Label the diagram in Figure 17.2.

(b) Colour the components of the epidermis.

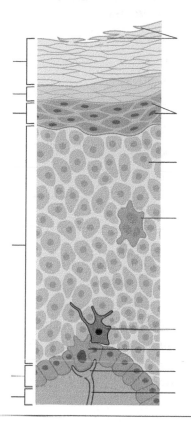

Figure 17.2 The layers of the epidermis.
Source: Peate and Nair, 2015. Reproduced with permission of John Wiley & Sons.

Question 5 Match the pairs.

Also known as a tactile cell	Keratinocytes
The most numerous cell in the skin	Merkel cell
Associated with immunity	Melanocyte
Located in the stratum basale	Langerhans cells

Question 6   Time yourself to unscramble these words.

Scrambled	Answer
YALEMCOTEN	
MUSTTAR	
LITECAT	
TUMMYINI	
SHALENRANG	
SLLEC	
NIPSMUSO	
RAYELS	

 Question 7
(a) Identify the various components of the pilosebaceous unit in Figure 17.3.

 (b) Colour in the various features.

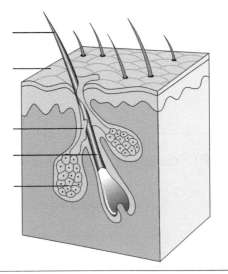

Figure 17.3   A pilosebaceous unit. *Source*: Nair and Peate, 2009. Reproduced with permission of John Wiley & Sons.

Question 8 Match the pairs.

Found on most surfaces of the body	Follicles
Accompanies hair follicles	Sebum
Hair follicles are found here	Sebaceous gland
A liquid substance exuded by the sebaceous glands	Hair
Most of the skin has these	Skin surface

Question 9 Time yourself to unscramble these words.

Scrambled	Answer
BEMUS	
CLIFSOLLE	
CABSESEOU	
RAIH	
LAIN	
CRETORRA	
BLUB	
TWEAS	

343

Question 10

(a) Figure 17.4 shows a sweat gland. Identify the component parts.

(b) Colour in the parts of the sweat gland.

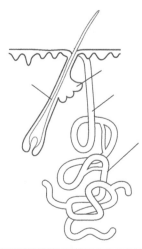

Figure 17.4 A sweat gland. *Source*: Nair and Peate, 2009. Reproduced with permission of John Wiley & Sons.

Question 11   Match the pairs.

Supplies lubrication to the skin	Apocrine gland (secretory portion)
Coiled glands, more prominent in localised sites such as pubic axillae	Hair follicle
Every pore is an opening for one of these	Sebaceous gland

Question 12   Time yourself to unscramble these words.

Scrambled	Answer
CUBIP	
EXALLIA	
OTRO	
SEXUPL	
SULVEL	
TARKEIN	
GAMPTENTINO	
FATSH	

Question 13   Figure 17.5 shows another appendage of the skin, the nail. Identify the various parts of the nail.

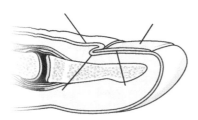
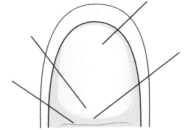

Figure 17.5   The nail. *Source*: Nair and Peate, 2009. Reproduced with permission of John Wiley & Sons.

Question 14   Match the pairs.

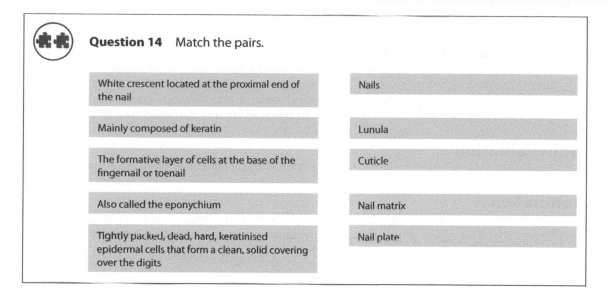

White crescent located at the proximal end of the nail	Nails
Mainly composed of keratin	Lunula
The formative layer of cells at the base of the fingernail or toenail	Cuticle
Also called the eponychium	Nail matrix
Tightly packed, dead, hard, keratinised epidermal cells that form a clean, solid covering over the digits	Nail plate

Question 15   Time yourself to unscramble these words.

Scrambled	Answer
NULALU	
ELICTUC	
TAXMIR	
LAHAPXN	
TASSNONEI	
COMYPHUNHIY	
LAIDST	
MIXORLAP	

The hair

Hair is made up of keratin, at the lower end is a bulb or root enclosed in a follicle that produces the hair, indented by a hair papilla, connective tissue and blood vessels. On the body only the palms of the hands, soles of the feet, nails, parts of the external genitalia, lips and nipples do not have hair.

Healing
The inflammatory response

Inflammation is an innate response to tissue damage. Increased blood flow explains redness and heat associated with inflammation. Capillaries within injured tissue dilate, becoming permeable; this is essential for an appropriate inflammatory response, providing an opportunity for some of the blood components (such as platelets) to be released into the damaged area.

Epithelialisation

Epithelialisation usually occurs in response to tissue damage, for example, after a wound has occurred.

Granulation

This is an essential physiological requirement for wound healing. Tissue granulation occurs in the proliferative phase of the process of wound healing, during which new, healthy tissue reforms and rebuilds the area of the wound.

Question 16 Figure 17.6 shows a summary of wound healing events. In the three phases identify:

- inflammation, and add comment
- granulation tissue formation, and add comment
- maturation, and add comment

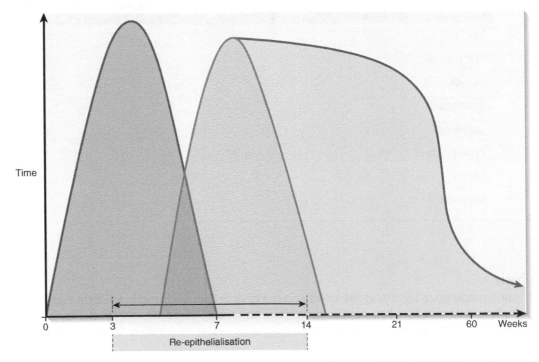

Figure 17.6 Summary of wound healing events. *Source*: Peate and Nair, 2015. Reproduced with permission of John Wiley & Sons.

Skin characteristics

Throughout the body the skin's characteristics vary; for instance, the head contains more hair follicles than anywhere else, while the soles of the feet have none. The thickness of the layers of the skin varies: the eyelids have the thinnest layer of epidermis and the palms of the hands and soles of the feet have the thickest. The dermis is at its thickest on the back. Skin type is another characteristic.

Question 17 Figure 17.7 considers six skin types. In the blank column (UV sensitivity and tendency to burn) make notes about how easily these types of skin may burn.

	Natural skin colour	UV sensitivity and tendency to burn
1	Very fair, pale white, often freckled	
2	Fair, white skin	
3	Light brown	
4	Moderate brown	
5	Dark brown	
6	Deeply pigmented, dark brown to black	

Figure 17.7 Skin types. *Source*: Peate and Nair, 2015. Reproduced with permission of John Wiley & Sons.

Snap shot

Capillary nail bed refill (also called the nail blanch test)

1. What is the purpose of the nail blanch test?
2. How is it performed?
3. What are the normal parameters?
4. What should you remove prior to performing the test?
5. Who should abnormalities be reported to?
6. Where should the outcome of the test be recorded?

Word search

G	L	Q	E	Z	T	O	X	M	E	P	I	D	E	R	M	I	S	E	N
K	U	G	K	N	V	A	C	F	T	M	U	B	E	S	K	E	W	W	A
F	N	Y	S	M	A	Q	S	U	O	E	C	A	B	E	S	N	J	S	T
Q	U	D	P	B	U	R	Q	A	P	M	Y	G	I	X	I	R	T	A	M
J	L	O	M	O	Y	I	B	D	J	B	C	L	N	Y	O	D	O	D	B
V	A	U	B	S	X	H	M	W	Z	A	B	R	P	J	F	J	L	U
T	C	E	B	L	M	H	I	C	E	X	R	A	G	R	L	S	A	R	U
N	M	N	E	S	V	X	P	Q	Y	M	T	K	R	U	B	N	L	E	M
R	Z	I	S	R	N	R	I	S	P	N	H	Y	U	W	G	I	V	F	G
I	B	R	O	M	D	S	G	K	E	N	O	A	T	E	Y	X	K	V	P
A	L	C	O	X	F	E	I	M	E	H	G	P	R	I	Q	F	P	M	E
H	J	O	G	A	G	L	U	L	Y	D	O	H	E	X	N	L	E	M	R
W	E	P	M	A	A	G	E	P	S	V	A	U	G	F	V	U	S	L	F
F	Q	A	C	W	E	K	O	K	M	N	E	N	R	J	V	Y	M	Z	U
K	J	N	C	T	R	D	I	Q	S	F	M	U	T	A	R	T	S	M	S
F	Y	A	N	E	E	N	R	H	M	A	G	P	E	I	C	J	T	C	I
I	Y	I	M	R	Y	U	I	W	S	O	A	C	V	W	F	L	E	U	O
B	I	L	M	S	E	T	Y	C	O	N	I	T	A	R	E	K	W	R	N
D	I	I	D	N	S	M	P	B	A	R	R	E	C	T	O	R	Y	V	I
L	S	E	T	Y	C	O	N	A	L	E	M	M	W	V	W	T	O	V	K

IMMUNITY	HAIR	MEMBRANE
PERFUSION	SKIN	LANGERHANS
APOCRINE	GOOSEBUMPS	LUNULA
EPIDERMIS	SEBUM	STRATUM
HYPODERMIS	MELANOCYTES	ARRECTOR
KERATINOCYTES	SEBACEOUS	MATRIX
INTEGUMENTARY	MERKEL	
NAIL	EPONYCHIUM	

Crossword

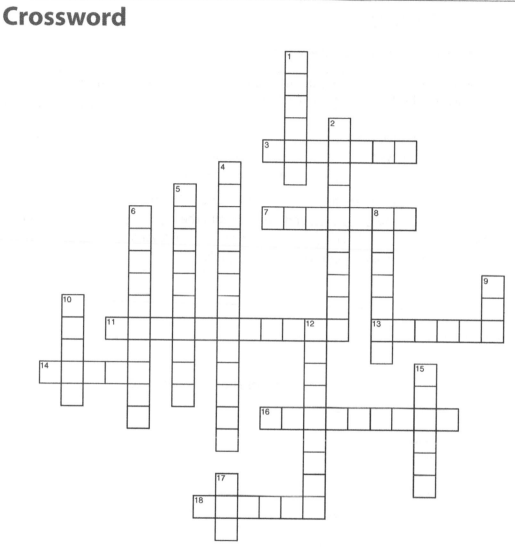

Across

3. The substance nails are made of
7. The phase of life when sebum glands are most active
11. Cells that produce the pigment melanin
13. Very fine, downy, non-pigmented type of hair
14. Secreted by the sebaceous glands
16. A chemical substance that serves as a stimulus to other individuals of the same species for one or more behavioural responses
18. The deepest part of the skin

Down

1. The shape of the apocrine glands
2. These cells are a part of the immune system
4. These cell types are organised in four layers
5. The accessory structures of the skin
6. The subcutaneous fascia
8. Pertains to touch
9. Number of distinct layers in the skin
10. Stratum
12. The thinnest aspect of the skin
15. The crescent shape at the base of the nail
17. The hormones that influence the manufacture of sebum

Fill in the blanks

Use the words in the box to complete the sentences:

adipose, chemical, connective, dermis, external, hypodermis, insulating, loss, organs, protecting, regions, subcutaneous, thermoregulation, under, vital, water

1. The skin carries out a number of _____ functions, including _____ the person against _____ physical, _____ and biological attack. It also prevents the _____ of excess _____ from the body and plays a central role in _____ .

2. The skin is one of the more versatile _____ of the body. The skin is composed of distinct _____ – the _____ and the epidermis. The _____ fascia (sometimes referred to as the _____) lies _____ the dermis. This layer of loose _____ and _____ tissue has an important _____ role.

350 Multiple choice questions

1. Which of the following is most likely to increase body temperature?

    (a) Dilation of the blood vessels in the skin
    (b) Shivering
    (c) Secretion of cerumen
    (d) Secretion of sebum

2. The stratum germinativum

    (a) Is an infectious skin disease
    (b) Gives rise to epidermal cells
    (c) Contains the blood vessels that nourish the hair
    (d) Is part of the hypodermis

3. The epidermis is nourished by

    (a) Inhaled air that diffuses into the pores
    (b) Blood vessels in the hair shafts
    (c) Blood vessels in the underlying dermis
    (d) Oxygen and glucose in the cerumen

4. Which of the following is true of the stratum corneum?

    (a) It always produces epidermal cells
    (b) It secretes keratin for making the skin supple
    (c) It is the dead layer sloughed off
    (d) It continuously secretes mucus

5. Which word best describes the function of the stratum germinativum?

    (a) Meiosis
    (b) Mitosis
    (c) Keratinisation
    (d) Thermogenesis

6. Secretion of the eccrine glands

    (a) Lubricates the hair shafts
    (b) Produces vernix caseosa protects the skin of the foetus
    (c) Lowers body temperature
    (d) Blocks the production of sebum

7. When does cyanosis occur?

    (a) The blood in the cutaneous blood vessels is unoxygenated
    (b) The reason is pyrexial
    (c) Cutaneous blood vessels dilate
    (d) All of the above

8. Which word relates to all the following: apocrine, sudoriferous, eccrine and sebaceous?

    (a) Sweat glands
    (b) Vellum
    (c) Mucus
    (d) Exocrine glands

9. Shivering thermogenesis

    (a) Increases body temperature
    (b) Is a decrease in body temperature
    (c) Is due to immobility
    (d) Is another word for rigor mortis

10. What are dermal papillae also known as?

    (a) Skin break down
    (b) Dermatitis
    (c) Friction ridges
    (d) None of the above

References

Nair, M. and Peate, I. (2009) *Fundamentals of Applied Pathophysiology: An Essential Guide for Nursing Students.* Oxford: John Wiley & Sons, Ltd.

Peate, I. and Nair, M. (2011) *Fundamentals of Anatomy and Physiology for Student Nurses.* Oxford: John Wiley & Sons, Ltd.

Peate, I. and Nair, M. (2015) *Anatomy and Physiology for Nurses at a Glance.* Oxford: John Wiley & Sons, Ltd.

Peate, I., Wild, K. and Nair, M. (eds) (2014) *Nursing Practice: Knowledge and Care.* Oxford: John Wiley & Sons, Ltd.

Tortora, G.J. and Derrickson, B.H. (2009) *Principles of Anatomy and Physiology*, 12th edn. Hoboken, NJ: John Wiley & Sons, Inc.

Answers

Chapter 1

1.

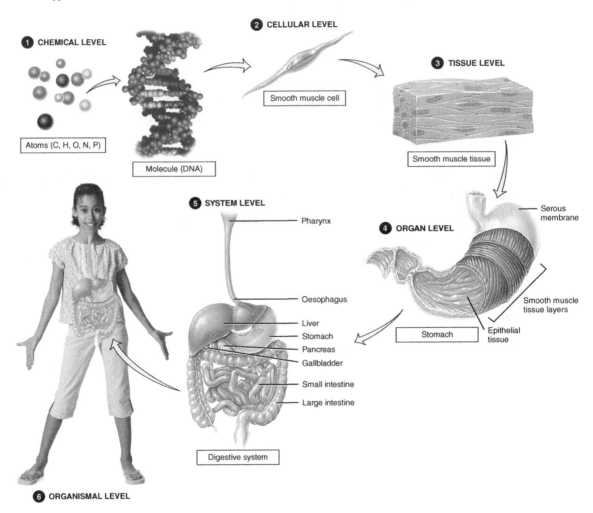

① CHEMICAL LEVEL

Atoms (C, H, O, N, P)

Molecule (DNA)

② CELLULAR LEVEL

Smooth muscle cell

③ TISSUE LEVEL

Smooth muscle tissue

④ ORGAN LEVEL

Stomach

Serous membrane

Smooth muscle tissue layers

Epithelial tissue

⑤ SYSTEM LEVEL

Pharynx

Oesophagus

Liver

Stomach

Pancreas

Gallbladder

Small intestine

Large intestine

Digestive system

⑥ ORGANISMAL LEVEL

Fundamentals of Anatomy and Physiology Workbook: A Study Guide for Nursing and Healthcare Students, First Edition. Ian Peate.
© 2017 John Wiley & Sons Ltd. Published 2017 by John Wiley & Sons Ltd.

2.

- The most abundant substance found in the body → Water
- Supplies the energy for the organism to fulfil all the essential characteristics compatible with life → Food
- Forms 20% of air, is used in the release of energy from the assimilated nutrients → Oxygen
- A form of energy that partially controls the rate at which metabolic reactions happen → Heat
- Two types of pressure that are required by an organism → Atmospheric and hydrostatic

3.

CHAOSTEMPRI → ATMOSPHERIC
SYPHIGOYLO → PHYSIOLOGY
SONGMAIR → ORGANISM
ATOMBLICE → METABOLIC

LAMIECHOBCANI → BIOMECHANICAL
REMYSCHIT → CHEMISTRY
AMTONYA → ANATOMY
UHNAM → HUMAN

4.

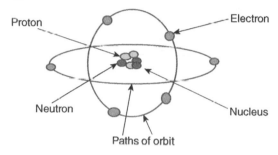

5.

- Always central → The nucleus
- The building blocks of life → Atoms
- Carry a positive electrical charge → Protons
- Carry a negative electrical charge → Electrons

6.

TORPON → PROTON
BORTI → ORBIT
CETRENLO → ELECTRON

VISITOPE → POSITIVE
VENEGIAT → NEGATIVE
THAP → PATH

LELSH → SHELL
DUBLINGI → BUILDING

7. Nitrogen has atomic number 7.

8.

The smallest particle of an element or compound → Molecule
The 'attractive' force that holds atoms together → Chemical bonds (ionic, covalent or polar/hydrogen)
Atoms with extra electrons or missing electrons → Ions

9.

BARCON → CARBON
RAGECH → CHARGE
BATSIYLIT → STABILITY

RATTYLENUI → NEUTRALITY
TROGENIN → NITROGEN
VACOLENT → COVALENT

CINIO → IONIC
DOGYRHEN → HYDROGEN

10.

Element	Chemical symbol	Metal	Non-metal
Iron	Fe	Yes	No
Hydrogen	H	No	Yes
Carbon	C	No	Yes
Nitrogen	N	No	Yes
Oxygen	O	No	Yes
Calcium	Ca	Yes	No
Potassium	K	Yes	No
Sodium	Na	Yes	No
Chlorine	Cl	No	Yes
Sulphur	S	No	Yes
Phosphoros	P	No	Yes

11.

1												13	14	15	16	17	18
1 H	2															1 H	2 He
3 Li	4 Be											5 B	6 C	7 N	8 O	9 F	10 Ne
11 Na	12 Mg	3	4	5	6	7	8	9	10	11	12	13 Al	14 Si	15 P	16 S	17 Cl	18 Ar
19 K	20 Ca	21 Sc	22 Ti	23 V	24 Cr	25 Mn	26 Fe	27 Co	28 Ni	29 Cu	30 Zn	31 Ga	32 Ge	33 As	34 Se	35 Br	36 Kr
37 Rb	38 Sr	39 Y	40 Zr	41 Nb	42 Mo	43 Tc	44 Ru	45 Rh	46 Pd	47 Ag	48 Cd	49 In	50 Sn	51 Sb	52 Te	53 I	54 Xe
55 Cs	56 Ba	71 Lu	72 Hf	73 Ta	74 W	75 Re	76 Os	77 Ir	78 Pt	79 Au	80 Hg	81 Tl	82 Pb	83 Bi	84 Po	85 At	86 Rn

☐ Metals   ☐ Metalloids   ☐ Non-metals

12.

- A pure substance made up of two or more elements chemically bonded together → A compound such as H_2O (water), NaCl (salt), CO_2 (carbon dioxide)
- They donate electrons (to other atoms to make molecules) → Metals
- They accept electrons (from donor atoms) → Non-metals
- They are neither metals nor non-metals – they are sometimes referred to as semi-metals → Metalloids
- $NaHCO_3$ → Sodium bicarbonate
- Potassium chloride → KCl

13.

MOPSITASU → POTASSIUM
DELTOILSAM → METALLOIDS
DUMPNOOCS → COMPOUNDS
LAMECHIC → CHEMICAL

TEEMLEN → ELEMENT
MYSOBL → SYMBOL
DROIPIEC → PERIODIC
RODNO → DONOR

14.

Type of electrolyte	Conduction of electrical current
Strong electrolytes	Conduct electrical current very well
Weak electrolytes	Conduct electrical current poorly
Non-electrolytes	Do not conduct electrical current

15.

Substance	pH
Milk	Acidic
Water	Neutral
Vinegar	Acidic
An orange	Acidic
Coconut water	Alkaline
Salt	Neutral
Ammonia	Alkaline
Tea	Acidic
Oven cleaner	Alkaline
Liquid used in car battery	Acidic
Blood	Neutral

355

16.

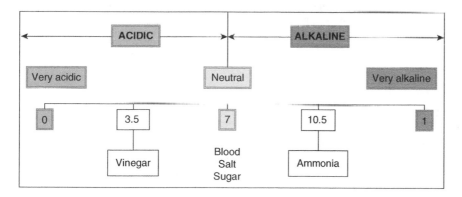

17.

- In a strong acid → nearly all the acid molecules form ions
- In a weak acid → only some of the acid molecules form ions
- The more OH⁻ ions (hydroxide ions) → the more alkaline an alkali will be
- The more OH⁻ ions → the higher the pH number
- The strength of an acid or alkali is shown using a scale of numbers called the pH scale → the numbers go from 0–14

18.

ECLULEMO → MOLECULE
SOSCIDIDATE → DISSOCIATED
NIMRALES → MINERALS
BLANCAE → BALANCE

AILLYTINKA → ALKALINITY
UNISTOOL → SOLUTION
DACICI → ACIDIC
TREAVICE → REACTIVE

19.

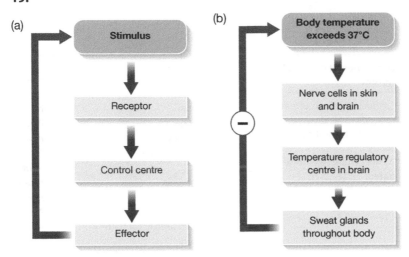

(a)

Stimulus

Receptor

Control centre

Effector

(b)

Body temperature
exceeds 37°C

Nerve cells in skin
and brain

Temperature regulatory
centre in brain

Sweat glands
throughout body

(−)

(c)

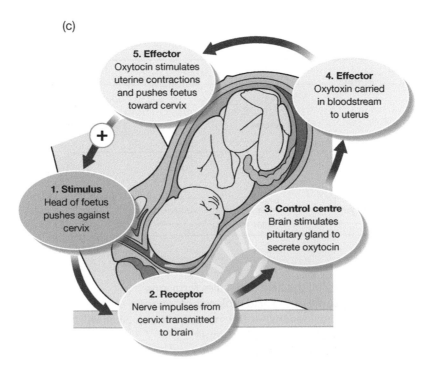

5. Effector
Oxytocin stimulates
uterine contractions
and pushes foetus
toward cervix

4. Effector
Oxytoxin carried
in bloodstream
to uterus

(+)

1. Stimulus
Head of foetus
pushes against
cervix

3. Control centre
Brain stimulates
pituitary gland to
secrete oxytocin

2. Receptor
Nerve impulses from
cervix transmitted
to brain

20.

- Certain nerve endings in the skin sense temperature change → they detect changes such as a sudden rise or drop in body temperature
- The control centre is → the brain (the hypothalamus in body temperature regulation)
- An effector is → a body system such as the skin, blood vessels or the blood that receives the information from the control centre, producing a response to the condition
- Homeostasis is → a state of balance within the body
- A stimulus is → something that can elicit or evoke a response in a cell, a tissue, or an organism. A stimulus can be internal or external
- A response is → a reaction to a specific stimulus

21.

LAXETERN → EXTERNAL

MEQUILIRIBU → EQUILIBRIUM

MASSIHOOTES → HOMEOSTASIS

TROFFECES → EFFECTORS

TROVEMENNIN → ENVIRONMENT

KCABDEEF → FEEDBACK

LOONTRC → CONTROL

LIMTUUSS → STIMULUS

22.

Quantity	Name	Symbol
Length	metre	m
Mass	kilogram	kg
Time	second	s
Current	ampere	A
Temperate	Kelvin	K
Amount of substance	mole	mol
Luminous intensity	candela	cd

Prefix	Symbol	Meaning	Scientific notation
tera	T	one million million	10^{12}
giga	G	one thousand million	10^{9}
mega	M	one million	10^{6}
kilo	k	one thousand	10^{3}
hecto	h	one hundred	10^{2}
deca	da	ten	10^{1}
deci	d	one tenth	10^{-1}
centi	c	one hundredth	10^{-2}
milli	m	one thousandth	10^{-3}

1 kilogram = 1000 grams

1 gram = 1000 milligrams

1 milligram = 10^{-3} grams

1 microgram = 10^{-6} grams

1 litre = 1000 millilitres

100 millilitre = 1 decilitre

1 millilitre = 1000 microlitres

Snap shot

Body temperature represents heat production and heat loss. If heat generated equals heat lost, the core body temperature will be stable and there will be a state of homeostasis.

1. The oral cavity. This site is considered reliable when the thermometer is placed posteriorly into the sublingual pocket. Electronic or disposable chemical thermometers may be used. Factors impacting on accuracy include recent ingestion of food or fluid, having a respiratory rate above 18 breaths per minute and smoking.

   Tympanic measurement. The tympanic thermometer senses reflected infrared emissions from the tympanic membrane via a probe placed in the external auditory canal. This method is minimally invasive and easy to perform. User error and poor technique can result in incorrect readings. Cerumen (ear wax) can impact negatively on the accuracy of readings.

   Axillary measurement. Temperature is measured at the axilla; the thermometer is placed centrally with the arm adducted close to the chest wall. This site should not be used to assess core body temperature, as there are no significant blood vessels in this area.

   Rectal temperature measurement. This is one of the most accurate methods for measuring the core temperature. It is time consuming and might, for some patients, be considered unfavourable. The presence of faecal matter prevents the thermometer from touching the wall of the bowel and could result in an inaccurate reading.

   Temporal artery measurement. The temporal artery thermometer is held over the forehead sensing infrared emissions radiating from the skin. This method has reliability and validity issues, it may underestimate body temperature.

2. Clinical indications for measuring body temperature include:
   - to ascertain a baseline temperature providing comparisons to be made with future recordings
   - to permit close observation in addressing hypothermia/hyperthermia
   - to observe and monitor patients for changes in their condition which could indicate infection
   - to monitor the outcomes of treatment
   - prior to and during a blood transfusion to monitor for signs of an undesired reaction.

3. Intrinsic factors include:
   - ovulation – an increase in body temperature
   - circadian rhythm – body temperature increases in the evening and in the early hours of morning this decreases
   - age
   - young and older people have inability to maintain equilibrium
   - exercise, results in an increase in body temperature
   - thyroid hormones increase metabolic rate and as such cause an increase in body temperature.

4. Core body temperature below 35 °C.

5. A rise in body temperature.

6. A core temperature above 40 °C and body temperature is out of control.

Word search

```
O  I  S  N  O  R  T  U  E  N  S  J  D  D  O  J  L  E  T  Z
J  E  J  H  W  S  A  L  E  L  E  C  T  R  O  N  F  L  M  R
M  K  Y  Y  L  F  V  W  R  R  E  L  F  S  L  O  I  E  C  W
S  F  R  A  F  J  M  B  Z  D  Q  S  S  G  C  N  S  M  Z  V
S  M  T  O  E  D  D  E  C  T  V  T  R  U  E  V  P  E  T  S
A  E  E  L  J  M  C  I  T  A  T  S  O  R  D  Y  H  N  H  P
M  T  G  F  G  W  V  A  X  A  A  C  I  D  H  J  O  T  S  U
C  A  D  C  B  U  O  E  Y  B  B  D  Q  S  G  E  M  C  N  F
K  L  S  A  I  E  F  K  C  Y  C  O  T  Q  X  L  E  W  O  W
E  L  E  C  T  R  I  C  I  T  Y  E  L  A  H  E  O  P  T  S
N  O  V  T  E  M  Q  I  C  N  U  R  U  I  T  C  S  K  O  U
I  I  E  X  A  Q  O  O  N  T  Y  L  C  I  C  T  T  C  R  M
L  D  H  O  M  E  O  S  T  A  S  I  S  Y  U  R  A  A  P  S
A  S  O  U  O  R  H  C  P  I  G  B  J  E  M  O  S  R  Y  I
K  P  M  O  T  A  V  J  X  H  M  H  W  N  O  L  I  B  L  N
L  T  Q  M  L  G  R  M  F  M  E  I  A  L  S  Y  S  O  S  A
A  Y  K  Y  K  B  Z  T  O  M  S  R  T  L  W  T  Y  N  G  G
Z  P  I  K  N  E  O  C  O  W  Z  I  I  M  Z  E  Y  I  O  R
B  S  G  M  E  F  X  Y  D  N  M  X  Y  C  C  S  U  I  E  O
F  B  C  O  T  B  B  I  R  E  T  A  W  Q  F  E  I  M  G  L
```

Crossword

Across
- 2. VALENCE
- 5. ALKALI
- 6. CATIONS
- 8. PHYSIOLOGY
- 9. HYDROGEN
- 13. ELECTRON
- 14. ATOM
- 16. OXYGEN
- 18. METALLOIDS

Down
- 1. ACID
- 3. NITROGEN
- 4. BASE
- 7. HOMEOSTASIS
- 10. PROTON
- 11. WATER
- 12. JOULE
- 15. ANIONS
- 17. CARBON

Fill in the blanks

1. Anatomy is the study of <u>structure</u> and physiology is the study of <u>function</u>. However, <u>structure</u> is always related to function because the structure determines the <u>function</u>, which in turn determines how the body/organ is <u>structured</u> – the two are <u>interdependent</u>.

2. The <u>body</u> is a very <u>complex</u> organism which consists of many components, starting with the smallest of them – the <u>atom</u> – and concluding with the <u>organism</u> itself.

3. Water is the most <u>abundant</u> substance in the <u>body</u>. Food supplies the <u>energy</u> for the <u>organism</u>. It also supplies the <u>raw</u> materials for <u>growth</u>. <u>Oxygen</u> forms 20% of <u>air</u> and is used in the release of <u>energy</u> from the assimilated nutrients. Heat is a form of <u>energy</u> that partly controls the <u>rate</u> at which <u>metabolic</u> reactions occur. There are two types of pressure that are required by an <u>organism</u>: <u>atmospheric</u> pressure, which is important in the process of <u>breathing</u>, and <u>hydrostatic</u> pressure, which keeps the <u>blood</u> flowing through the body.

4. The smallest building block of the body is the <u>atom</u>. An atom consists of <u>electrons</u>, <u>neutrons</u> and <u>protons</u>. Carbon is a very important <u>atom</u> for life forms, as we are all <u>carbon-based</u> entities. A <u>molecule</u> is the smallest particle of an <u>element</u> or compound which exists <u>independently</u>. It contains <u>atoms</u> that have bonded together. The formation of chemical bonds also results in the release of <u>energy</u> previously contained in the <u>atoms</u>.

5. An ion is an atom or a <u>molecule</u> in which the total number of <u>electrons</u> is not <u>equal</u> to the total number of <u>protons</u> – hence the atom or molecule has a net <u>positive</u> or negative electrical <u>charge</u>.

6. Electrolytes are substances that move to <u>oppositely</u> charged electrodes in <u>fluids</u>. If <u>molecules</u> that are bonded together <u>ionically</u> are dissolved in water within the body <u>cells</u>, they undergo a process where the <u>ions</u> separate; they become <u>dissociated</u>. These ions are now known as <u>electrolytes</u>.

7. A chemical <u>element</u> is a <u>pure</u> chemical substance which cannot be <u>broken</u> down into anything simpler by <u>chemical</u> means. Metals <u>conduct</u> heat and electricity. Non-metals are <u>poor</u> conductors of heat and electricity. Metalloids are neither <u>metals</u> nor non-metals – they are sometimes referred to as <u>semi-metals</u>.

8. An <u>acid</u> is any substance which donates <u>hydrogen</u> ions (H^+) into a solution. An <u>alkali</u> (also known as a <u>soluble</u> base) is any substance which donates <u>hydroxyl</u> <u>ions (OH⁻)</u> into a solution or accepts $H^±$ ions from a solution. Solutions with a <u>pH</u> lower than 7 are <u>acids</u>, and those with a <u>pH</u> greater than <u>7</u> are <u>bases/alkaline</u>. The further away from a pH of 7 a solution becomes the more <u>acidic</u> or alkaline it is.

9. Homeostasis is the body's attempt to maintain a <u>stable</u> internal <u>environment</u> by achieving <u>balance</u>. The body is normally able to achieve a relatively stable internal <u>environment</u> even though the <u>external</u> environment is constantly <u>changing</u>.

Multiple choice answers

1. (c), 2. (a), 3. (d), 4. (d), 5. (b), 6. (c), 7. (c), 8. (d), 9. (a), 10. (a)

Chapter 2

1.

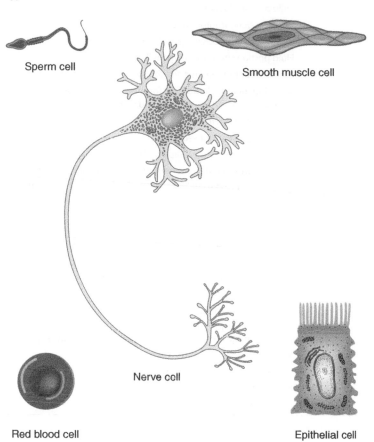

Sperm cell

Smooth muscle cell

Nerve cell

Red blood cell

Epithelial cell

2.

Components	Functions
Centrioles	Cellular reproduction
Chromatin	Contains genetic information
Cilia	Move fluid or particles over the surface of the cell
Cytoplasm	Fluid portion supporting organelles
Cytoskeleton	Provides support and is a site for specific enzymes
Endoplasmic reticulum (rough and smooth)	Many functions including site for protein transportation, modification of drugs and synthesis of lipids and steroids
Glycogen granules	Stores for glycogen
Golgi complex	Packages proteins for secretion
Intermediate filament	Helps to determine the shape of the cell
Lysosomes	Break down and digest harmful substances. In normal cells, some of the synthesised proteins may be faulty – lysosymes are responsible for their removal
Microfilaments	Provides structural support and cell movement
Microtubules	Provide conducting channels through which various substances can move through the cytoplasm. Provide shape and support for cells
Microvilli	Increase cell surface; site for secretion, absorption and cellular adhesion
Mitochondria	Energy producing sites of the cell. Mitochondria are self-replicating
Nucleolus	Site for the formation of ribosomes
Nucleus	Contains genetic information
Peroxisomes	Carry out metabolic reactions. Site for the destruction of hydrogen peroxide. Protect the cell from harmful substances, for example, alcohol and formaldehyde
Plasma membrane	Regulates movement of substances in and out of the cell
Ribosomes	Sites for protein synthesis
Secretory vesicles	Secrete hormones and neurotransmitters

3.
- Humans are → multicellular
- Some organisms such as bacteria are → unicellular
- Fluid and electrolytes are constantly moved between → the intracellular and extracellular compartments
- The basic structural, functional and biological unit of all known living organisms → is the cell
- For cells to survive → there are various fundamental chemical activities occurring within the cell, for example, cellular growth, metabolism and reproduction
- One of the four basic aspects associated with the cell is → the cell membrane

4.

MAGICMOSRONIR → MICROORGANISM
CEARILUNLLU → UNICELLULAR
BRACEITA → BACTERIA
BREENMAM → MEMBRANE

YOKCROPARTI → PROKARYOTIC
BOTEMMLISA → METABOLISM
TEXUALLRACELR → EXTRACELLULAR
OBLIOGICAL → BIOLOGICAL

5.

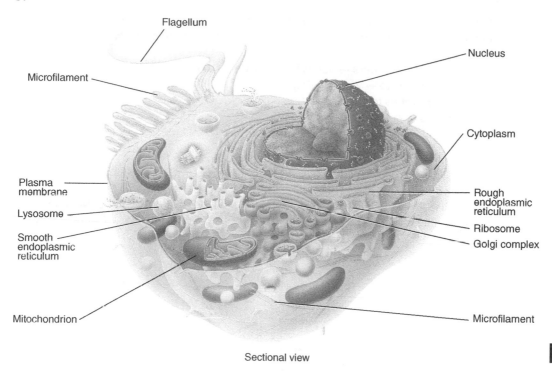

Flagellum

Microfilament

Nucleus

Cytoplasm

Plasma membrane

Rough endoplasmic reticulum

Lysosome

Smooth endoplasmic reticulum

Ribosome

Golgi complex

Mitochondrion

Microfilament

Sectional view

6.

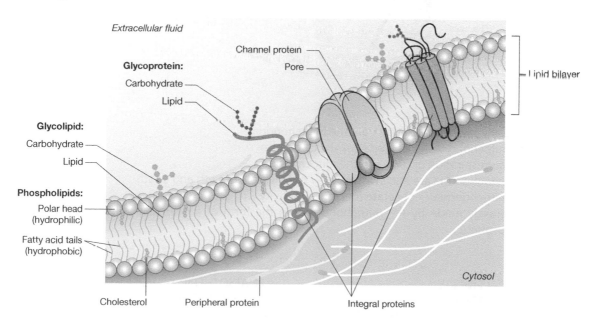

Extracellular fluid

Channel protein

Pore

Glycoprotein:

Carbohydrate

Lipid

Lipid bilayer

Glycolipid:

Carbohydrate

Lipid

Phospholipids:

Polar head (hydrophilic)

Fatty acid tails (hydrophobic)

Cytosol

Cholesterol

Peripheral protein

Integral proteins

7.

- Cell membrane → separates and protects a cell from its surrounding environment
- Cell membranes are made up mostly from → a double layer of proteins and lipids (fat-like molecules)
- Cell membrane thickness → varies from 7.5 nm to 10 nm
- Hydrophilic refers to → water loving
- Hydrophobic refers to → water hating
- The bilayer is → self-sealing

8.

CYPRHOHILID → HYDROPHILIC
LAYBIER → BILAYER
POPPIDHOHSLIS → PHOSPHOLIPIDS
POCYGLOTREINS → GLYCOPROTEINS

SECLUMOLE → MOLECULES
PIDIL → LIPID
BLEEPMEMIRA → IMPERMEABLE
DRATYOBHECARS → CARBOHYDRATES

9.

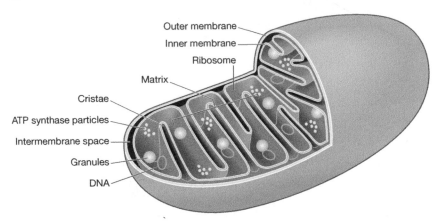

10.

- The cell's power producers → are the mitochondria
- The mitochondria are located in → the cytoplasm
- Cellular respiration occurs → in the mitochondrion
- The mitochondria are also involved in → cell division, growth and death
- The mitochondria → generate fuel for cell activity
- The energy made by the mitochondria is in the form of a chemical called → adenosine triphosphate

11.

RENGEY → ENERGY
ROWEP → POWER
CHOMDRIAINOT → MITOCHONDRIA
DENISEAON → ADENOSINE

PHATSOTHERIP → TRIPHOSPHATE
CIHOOTMINDRON → MITOCHONDRION
RATIONSPIRE → RESPIRATION
SCHOOLLETER → CHOLESTEROL

12.

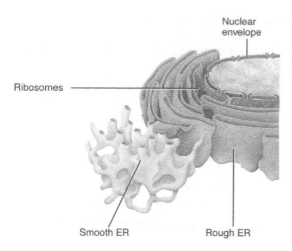

13.

- The endoplasmic reticulum → is an organelle of the cell
- The endoplasmic reticulum → works closely with the Golgi apparatus
- Cells with large amount of endoplasmic reticulum → are found in the pancreas and liver
- Rough endoplasmic reticulum → has ribosomes attached to its surface
- Smooth endoplasmic reticulum → is a smooth network without any ribosomes
- The smooth endoplasmic reticulum is found → in abundance in mammalian liver and gonad cells

14.

RANGELELO → ORGANELLE
TRICULUME → RETICULUM
COFIXTATIONIDE → DETOXIFICATION
CLASPENDOMI → ENDOPLASMIC

BROOMEISS → RIBOSOMES
GROUH → ROUGH
DANGO → GONAD
GIGOL → GOLGI

15.

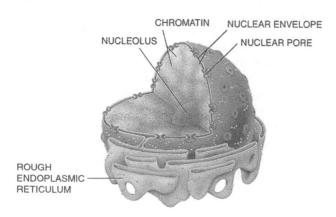

16.

- The genetic information of cell is packaged in the form of → chromatin
- The nucleus is a characteristic feature of → most eukaryotic cells
- One of the key functions of the cell nucleus → is deoxyribonucleic acid (DNA) replication
- Within the cell nucleus is the → nucleolus
- There is no membrane surrounding the nucleolus → it sits in the nucleus
- The nucleolus makes → ribosomal subunits from proteins and ribosomal RNA (rRNA)

17.

GEENCIT → GENETIC
SLUCNUE → NUCLEUS
MOMOCHORES → CHROMOSOME
TAPECLIRION → REPLICATION

LYCEC → CYCLE
CLOUNLUSE → NUCLEOLUS
TINPORES → PROTEINS
ROACHMTIN → CHROMATIN

18.

- Cytoplasm is some times referred to as → cytosol
- The cytoplasm is composed of over → 80% water
- The cell's organelles are suspended and held together by a → fatty membrane
- The cell membrane anchors to → the cytoskeleton
- Membrane proteins are categorised as → integral or peripheral proteins
- Some protein molecules in the cell membrane → carry out metabolic reactions near the inner surface of the cell membrane

19.

SYCTOOL → CYTOSOL
PYSCOLMATIC → CYTOPLASMIC
ELACTRLINULAR → INTRACELLULAR
TOOTSYKELCEN → CYTOSKELETON

TATYF → FATTY
PHEEPRALIR → PERIPHERAL
GRAINLET → INTEGRAL
SCIVSOU → VISCOUS

Snap shot
Intravenous electrolyte administration

Intravenous solutions are used for a variety of reasons as sources of electrolyte replacement, calories and water for hydration. The dosage is prescribed by a doctor and is related to age, weight, the patient's clinical condition and laboratory results. Frequent assessment of laboratory blood analysis along with clinical assessment is essential to monitor changes in blood glucose and electrolyte concentrations, and fluid and electrolyte balance, during prolonged intravenous therapy. Some intravenous additives may be incompatible with each other, and the nurse should always consult with the pharmacist to determine the compatibility of additives.

Fluid and electrolyte preparations are the most commonly prescribed medications in hospitals and appropriate fluid therapy depends on an understanding of the underlying physiology and pathophysiology and a consideration of external and internal fluid balance.

Word search

```
F  O  J  M  W  V  P  R  O  K  A  R  Y  O  T  I  C  S  Z  X
B  G  I  A  E  U  H  B  X  S  J  W  N  X  V  X  E  C  H  O
G  N  M  E  D  T  I  S  U  W  V  H  C  N  H  M  K  U  M  J
A  S  V  O  L  L  A  E  V  E  A  N  Y  P  O  R  L  S  T  Q
Q  I  C  K  A  B  L  B  M  F  Y  O  I  S  Z  O  I  Z  K  L
X  T  R  Y  P  C  A  U  O  H  T  O  O  T  R  N  J  P  T  N
E  L  E  E  U  P  L  E  M  L  Y  B  R  E  A  E  B  V  P  D
J  R  O  N  T  U  V  G  M  M  I  D  T  G  Y  M  F  C  Y  N
T  S  I  C  C  Q  A  M  R  X  S  R  Q  A  X  O  G  U  M
M  V  N  I  Z  Y  A  L  G  G  E  O  M  O  X  N  Y  R  C  Y
N  F  T  R  S  N  D  B  V  L  O  P  R  F  P  G  I  J  H  F
P  E  H  F  H  K  R  S  O  R  B  H  M  G  R  H  E  S  Z  C
R  A  I  R  D  N  O  H  C  O  T  I  M  I  A  K  I  D  M  X
N  R  Y  T  E  Q  C  I  F  K  R  M  T  G  Z  N  I  L  W  E
L  D  P  O  H  B  M  L  Z  M  N  Z  X  A  N  T  E  W  I  J
E  N  N  T  U  N  I  C  E  L  L  U  L  A  R  T  T  L  Z  C
B  A  U  S  U  L  O  E  L  C  U  N  V  W  L  T  C  S  L  W
Z  C  I  T  O  Y  R  A  K  U  E  S  V  G  H  P  D  E  J  E
P  U  S  N  I  E  T  O  R  P  O  C  Y  L  G  K  B  N  V  E
Z  H  Y  D  R  O  P  H  O  B  I  C  I  R  Q  L  K  N  K  N
```

Crossword

Across

3. ROUGH
7. PROKARYOTIC
10. MITOCHONDRIA
14. MULTICELLULAR
16. CYTOPLASM
17. NUCLEOLUS
18. HYDROPHOBIC

Down

1. WATER
2. MICROFILAMENTS
4. GOLGI
5. CYTOSKELETON
6. EUKARYOTIC
8. CHROMATIN
9. UNICELLULAR
11. HYDROPHILIC
12. SMOOTH
13. NUCLEUS
15. CYTOSOL
16. CELLS

Fill in the blanks

1. The basic structural, <u>functional</u> and <u>biological</u> units of all known <u>living</u> organisms are cells. Humans are <u>multicellular</u>, this is in comparison to some organisms such as <u>bacteria</u> (unicellular). Cells take in <u>nutrients</u>, convert these nutrients into <u>energy</u>, carry out specialised functions and <u>reproduce</u> as necessary.

2. Water, <u>electrolytes</u> and <u>nutrients</u> move in and <u>out</u> of a cell through the use of a <u>transport</u> system. Fluid and <u>electrolytes</u> are constantly moved between the <u>intracellular</u> and extracellular compartments, ensuring that the <u>cells</u> have a <u>constant</u> supply of <u>electrolytes</u>, for example, sodium, chloride, <u>potassium</u>, magnesium, phosphates, <u>bicarbonate</u> and calcium, required for cellular <u>function</u>.

3. The cell <u>membrane</u> separates and <u>protects</u> a cell from its surrounding environment and is primarily made up of a <u>double</u> layer of <u>proteins</u> and <u>lipids</u>. Within this membrane are embedded a variety of other <u>molecules</u> acting as channels and pumps, transporting different molecules <u>into</u> and <u>out</u> of the cell. The cell membrane can vary in <u>thickness</u>.

4. The cell's <u>power</u> producers are the <u>mitochondria</u>, which convert <u>energy</u> into a form usable by the cell. They also produce <u>cholesterol</u>. The mitochondria are located in the <u>cytoplasm</u>; they generate the <u>fuel</u> needed for the cell's various <u>activities</u>. Mitochondria are also concerned with other cell processes, for example cell <u>division</u> and <u>growth</u>, and also cell <u>death</u>.

5. The <u>endoplasmic</u> reticulum is an <u>organelle</u> of cells. The endoplasmic <u>reticulum</u> is classified into <u>two</u> types, <u>rough</u> endoplasmic reticulum and <u>smooth</u> endoplasmic reticulum. Rough endoplasmic reticulum is studded with <u>ribosomes</u> on the cytosolic <u>face</u>. Rough endoplasmic reticulum is mainly found in <u>hepatocytes</u> where protein <u>synthesis</u> occurs <u>actively</u>. Smooth endoplasmic reticulum is a smooth network <u>without</u> any ribosomes. The smooth endoplasmic reticulum is associated with <u>lipid</u> and <u>carbohydrate</u> metabolism and <u>detoxification</u>.

6. The cell <u>nucleus</u> is a double <u>membrane-bound</u> <u>organelle</u> and contains the genetic <u>information</u> of the cell packaged in the form of <u>chromatin</u>. The nucleus is a characteristic feature of most <u>eukaryotic</u> cells. The nucleus is said to be one of the most <u>important</u> structures of eukaryotic cells. It serves the function of <u>information</u> <u>storage</u>, <u>retrieval</u> and <u>duplication</u> of genetic information.

7. Cytoplasm is the substance that fills the <u>cell</u>. It is composed of <u>80%</u> water and is usually <u>clear</u> in colour. Cytoplasm is the substance of life in which all of the cell's <u>organelles</u> are <u>suspended</u> and held together by a <u>fatty</u> membrane. It is found inside the cell <u>membrane</u>, surrounding the <u>nuclear</u> envelope and the <u>cytoplasmic</u> organelles.

Multiple choice answers

1. (c), 2. (d), 3. (a), 4. (c), 5. (a), 6. (c), 7. (b), 8. (d), 9. (c), 10. (a)

Chapter 3

1.

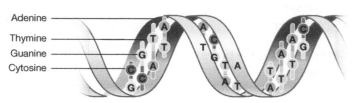

Adenine
Thymine
Guanine
Cytosine

2.

A	G	C	A	G	G	A	T	T
↓	↓	↓	↓	↓	↓	↓	↓	↓
T	C	G	T	C	C	T	A	A

3.

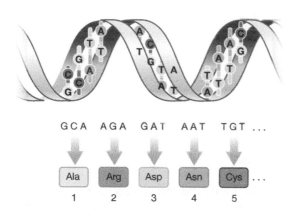

GCA   AGA   GAT   AAT   TGT . . .

↓   ↓   ↓   ↓   ↓

| Ala | Arg | Asp | Asn | Cys | . . . |

1   2   3   4   5

4.

- Genes are → sections of deoxyribonucleic acid (DNA)
- The sections of DNA → are carried within our chromosomes
- Guanine always pairs with → cytosine
- Genes resemble regions within DNA → a molecule that is made up of a chain of four different types of nucleotides
- The four nucleotides are also known → as the bases
- Adenine always pairs with → thymine

5.

SEENITGC → GENETICS
RUEOXIDYBONCLICE → DEOXYRIBONUCLEIC
MULEECOL → MOLECULE
DENISECLOUT → NUCLEOTIDES

ELIXH → HELIX
SYNITECO → CYTOSINE
NINAGUE → GUANINE
HYMINTE → THYMINE

6.

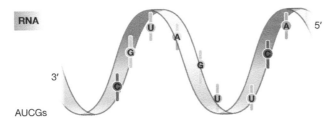

7.

- RNA → differs from DNA – it is single-stranded
- The base uracil is used instead of → thymine
- Cells have → three different RNAs
- Messenger RNA (mRNA) → determines the amino acid composition of proteins
- Ribosomal RNA (rRNA) → combines with proteins imported from the cytoplasm to make the ribosome
- Transfer RNA (tRNA) → is responsible for matching the code of the mRNA with amino acids

8.

DANSTR → STRAND
CLIECNUBIRO → RIBONUCLEIC
LAMBSOOIR → RIBOSOMAL
CLUIAR → URACIL

GESSERMEN → MESSENGER
FRANTRES → TRANSFER
DECO → CODE
NOAIM → AMINO

9.

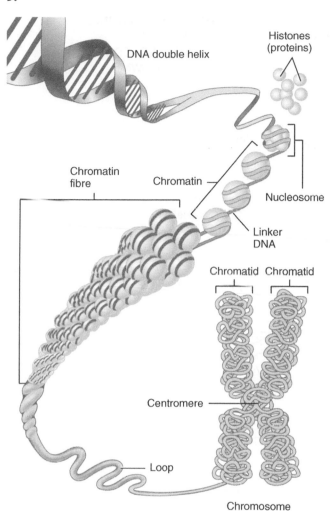

DNA double helix

Histones
(proteins)

Chromatin
fibre

Chromatin

Nucleosome

Linker
DNA

Chromatid Chromatid

Centromere

Loop

Chromosome

10.

- Chromosomes are thread-like structures of DNA → found inside the nucleus of a cell
- Each chromosome is made of → protein and a single molecule of DNA
- For organisms to grow and function properly → cells have to constantly divide to produce new cells, replacing old, worn-out cells
- Changes in the number or structure of chromosomes in new cells → can lead to serious problems
- Those with Down syndrome have → three copies of chromosome 21
- The constricted region of linear chromosomes is known → as the centromere

11.

CHOOSERMOM → CHROMOSOME
SCROTEMREEN → CENTROMERES
PLACTEIER → REPLICATE
THROMCAID → CHROMATID

THISONES → HISTONES
XILEH → HELIX
DIEPCO → COPIED
OWND → DOWN

12.

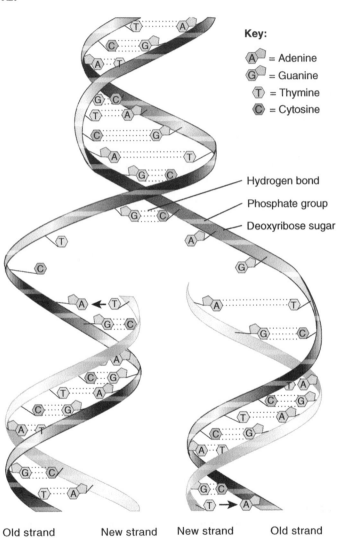

Key:

Ⓐ = Adenine
Ⓖ = Guanine
Ⓣ = Thymine
Ⓒ = Cytosine

Hydrogen bond
Phosphate group
Deoxyribose sugar

Old strand   New strand   New strand   Old strand

13.

- In order to synthesise proteins → the genetic information encoded in the DNA has to be translated
- The first thing that needs to happen during protein production is → that the DNA has to separate in order to allow for all of the genetic information in a region of DNA to be copied on to RNA
- When the information has been transcribed → the RNA attaches to a ribosome where the information contained in the RNA is translated into a corresponding sequence of amino acids, forming a new protein molecule
- In transcription → the genetic information contained in the DNA is transcribed into the RNA
- the DNA serves as a template for copying the information → into a complementary sequence of codons
- Ribosomes consist of → two parts, a large subunit and a small subunit

14.

EGENCIT → GENETIC

THISSENYS → SYNTHESIS

PRATTSCRINION → TRANSCRIPTION

NATIONSRLAT → TRANSLATION

MEALPETT → TEMPLATE

BUUSTIN → SUBUNIT

LIARBOOMS → RIBOSOMAL

DEEDCON → ENCODED

15. Stages of mitosis:

1. Prophase
2. Metaphase
3. Anaphase
4. Telophase

16. Stages of meiosis:

1. Meiosis I
2. Meiosis II

17. Stages of meiosis I:

1. Prophase I
2. Metaphase I
3. Anaphase I
4. Telophase I

18. Stages of meiosis II:

1. Prophase II
2. Metaphase II
3. Anaphase II
4. Telophase II

19.

- The process of gene transference can be divided into → two stages
- Mitosis describes → the process by which the nucleus of a cell divides to create two new nuclei, each containing an identical copy of DNA
- Meiosis is → the process by which certain sex cells are created
- The spermatozoa of the male and the ova of the female go through the process of → meiosis
- During the interphase that precedes meiosis I → the chromosome of the diploid starts to replicate
- In meiosis II, both of the cells produced in meiosis I → further divide again

20.

LIPIDOD → DIPLOID
LICEUN → NUCLEI
HAAPENAS → ANAPHASE
STEALHOPE → TELOPHASE

STOMACHRID → CHROMATIDS
FENCESRENTAR → TRANSFERENCE
CLIPARTIONE → REPLICATION
SHAPERENTI → INTERPHASE

Snap shot

Cystic fibrosis causes thick and sticky secretions in the lungs and the digestive system, leading to infection, inflammation, lung damage, respiratory failure, malabsorption, malnutrition and poor growth, as well as liver problems, diabetes and potential bowel obstruction.

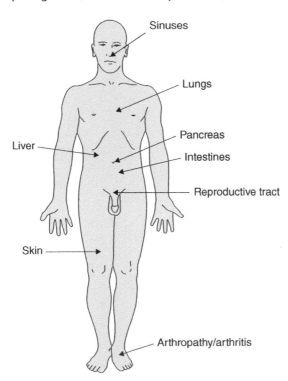

Sinuses

Lungs

Liver

Pancreas

Intestines

Reproductive tract

Skin

Arthropathy/arthritis

Word search

G	Q	T	H	Y	M	I	N	E	J	E	B	X	R	R	J	E	H	B	J
V	N	J	K	F	I	N	T	E	R	P	H	A	S	E	C	V	P	A	V
R	B	P	F	C	E	N	T	R	O	M	E	E	I	J	Z	K	M	T	D
O	E	B	N	L	T	M	I	T	O	S	I	S	A	M	L	T	N	I	E
U	N	F	N	O	I	T	P	I	R	C	S	N	A	R	T	P	R	N	O
M	I	S	N	L	X	I	L	E	H	H	E	T	A	Z	V	Y	D	U	X
R	S	C	X	C	S	X	D	E	O	X	Y	R	I	B	O	S	E	B	Y
I	O	S	C	I	N	E	B	F	W	B	I	K	M	K	N	S	G	U	R
Z	T	I	T	E	L	V	M	P	C	S	E	N	U	C	H	N	X	S	I
O	Y	S	S	L	S	E	N	O	T	S	I	H	H	L	B	U	S	N	B
E	C	O	C	C	A	B	N	L	S	V	J	C	G	O	J	C	D	K	O
M	P	I	I	U	H	M	B	I	E	O	H	U	P	N	N	L	A	I	N
O	R	E	T	N	X	T	I	O	N	R	M	I	R	E	T	E	S	D	U
S	O	M	E	O	C	G	T	N	O	A	O	O	H	A	I	O	V	T	C
O	T	O	N	B	D	A	Y	M	O	S	U	Q	R	U	C	T	V	P	L
E	E	A	E	I	N	R	A	Q	V	E	F	G	U	H	Y	I	X	Y	E
L	I	P	G	R	Y	T	E	N	I	N	E	D	A	P	C	D	L	E	I
C	N	K	R	G	I	B	A	G	Y	E	K	P	P	D	L	E	B	Y	C
U	Q	Y	U	D	M	P	D	G	N	G	K	V	X	Q	V	S	J	H	D
N	W	R	S	K	A	U	W	F	G	L	A	T	H	W	S	G	A	R	L

Crossword

Across
2. BASES
6. CHROMOSOMES
7. TERMINATOR
9. THREE
10. PENTOSE
12. FOUR
13. HYDROGEN
15. INHERITED
16. INTERPHASE
18. TELOPHASE
19. MEIOSIS
20. THYMINE

Down
1. MITOSIS
3. TRANSCRIPTION
4. CENTROMERE
5. CYTOSINE
8. CELL
11. ONE
14. GENES
17. HISTONES

Fill in the blanks

1. Genetics is the branch of science dealing with how we <u>inherit</u> physical and <u>behavioural characteristics</u> (traits); these also include <u>medical</u> conditions, and many health problems are linked to <u>genes</u>. Each cell in the human body contains approximately 25 000 to 35 000 <u>genes</u>.

2. Genes are sections of <u>deoxyribonucleic</u> acid (DNA) that are carried within the <u>chromosomes</u>. Genes contain particular sets of instructions that are related functions including <u>growth</u>, development, <u>reproduction</u>, functioning and <u>ageing</u>. Without <u>genes</u> life would be <u>unsustainable;</u> our genes make us what we are. All of our <u>genes</u> are inherited from our parents, who in turn <u>inherited</u> theirs from their <u>parents</u>.

3. DNA makes all the basic units of <u>hereditary</u> material, these control cellular structure and direct <u>cellular</u> activities. The ability of the <u>DNA</u> to <u>replicate</u> itself provides the basis of hereditary <u>transmission</u>.

4. The four <u>nucleotides</u> (the bases) are very particular as to which other <u>base</u> they <u>pair</u> with. Adenine always pairs with <u>thymine</u> and guanine always pairs with <u>cytosine</u>.

5. RNA is different from <u>DNA</u>. RNA is <u>single-stranded</u>, the sugar is the <u>pentose</u> sugar and contains the <u>pyrimidine</u> base <u>uracil</u> (U) instead of <u>thymine</u>. Cells have three different RNAs: <u>messenger</u> RNA (mRNA), <u>ribosomal</u> RNA (rRNA) and <u>transfer</u> RNA (tRNA).

6. Chromosomes are thread-like structures of <u>DNA</u> found inside the <u>nucleus</u> of a <u>cell</u>; each is made of <u>protein</u> and a single molecule of DNA. The unique structure of <u>chromosomes</u> keeps DNA tightly wrapped around spool-like <u>proteins;</u> these are called <u>histones</u>. Human body cells have <u>46</u> chromosomes, <u>23</u> inherited from each parent. DNA contains the specific <u>instructions</u> that make each living creature <u>unique</u>.

7. Protein production and all the genetic instructions for making <u>proteins</u> are found in <u>DNA</u>. In order to <u>synthesise</u> these proteins, the genetic information <u>encoded</u> in the <u>DNA</u> has to be <u>translated</u> first. A complex series of reactions occurs, information contained in <u>RNA</u> is <u>translated</u> into a corresponding specific sequence of <u>amino</u> acids in a newly produced <u>protein</u> molecule – <u>transcription</u> and translation.

8. Genetic information is <u>transferred</u> from <u>cells</u> to new cells and also from <u>parents</u> to their <u>children</u>. For the body to <u>grow</u> and for the <u>replacement</u> of body cells that have <u>died</u>, cells have to <u>reproduce</u> themselves. However, to prevent <u>genetic</u> information from getting lost during <u>reproduction</u> they must be able to reproduce themselves <u>accurately;</u> cells do this by <u>cloning</u> themselves. Gene <u>transference</u> can be divided into two stages: <u>mitosis</u> and <u>meiosis</u>.

Multiple choice answers

1. (d), 2. (a), 3. (b), 4. (c), 5. (a), 6. (c), 7. (c), 8. (a), 9. (b), 10. (c)

Chapter 4

1.

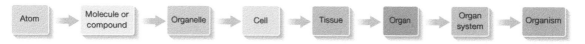

2.

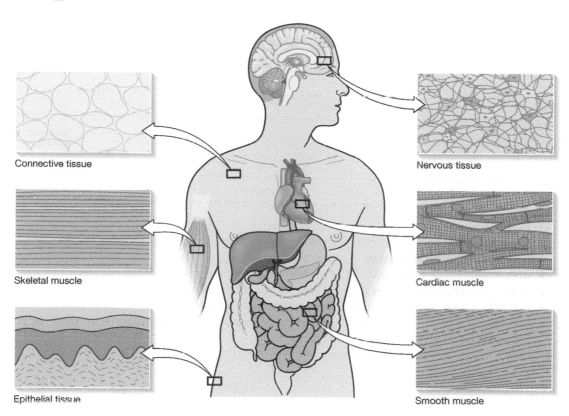

3.

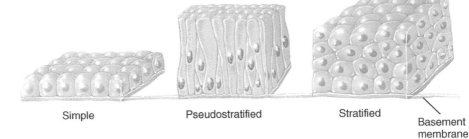

Arrangement of layers

Simple   Pseudostratified   Stratified   Basement membrane

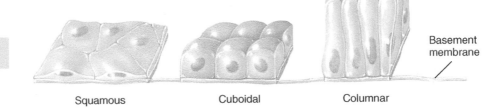

Cell shape

Squamous   Cuboidal   Columnar   Basement membrane

4.

- The overall function of the epithelium is → to provide protection and impermeability
- Epithelial tissue is classified by → shape and depth
- In epithelial tissue there is usually → a basement membrane on which the cells lie
- The intracellular substance is minimal and → the cells are closely packed
- Epithelial tissue may be → simple, pseudostratified or stratified
- Epithelial tissue is located in the → covering of external and internal surfaces, the hollow organs, tubes and glands

5.

DSLANG → GLANDS

SUESIT → TISSUE

NAMEBERM → MEMBRANE

GROANS → ORGANS

FAIRTSTIED → STRATIFIED

CURATENLLILAR → INTRACELLULAR

VEINCONECT → CONNECTIVE

KEELSLAT → SKELETAL

6.

Cell	Description
Adipocytes	Adipocytes are fat cells, they store triglycerides (fats)
Primary blast cells	Primary blast cells continually secrete ground substance and produce mature connective tissue cells
Macrophages	Form part of the body's immune system. Engulf invading substances
Plasma cells	Form part of the body's immune system. Produce antibodies
Mast cells	Form part of the body's immune system. Produce histamine, promoting vasodilation during the inflammatory response
Leucocytes	Form part of the body's immune system. White blood cells are not usually found in substantial numbers in connective tissue; they migrate into connective tissue during inflammation

7.

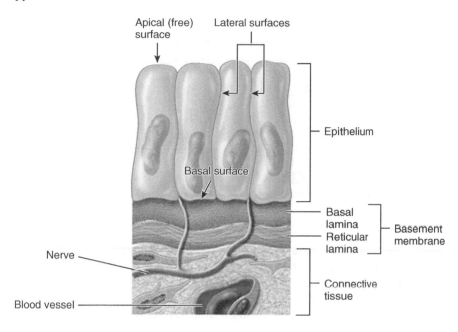

Apical (free) surface
Lateral surfaces
Epithelium
Basal surface
Basal lamina
Reticular lamina
Basement membrane
Nerve
Connective tissue
Blood vessel

8.

- This is the most abundant type of tissue → connective
- The cells of the connective tissue → secrete substances composed of extracellular material
- Important biological features of the connective tissues include → substance transportation, protection of the organism and insulation
- The usual function of connective tissue → is to fill empty spaces among other body tissues
- The matrix of areolar connective tissue → is semi-solid
- Connective tissue → is not present on body surfaces

9.

TAILSUNION → INSULATION
THUMPLEEII → EPITHELIUM
RAREALO → AREOLAR
ELECTLAXRULAR → EXTRACELLULAR

AGENLOLC → COLLAGEN
MRTAXI → MATRIX
NOTICEPROT → PROTECTION
SPORTUP → SUPPORT

10.

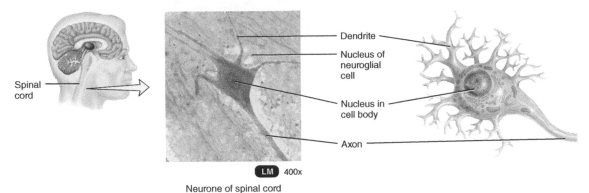

LM 400x

Neurone of spinal cord

11.

- The function of the nervous tissue is → to receive and transmit neural impulses
- Within the nervous system there are two types of tissue → excitable cells and non-excitable cells
- Nervous tissue is composed of → neurones and glial cells
- The neuroglial cells → support the neurones
- The neurones → initiate, receive, conduct and transmit information
- Axons frequently terminate → at a synapse

12.

PSYNASE → SYNAPSE
RENUOGALLI → NEUROGLIAL
SONENURE → NEURONES
PLUMSEIS → IMPULSES

TINDREED → DENDRITE
ANOX → AXON
MISSISTRANON → TRANSMISSION
TAXIBLEEC → EXCITABLE

13.

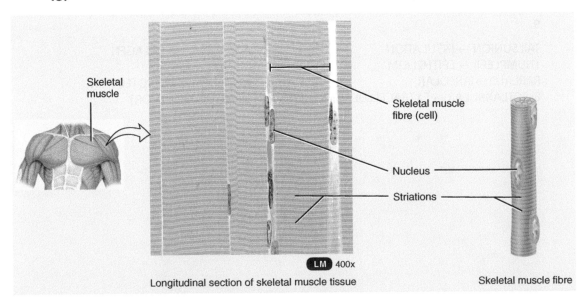

LM 400x

Longitudinal section of skeletal muscle tissue

Skeletal muscle fibre

14.

- Skeletal muscle is found → adjacent to the skeleton
- Skeletal muscle is also known as → striated muscle
- Muscle tissues are composed of cells that → permit contractions and as such they generate movement
- Muscle tissue contains → long muscle fibres
- Skeletal muscle also has → protective functions
- Skeletal muscle is usually attached to bone → by tendons

15.

SONTEND → TENDONS

TIRADEST → STRIATED

TRAINSCONTCO → CONTRACTIONS

NOTLEEKS → SKELETON

URNAVYLOT → VOLUNTARY

VASERIC → VISCERA

SELVESS → VESSELS

NOBE → BONE

16.

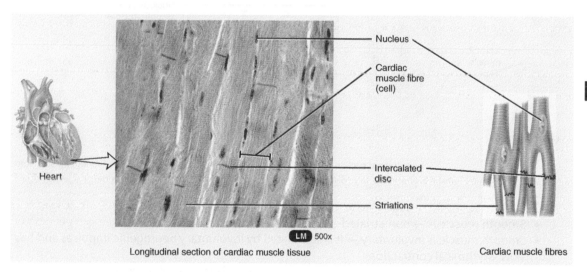

Longitudinal section of cardiac muscle tissue

Cardiac muscle fibres

17.

- Cardiac muscle is a specialised type of muscle with the muscle fibres interlocking → ensuring as one aspect of the muscle is stimulated all other stimulated fibres will contract sequentially
- Cardiac muscle is → not under voluntary control
- The special cells of the sino-atrial node have the responsibility for sending out impulses that → result in cardiac contraction, cardiac muscle provides the driving force of contraction
- Each cardiac muscle fibre contains → a single nucleus and is striated
- When the muscle fibres contract, myosin → pulls the actin filaments together to shrink the muscle cell making it contract
- Cardiac muscle tissue is able to → set its own contraction rhythm as a result of pacemaker cells

18.

MAKEPEACR → PACEMAKER
SYNIMO → MYOSIN
FAILSNETM → FILAMENTS
CINTELOKRING → INTERLOCKING

DONE → NODE
TRANCCOTION → CONTRACTION
LACENDIRATTE → INTERCALATED
TINCA → ACTIN

19.

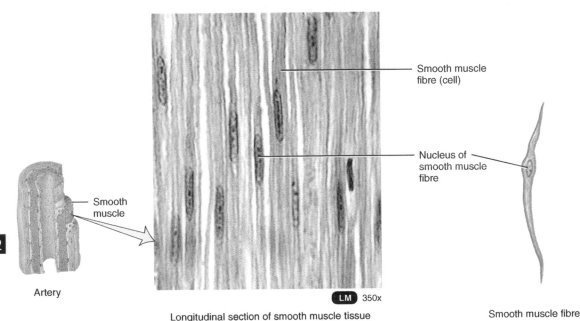

Smooth muscle fibre (cell)

Nucleus of smooth muscle fibre

Smooth muscle

Artery

LM 350x

Longitudinal section of smooth muscle tissue

Smooth muscle fibre

20.

- Smooth muscle is → non-striated
- Smooth muscle is involuntary → it is stimulated by involuntary neurogenic impulses and has slow, rhythmical contractions
- It is held together by → connective tissue with bands of elastic protein wrapped around them
- Smooth muscle is found → in the walls of hollow internal structures and vessels
- Smooth muscle tends to → have greater elasticity than striated muscle
- Contraction of smooth muscle is caused by the sliding of → myosin and actin filaments over each other

21.

GENIOCRENU → NEUROGENIC
TRAYVILNOUN → INVOLUNTARY
SPUMESIL → IMPULSES
THOOMS → SMOOTH

SLEVESS → VESSELS
LICESAT → ELASTIC
NOTICVENCE → CONNECTIVE
LIDSE → SLIDE

22.

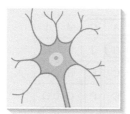

Nerve cell

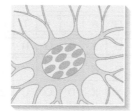

Bone cell

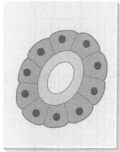

Gland cell

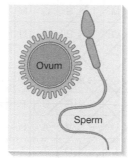

Reproductive cells

Snap shot

Stage 1. **Non-blanchable erythema.** Sores are not open wounds. The skin may be painful; there are no breaks or tears. The skin appears reddened and does not blanch. In people with dark skin, the area may appear to be a different colour than the surrounding skin; it may not look red. Skin temperature is often warmer. The stage 1 sore can feel either firmer or softer than the surrounding area.

Stage 2. **Partial thickness.** The skin breaks open, wears away, or forms an ulcer. This is usually tender and painful. The sore expands into deeper layers of the skin. It can look like an abrasion, a blister or a shallow crater in the skin. This stage may look like a blister filled with clear fluid. At this stage, skin may be damaged beyond repair or may die.

Stage 3. **Full-thickness skin loss.** The sore gets worse and extends into the tissue beneath the skin, forming a small crater. Fat may show in the sore, but not muscle, tendon or bone. Slough may be present but does not obscure the depth of tissue loss.

Stage 4. **Full-thickness tissue loss.** The pressure sore is very deep, reaching into muscle and bone and causing extensive damage. Damage to deeper tissues, tendons and joints can occur.

In stages 3 and 4 there may be little or no pain as a result of significant tissue damage. Serious complications, such as osteomyelitis, osteitis or sepsis can occur if pressure sores progress.

Word search

```
R B J H K N Z E H E G A L I T R A C V I
O E Y F I Q U X E R U T C U R T S J I Q
D R X S S S L E D B P R R Y Y V C E E P
A T O T T U R A E O X X D O U Z C P G O
T Y U A R R O Z D X O Z K J K B U I R S
M V G L C A A M K I M L S O M P Z T R T
B M R A L T C T A O O I B G U S N H D N
D K A T A G I E I U C B N B I O E E E E
X S N Y I N N N L F Q O U M L C R L N M
R T M T L E S D N L I S G C E A V I D A
N R U I E D K T D T U E V A H I O A R L
R I L S H Q E L A A L D T T D U L I I I
C A O S T S L R B E T N A K I R S Y T F
F T C U I T E L V Y E S I R P A G D E U
C E Q E P N T B M U H T M P E C Q C S T
Q D U L E Y A W R P E V I T C E N N O C
J N I G E J L O N C B Z H Y D M X J R T
Z B E I F D N A Z O H T O O M S X T R V
U R O S J E C K N M A T R I X F C R B I
D S Y U S I M E Y J W A C W J T X O F F
```

Crossword

Across
1. TISSUE
3. RENEWAL
5. FORCE
7. CONNECTIVE
8. MACROPHAGES
13. BLOOD
14. ADIPOCYTES
16. DEPTH
17. STRIATED
18. GLIAL
19. FOUR
20. NEURONES
21. SYNAPSE

Down
2. SKELETON
4. IMPERMEABILITY
6. NERVOUS
8. MUSCLE
9. CARDIAC
10. SLIDE
11. SARCOMERES
12. ELASTICITY
15. TENDONS

Fill in the blanks

1. Cells vary in their <u>shape</u>, size and <u>life</u> span; they can, however, be <u>categorised</u> subject to their <u>structure</u> and <u>functions</u>. Groups of <u>cells</u> that have similar structure and <u>function</u> are known as <u>tissue</u>; there are <u>four</u> separate types of tissue within the human body.

2. Epithelial tissue is <u>located</u> in the <u>covering</u> of external and <u>internal</u> surfaces of the body, <u>hollow</u> organs and <u>tubes</u> and also in the <u>glands</u>. The overall function of the epithelium is to <u>provide</u> protection and <u>impermeability</u> or selective <u>permeability</u> to the covered <u>structure</u>. The cells are closely <u>packed</u> and the <u>intracellular</u> substance is <u>minimal</u>. There is usually a basement <u>membrane</u> on which the cells lie. Epithelial tissue may be <u>simple</u>, pseudostratified or <u>stratified</u>, with cell <u>shapes</u> squamous, <u>cuboidal</u> and <u>columnar</u>.

3. There are a number of <u>varieties</u> of connective tissue; it is the most <u>abundant</u> type of tissue. The usual function of <u>connective</u> tissue is to fill <u>empty</u> spaces among other body tissues. The cells of connective tissue <u>secrete</u> substances <u>composed</u> of extracellular <u>material</u>, providing significant <u>spacing</u> between these <u>cells</u>.

4. Nervous <u>tissue</u> is composed of <u>neurones</u> and <u>glial</u> cells. The function is to <u>receive</u> and to also <u>transmit</u> neural <u>impulses</u>. Within the nervous system there are <u>two</u> types of cell: <u>excitable</u> cells, which <u>initiate</u>, receive, <u>conduct</u> and transmit information, and non-excitable cells, the <u>neuroglial</u> cells, which <u>support</u> the neurones. The basic unit of nervous tissue is the neurone, made up of <u>two</u> main parts, the <u>cell</u> body, that contains the neurone's nucleus, <u>cytoplasm</u> and other <u>organelles</u>, and the axon.

5. Muscle tissues are composed of cells that permit <u>contractions</u> and as such they generate <u>movement</u>. The function of the <u>muscle</u> tissue is to <u>pull</u> bones (skeletal <u>striated</u> muscle), to <u>contract</u> and move <u>viscera</u> and <u>vessel</u> walls (<u>smooth</u> muscle) and also to make the heart <u>beat</u> (cardiac <u>striated</u> muscle). Muscle tissue is found where there is a need for <u>movement</u> and <u>maintenance</u> of <u>posture</u>. Muscle tissues contract in <u>response</u> to nerve, <u>nerve</u>-like or hormonal <u>stimulation</u>.

Multiple choice answers

1. (c), 2. (a), 3. (d), 4. (a), 5. (a), 6. (b), 7. (d), 8. (b), 9. (c), 10. (b)

Chapter 5

1.

Structure of axial skeleton	Number of bones	Number of bones	Structure of appendicular skeleton
• Skull			• Pectoral (shoulder) girdles
– Cranium	8	2	– Clavicle
– Face	14	2	– Scapula
• Hyoid	1		• Upper limbs
• Auditory ossicles	6	2	– Humerus
		2	– Ulna
• Vertebral column	26	2	– Radius
• Thorax		16	– Carpals
– Sternum	1	10	– Metacarpals
– Ribs	24	28	– Phalanges
Number of bones	**80**		• Pelvic (hip) girdle
		2	– Hip, pelvic, or coxal bone
			• Lower limbs
		2	– Femur
		2	– Patella
		2	– Fibula
		2	– Tibia
		14	– Tarsals
		10	– Metatarsals
		28	– Phalanges
		126	**Number of bones**

Total bones in an adult skeleton = 206

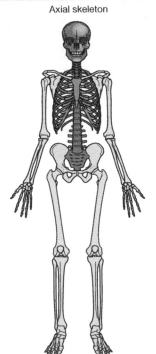

Axial skeleton

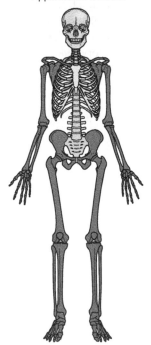

Appendicular skeleton

2.

Function	Description
Support	Without the skeleton the body would be jelly-like and would not be able to stand up. Bones provide the body with its shape/form. The skeletal system offers structural support for the body providing a bony framework for the attachment of soft tissues and organs
Movement	The skeleton allows and enables movement. Bones act as levers providing the transmission of muscular forces. Through leverage, a number of bones change the extent and direction of the forces generated by skeletal muscles, via the tendons and ligaments. These movements range from intricate, for example, the ability to write, the ability to coordinate fine movement, to gross movement, such as the ability to change body posture. The skeleton along with muscles allows breathing to occur. Through articulation movement becomes possible
Minerals and lipid store	Bones store minerals such as calcium, magnesium and phosphorus; calcium is the most abundant mineral in the body. The bone has the ability to release stored minerals in response to demand. When the amount of calcium in the blood is high, calcium can be deposited in the bones. This provides an internal homeostasis regulated by hormones. Lipids are also stored in the yellow marrow of some bones; they can be stored or released depending on needs
Protection	Bone is a rigid structure, protecting most of the soft tissues of the body and internal organs – the skull protects the brain, the sternum and ribs protect the lungs and heart, the spinal cord is protected by the vertebrae, the orbit protects the eyes and the periosteum protects the red bone marrow. The pelvis shields and protects delicate internal abdominal digestive and reproductive organs
Blood cell production	Some bones produce red and white blood cells (haematopoiesis). Haematopoiesis occurs mainly in red bone marrow, which fills the internal cavity of most bones

3.

- When old bone dies → new bone is being reconstructed
- Bones are made up of → a number of different tissues and this includes bone tissue
- The skeleton provides the body with → shape and the power to move
- The skeletal system is comprised → of bones, ligaments and tendons
- Infants are born with large amounts of cartilage → they have more bones than adults
- The skeleton is divided into two parts for classification purposes → the axial skeleton and the appendicular skeleton

4.

CILOBATEM → METABOLIC
NOTJIS → JOINTS
CIRULATETA → ARTICULATE
NILGASTEM → LIGAMENTS

NODESNT → TENDONS
LIMERANS → MINERALS
SIFISOOTCAIN → OSSIFICATION
USEF → FUSE

5.

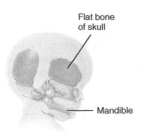

Flat bone
of skull

Mandible

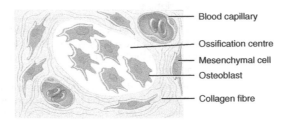

Blood capillary

Ossification centre

Mesenchymal cell

Osteoblast

Collagen fibre

1 Development of ossification centre

Osteocyte in lacuna

Canaliculus

Osteoblast

Newly calcified bone
matrix

2 Calcification

Mesenchyme
condenses

Blood vessel

Spongy bone
trabeculae

Osteoblast

3 Formation of trabeculae

Periosteum

Spongy bone tissue

Compact bone tissue

4 Development of the periosteum

6.

Stage	Activity
One	Initial bone formation in utero
Two	Bone growth during infancy, childhood and adolescence
Three	Replacement of old bone with new bone (bone remodelling) – occurring throughout a person's life
Four	Repair of bone fractures that may occur throughout a person's life

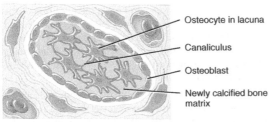

7.

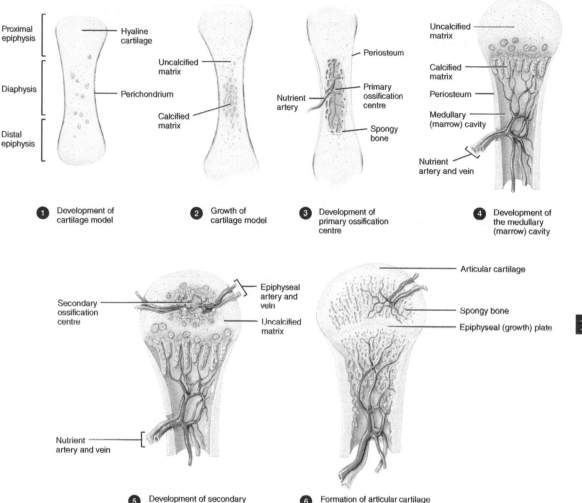

① Development of cartilage model

② Growth of cartilage model

③ Development of primary ossification centre

④ Development of the medullary (marrow) cavity

⑤ Development of secondary ossification centre

⑥ Formation of articular cartilage and epiphyseal plate

8.

- Intramembranous and endochondral ossification are → embryonic processes of bone formation
- Intramembranous ossification occurs → primarily during the initial formation of the flat bones of the skull, mandible and clavicles
- In intramembranous ossification the bone is formed from → mesenchyme connective tissue
- Endochondral ossification → is key for the formation of long and short bones
- Natural healing of small bone fractures → is associated with endochondral ossification
- The second stage of bone formation is associated with → bone growth during infancy, childhood and adolescence

9.

NOODLEDRANCH → ENDOCHONDRAL
FOSISIACTION → OSSIFICATION
INTROREMABAMNUS → INTRAMEMBRANOUS
BRICYOMEN → EMBRYONIC

SYPHIPEALE → EPIPHYSEAL
MYCHEMESEN → MESENCHYME
BRUTALEACE → TRABECULAE
SYPHISAID → DIAPHYSIS

10.

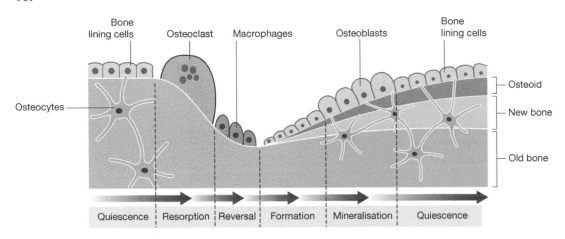

11.

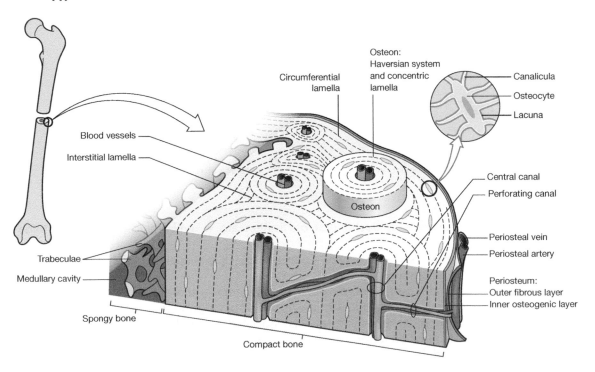

12.

Cell	Description	Responsible for
Osteoblasts	Bone-forming cells found near the surface of bones, making osteoid, consisting chiefly of collagen. The osteoid becomes mineralised, forming bone	Production of bone
Osteocytes	These are osteoblasts that are no longer on the surface of the bone, but are instead found in lacunae between the lamellae in bone	Maintenance of bone
Osteoclasts	The cells that breakdown and reabsorb bone, stem from monocytes and macrophages	Resorption of bone

13.

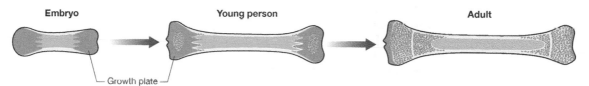

14.

- Remodelling takes place → at different rates in different parts of the body
- Bone is dynamic → it is continuously built, broken down and rebuilt
- A fine balance must exist between → the breakdown and build up of bone
- If bone is built up too quickly → an abnormally thick and heavy bone will be formed
- Weak bone, as a result of too much calcium or bone tissue loss, can result in → bone that breaks easily
- Bone resorption and formation is known as → remodelling

15.

GOLDLEMINER → REMODELLING
SORPITONER → RESORPTION
STOOLESTABS → OSTEOBLASTS
STOOLSTACES → OSTEOCLASTS
MALCUIC → CALCIUM

LOCLAGEN → COLLAGEN
SHIVERAAN → HAVERSIAN
SEVERRAL → REVERSAL

16.

Fracture occurs

↓

Phagocytes begin their work by removing dead bone tissue

↓

Chondroblasts form fibrocartilage at the site of fracture

↓

The fibrocartilage is converted to spongy bone tissues by the action of osteoblasts

↓

Bone remodelling occurs

↓

Dead bone is absorbed by the action of osteoclasts

↓

Spongy bone is converted to compact bone

17.

Type of bone	Description	Example
Long	These bones are often curved, assisting with strength; longer and wider than other bones, they consist of a shaft and a variable number of extremities	Femur, tibia, fibula, humerus, ulna and radius
Short	Described as cube-shaped, with about the same length and width. Primary function is to provide support and stability with little movement	Carpals and tarsals
Flat	Strong, flat plates of bone, key functions are to provide protection to the vital organs as well as being a base for muscular attachment	Scapula, sternum, cranium, os coxae, pelvis and ribs
Irregular	These bones do not fall into any other category, due to their non-uniform shape	Vertebrae, sacrum and mandible
Sesamoid	These are mostly short or irregular bones, embedded in a tendon	Patella, pisiform and the two small bones at the base of the first metatarsal

18.

Figure 5.8 A long bone.
Figure 5.9 A short bone.
Figure 5.10 A flat bone.
Figure 5.11 An irregular bone.
Figure 5.12 A sesamoid bone.
See answer 19. for completed labels.

19.

Name of bone	Bone
Long bone	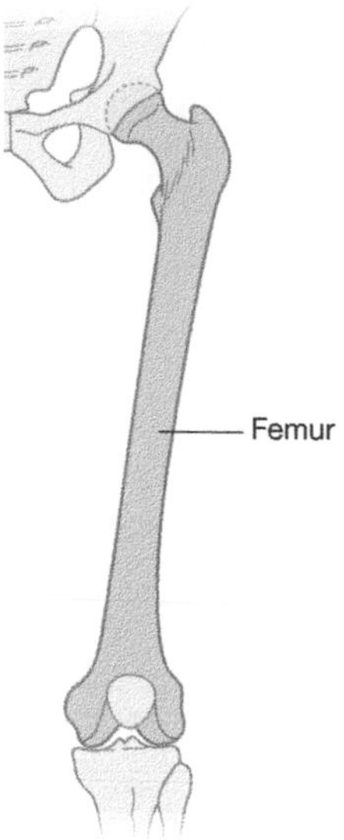 Femur
Short bone	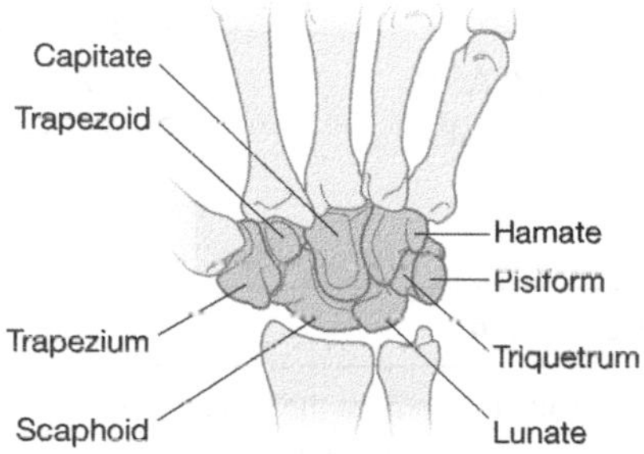 Capitate, Trapezoid, Hamate, Pisiform, Trapezium, Triquetrum, Scaphoid, Lunate
Flat bone	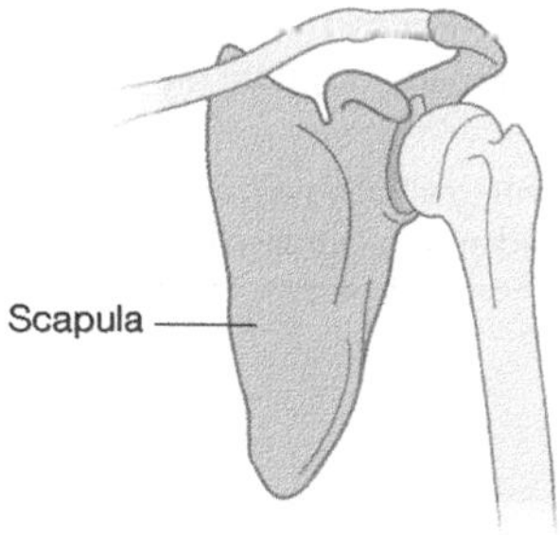 Scapula

(Continued)

(*Continued*)

Name of bone	Bone
Irregular bone 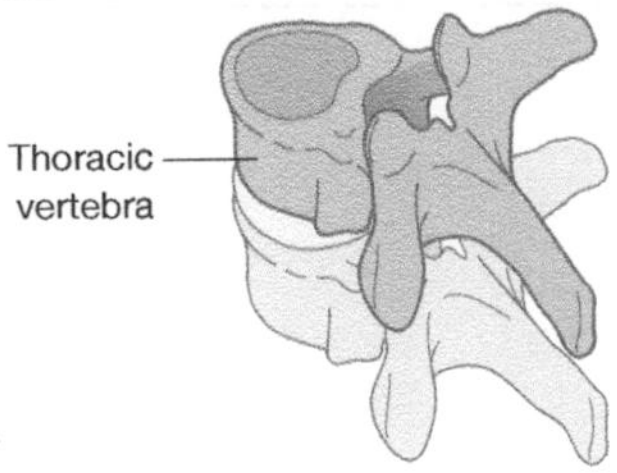
Thoracic vertebra
Sesamoid bone 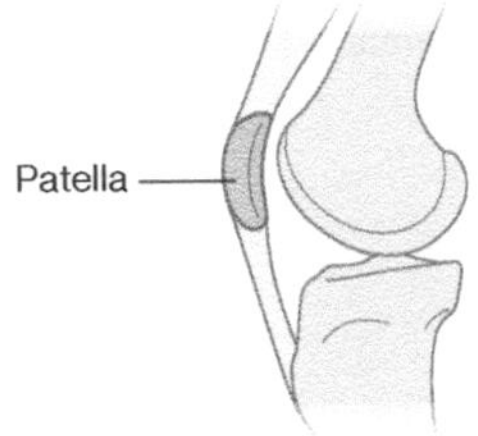
Patella |

20.

MACAPRETALS → METACARPALS

SOSIMADE → SESAMOID

DOBLASTSCROHN → CHONDROBLASTS

IBROCLEARAFITG → FIBROCARTILAGE

FURCREAT → FRACTURE

PYONGS → SPONGY

MOCAPCT → COMPACT

DIHYO → HYOID

21.

Movement	Description
Flexion	Reducing the angle at the joint, e.g. bending the knee or elbow
Extension	Increasing the angle at the joint, e.g. straightening the knee or elbow
Adduction	Moving the body part towards the centre of the body, e.g. bringing one leg in towards the other
Abduction	Moving the body part away from the centre of the body, e.g. taking one leg away from the other
Rotation	Turning or twisting a body part, either clockwise (external or lateral) or anticlockwise (internal or medial), e.g. turning the leg to point the toes outwards

22.

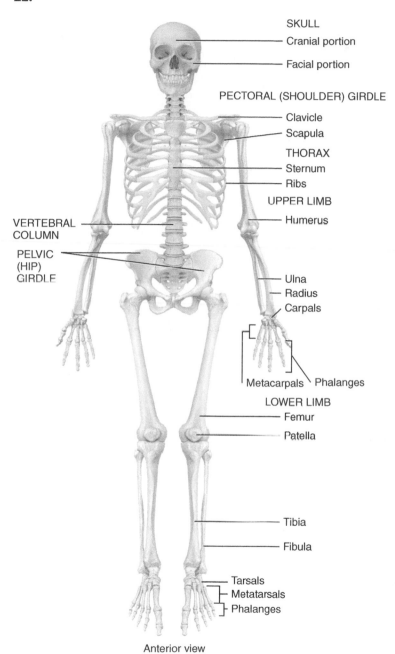

SKULL
— Cranial portion
— Facial portion

PECTORAL (SHOULDER) GIRDLE
— Clavicle
— Scapula
THORAX
— Sternum
— Ribs
UPPER LIMB
— Humerus

VERTEBRAL
COLUMN

PELVIC
(HIP)
GIRDLE

— Ulna
— Radius
— Carpals

Metacarpals — Phalanges

LOWER LIMB
— Femur
— Patella

Tibia

Fibula

Tarsals
Metatarsals
Phalanges

Anterior view

23.

Type of joint	Examples		Structure
Hinge	Elbow, knee	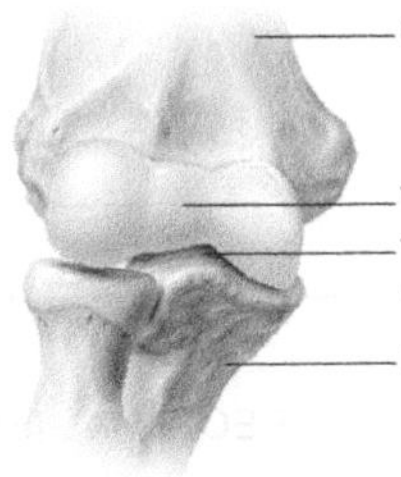 Humerus / Trochlea / Trochlear notch / Ulna	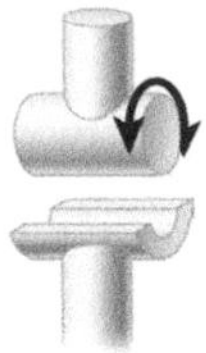
Pivot	Radius and ulna, the atlas and axis	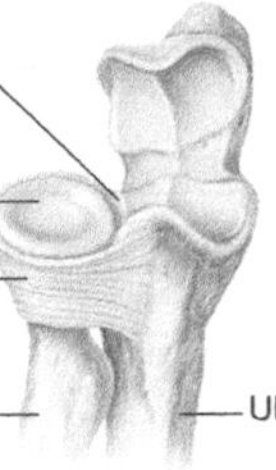 Radial notch / Head of radius / Annular ligament / Radius / Ulna	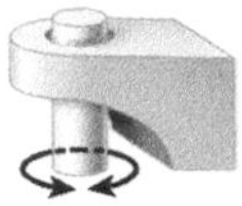
Ball and socket	Hip, shoulder	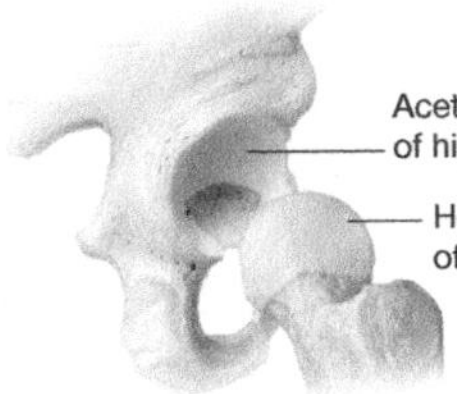 Acetabulum of hip bone / Head of femur	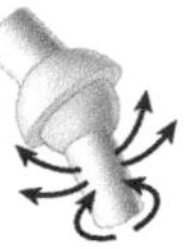
Saddle	The carpometacarpal joints of the thumb	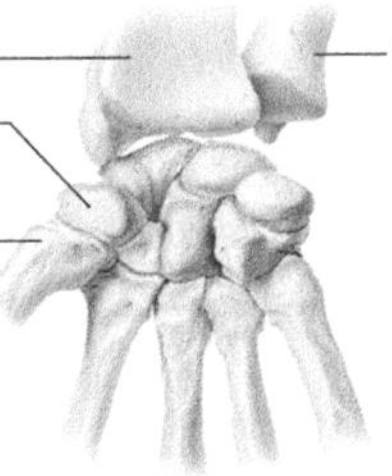 Radius / Ulna / Trapezium / Metacarpal of thumb	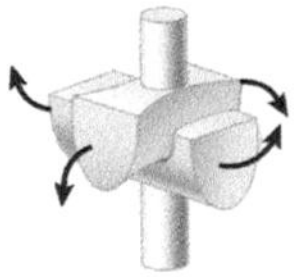
Condyloid	The radiocarpal and metacarpophalangeal joints of the hand	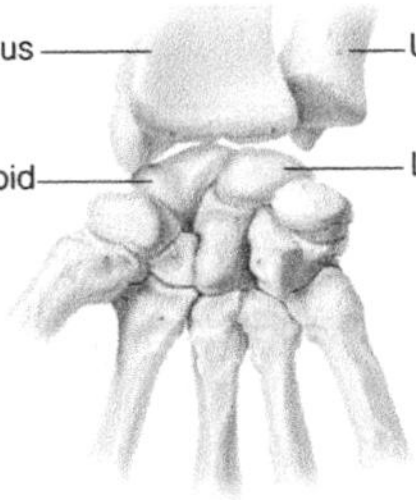 Radius / Ulna / Scaphoid / Lunate	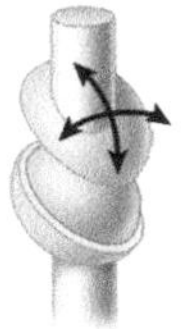
Gliding	Intertarsal and intercarpal joints of the hands and feet	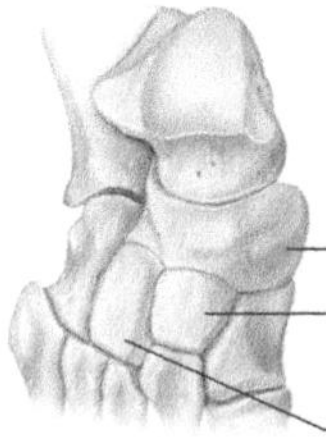 Navicular / Second cuneiform / Third cuneiform	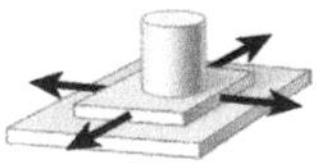

396

24.

SEXTONIEN → EXTENSION

SOURFIB → FIBROUS

NOILSAVY → SYNOVIAL

MASSDOIE → SESAMOID

TOESCK → SOCKET

HONEYSDROSSCN → SYNCHONDROSES

GEHIN → HINGE

LADDES → SADDLE

Snap shot

Adults aged between 19 and 64 are advised to do at least 150 minutes (2 hours and 30 minutes) of moderate-intensity aerobic activity, such as cycling or fast walking every week.

Weight-bearing exercise and resistance exercise are especially important for improving bone density and helping to prevent osteoporosis. As well as aerobic exercise, adults should be encouraged to carry out muscle-strengthening activities on two or more days each week by working all the major muscle groups, these include the legs, hips, back, abdomen, chest, shoulders and arms.

If the person has been diagnosed with osteoporosis, they should be advised to talk to the practice nurse, the GP or health specialist prior to starting a new exercise programme. Physical activity for adults includes:

- strength exercises
- balance exercises
- flexibility exercises
- sitting exercises.

Weight-bearing exercises

Weight-bearing exercises are exercises where the feet and legs support the person's weight. High-impact weight-bearing exercises include running, skipping, dancing, aerobics and even jumping up and down on the spot. These are all useful ways to strengthen the muscles, ligaments and joints.

When exercising, the person should be advised to wear footwear that provides their ankles and feet with adequate support, for example, trainers or walking boots.

People over 60 years of age can also benefit from regular weight-bearing exercise. This includes brisk walking, keep-fit classes or a game of tennis. Swimming and cycling, however, are not classed as weight-bearing exercises.

Resistance exercises

Resistance exercises use muscle strength, where the action of the tendons pulling on the bones gives a boost to bone strength. Examples include press-ups, weightlifting or using weight equipment at a gym.

The nurse should always undertake a full assessment of the person prior to engaging in or encouraging the person to take on any exercise, exercise classes or gym activity.

Word search

H	Z	N	X	U	O	M	U	S	C	L	E	S	E	L	J	N	S	M	L
F	T	K	F	N	H	O	F	G	S	D	I	P	I	L	M	O	E	G	T
Y	X	Y	U	S	C	C	G	P	G	W	J	K	O	P	L	I	T	R	T
S	L	G	S	E	A	G	J	X	A	N	T	R	K	F	O	T	Y	X	S
S	W	L	I	T	R	D	O	N	P	S	N	Z	V	X	M	A	C	E	G
T	J	B	S	Y	T	H	W	T	D	U	O	S	E	H	J	C	O	N	C
S	F	W	A	C	I	A	P	Z	H	O	T	C	V	O	D	I	E	D	P
A	U	P	T	O	L	E	K	W	P	N	E	L	J	E	B	F	T	O	X
L	J	L	S	E	A	M	A	V	R	A	L	E	P	T	Y	I	S	C	U
B	E	I	O	T	G	A	L	Q	R	R	E	V	S	A	B	S	O	H	T
O	X	G	E	S	E	T	T	Z	U	B	K	E	M	L	S	S	J	O	Y
E	Z	A	M	O	W	O	O	Z	U	M	S	R	M	U	C	O	R	N	A
T	Y	M	O	L	S	P	V	U	Z	E	M	A	B	C	K	L	N	D	N
S	M	E	H	A	E	O	W	A	N	M	U	G	A	I	M	A	S	R	M
O	J	N	R	I	S	I	C	G	S	A	I	E	G	T	I	R	J	A	J
Q	S	T	R	X	A	E	I	H	Q	R	C	S	C	R	S	E	G	L	C
A	N	S	A	A	M	S	A	E	V	T	L	Z	Y	A	H	N	T	C	H
D	U	N	D	K	O	I	L	W	W	N	A	D	B	S	E	I	W	N	S
U	S	I	E	N	I	S	P	L	M	I	C	W	Z	L	Q	M	X	E	C
E	D	V	G	S	D	G	Q	A	P	P	E	N	D	I	C	U	L	A	R

Crossword

Across
3. CARTILAGE
6. ORGANS
12. RECONSTRUCTED
15. THREE
16. EMBRYONIC
18. OSTEOBLASTS
19. HAEMATOPOIESIS
20. CALCIUM

Down
1. RED
2. BONES
4. APPENDICULAR
5. SECOND
7. ARTICULATION
8. INTRAMEMBRANOUS
9. TRABECULAR
10. REMODELLING
11. OSTEOCYTES
13. YELLOW
14. OSTEON
17. VERTEBRAE

Fill in the blanks

1. The <u>skeleton</u> permits <u>movement</u>; bones act as <u>levers</u> providing the <u>transmission</u> of muscular <u>forces</u> that are <u>generated</u> by skeletal <u>muscles</u>, through the <u>work</u> of the <u>tendons</u> and the <u>ligaments</u>. Movement becomes possible through <u>articulation</u>.

2. Tendons are <u>fibrous</u> connective <u>tissue</u> attaching <u>muscle</u> to <u>bone</u>; they help to move the <u>bone</u> or structure. Ligaments are <u>fibrous</u> connective <u>tissues</u> attaching <u>bones</u> to bones, holding structures together and keeping them <u>stable</u>.

3. Different types of <u>joints</u> provide different <u>types</u> of <u>movement</u>; the <u>shoulder</u> joint, for example, moves in more ways than the <u>knee</u> does.

4. Reducing the <u>angle</u> at the joint, <u>bending</u> the knee or <u>elbow</u>, is <u>flexion</u>. <u>Increasing</u> the angle at the joint, for example, <u>straightening</u> the <u>knee</u> or elbow, is <u>extension</u>. Moving the <u>body</u> part <u>towards</u> the centre of the body, for example bringing one leg in towards the other, is <u>adduction</u>. Moving the body part <u>away</u> from the <u>centre</u> of the body, taking one <u>leg</u> away from the other, is <u>abduction</u>. <u>Turning</u> or <u>twisting</u> a body part, either clockwise or <u>anti-clockwise</u>, for example, <u>turning</u> the <u>leg</u> to point the <u>toes</u> outwards, is <u>rotation</u>.

Multiple choice answers

1. (b), 2. (c), 3. (c), 4. (d), 5. (a), 6. (a), 7. (d), 8. (b), 9. (d), 10. (d)

Chapter 6

1.

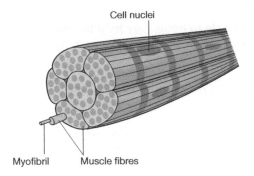

Cell nuclei

SKELETAL MUSCLE

Myofibril   Muscle fibres

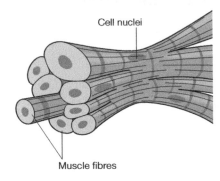

Cell nuclei

SMOOTH MUSCLE

Muscle fibres

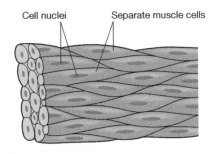

Cell nuclei   Separate muscle cells

CARDIAC MUSCLE

2.

	Skeletal muscle	Smooth muscle	Cardiac muscle
Location	Attached to bones or the skin (facial muscles only)	Found in the walls of hollow visceral organs and blood vessels	Located in the walls of the heart
Cell type	Single, long cylindrical cells	Single, narrow, rod-shaped cells	Branching chains of cells
Striation/ non-striation	Striated, multinucleated cells	Non-striated, uninucleated cells	Non-striated, uninucleated cells
Control	Voluntary control	Involuntary control	Involuntary control

3.

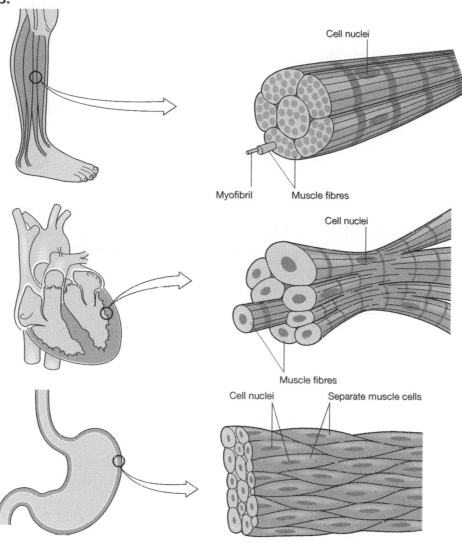

4.

Property	Description
Excitability (irritability)	The ability to receive and respond to stimuli via generation of an electrical pulse which results in contraction of the muscle cells
Contractility	Ability to shorten
Extensibility	Ability to be stretched or extended
Elasticity	The capability of a muscle fibre to recoil and resume its resting length

5.

LICROE → RECOIL
GENERY → ENERGY
TEENSTIBLIXIY → EXTENSIBILITY
BRITRIITILAY → IRRITABILITY

NATIONCORTC → CONTRACTION
COMINTOLOO → LOCOMOTION
VOMMENTE → MOVEMENT
LYNDACIRCIL → CYLINDRICAL

6.

Periosteum

Tendon

Epimysium

Bone

Perimysium

Fascicle

7.

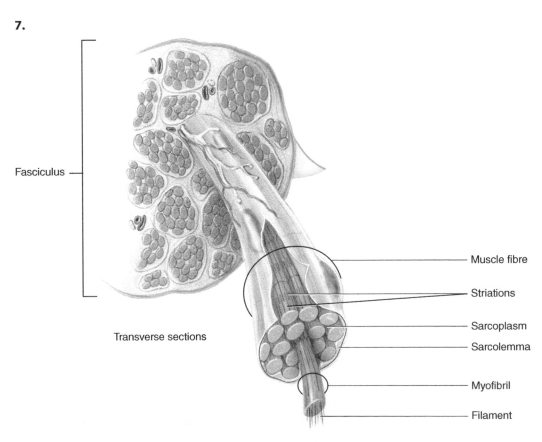

Fasciculus

Transverse sections

Muscle fibre

Striations

Sarcoplasm

Sarcolemma

Myofibril

Filament

8.

- Muscles contain other types of tissues, for example, blood vessels, connective and nervous tissue → they are considered to be organs
- Each cell in skeletal muscle tissue is a single muscle fibre → they contain hundreds of nuclei
- Microscopically, skeletal muscle cells appear cylindrical in shape → they have a distinctive banded appearance and lie parallel to each other
- Each muscle fibre is covered by a plasma membrane, the sarcolemma, and contain cylindrical structures. the myofibrils. These are → suspended inside the muscle fibre, extending along its length
- The myofibrils play a central role in the muscle contraction mechanism → they contain two types of protein filaments
- Extending across each of the thick filaments within the sarcomere is a dark area known as → the A band in the centre of which is a narrow H zone

9.

SELFICCAS → FASCICLES

FOYLISBRIM → MYOFIBRILS

CAROLEMMAS → SARCOLEMMA

SYDNEMOMIU → ENDOMYSIUM

YEMIMPUSI → EPIMYSIUM

PURIMSMIEY → PERIMYSIUM

TRAINCSEE → CISTERNAE

BOYGOMLIN → MYOGLOBIN

10.

Fibre	Description
Slow oxidative (SO)	Small, dark-red fibres that generate ATP by aerobic respiration, make up approximately 50% of skeletal muscle, capable of slow, prolonged contractions, not easily fatigued
Fast oxidative–glycolytic (FOG)	Medium, dark-red fibres, also generate ATP by aerobic respiration. Due to their high glycogen content also able to generate ATP by anaerobic glycolysis. FOG fibres contact and relax more quickly than SO fibres
Fast glycolytic (FG)	Large white fibres that generate ATP mainly by anaerobic glycolysis, providing the most rapid and powerful muscle contractions but they easily fatigue

11.

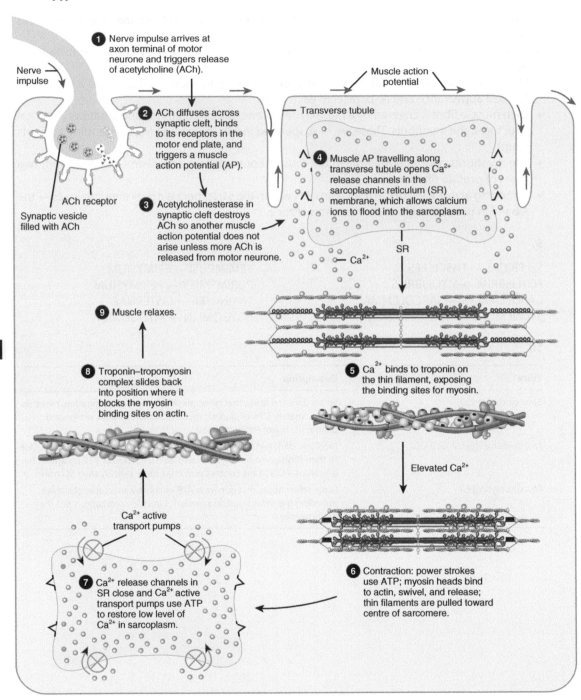

1. Nerve impulse arrives at axon terminal of motor neurone and triggers release of acetylcholine (ACh).

Nerve impulse

ACh receptor

Synaptic vesicle filled with ACh

2. ACh diffuses across synaptic cleft, binds to its receptors in the motor end plate, and triggers a muscle action potential (AP).

3. Acetylcholinesterase in synaptic cleft destroys ACh so another muscle action potential does not arise unless more ACh is released from motor neurone.

Muscle action potential

Transverse tubule

4. Muscle AP travelling along transverse tubule opens Ca^{2+} release channels in the sarcoplasmic reticulum (SR) membrane, which allows calcium ions to flood into the sarcoplasm.

Ca^{2+}

SR

9. Muscle relaxes.

8. Troponin–tropomyosin complex slides back into position where it blocks the myosin binding sites on actin.

5. Ca^{2+} binds to troponin on the thin filament, exposing the binding sites for myosin.

Elevated Ca^{2+}

Ca^{2+} active transport pumps

7. Ca^{2+} release channels in SR close and Ca^{2+} active transport pumps use ATP to restore low level of Ca^{2+} in sarcoplasm.

6. Contraction: power strokes use ATP; myosin heads bind to actin, swivel, and release; thin filaments are pulled toward centre of sarcomere.

12.

- Acetylcholine when released → causes changes to the sarcolemma, triggering contraction of the muscle fibre
- As a nerve impulse reaches the axon terminals → acetylcholine is released into the synaptic cleft
- The synaptic cleft → and motor end plate contain acetylcholinesterase
- The motor neurone and the muscle fibres it controls are known as → a motor unit
- The densely branched motor neurone axons mean that → one motor neurone axon can connect and control many muscle fibres
- Skeletal muscle contracts in response to → stimulation by muscle action potential

13.

SLUMPIE → IMPULSE

PSYICTAN → SYNAPTIC

FELTC → CLEFT

ACEHYLINECOLT → ACETYLCHOLINE

TOONCRACTIN → CONTRACTION

LATENTPOI → POTENTIAL

UJONCITO → JUNCTION

SLITMANER → TERMINALS

14.

Character/Term	Definition	Example
DIRECTION	Across	Transversus abdominis
Transverse	Diagonal	External oblique
Oblique	Straight	Rectus abdominis
Rectus		
SHAPE	Trapezoid	Trapezius
Trapezius	Triangular	Deltoid
Deltoid	Circular	Obicularis oculi
Obicularis	Diamond-shaped	Rhomboideus
Rhomboid	Flat	Platysma
Platys		
SIZE	Larger	Pectoralis major
Major	Smaller	Pectoralis minor
Minor	Largest	Gluteus maximus
Maximus	Smallest	Gluteus minimus
Minimus	Longest	Adductor longus
Longus	Widest	Latissimus dorsi
Latissimus		
NUMBER OF ORIGINS	Two origins	Biceps brachii
Biceps	Three origins	Triceps brachii
Triceps	Four origins	Quadriceps femoris
Quadriceps		

15.

- Head and neck
- Upper limbs (shoulder, arm and hand)
- Trunk (thorax and abdomen)
- Lower limbs (hip, pelvis/thigh and leg)

See answer to question 16 for further information on the muscles in posterior and anterior views.

16.

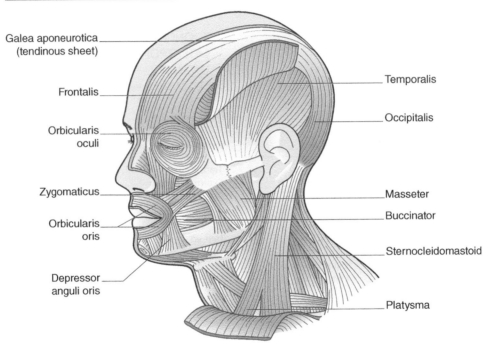

An anterior and lateral view

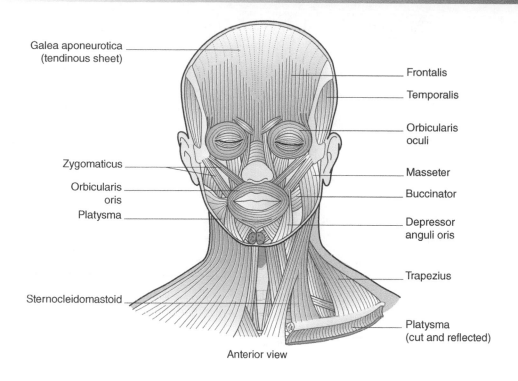

Galea aponeurotica
(tendinous sheet)

Frontalis

Temporalis

Orbicularis
oculi

Zygomaticus

Masseter

Orbicularis
oris

Buccinator

Platysma

Depressor
anguli oris

Trapezius

Sternocleidomastoid

Platysma
(cut and reflected)

Anterior view

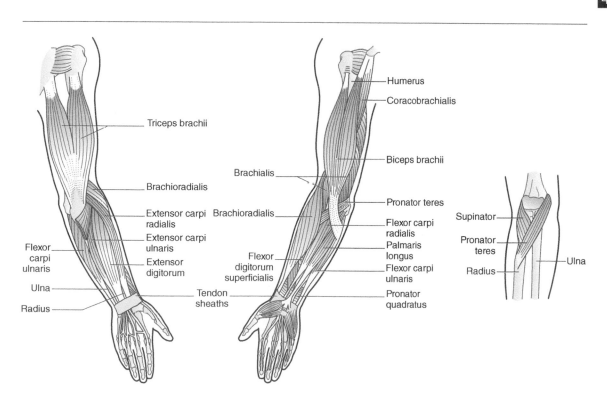

Triceps brachii

Humerus

Coracobrachialis

Brachioradialis

Biceps brachii

Brachialis

Extensor carpi
radialis

Brachioradialis

Pronator teres

Extensor carpi
ulnaris

Flexor carpi
radialis

Flexor
carpi
ulnaris

Extensor
digitorum

Flexor
digitorum
superficialis

Palmaris
longus

Supinator

Pronator
teres

Ulna

Flexor carpi
ulnaris

Radius

Radius

Tendon
sheaths

Pronator
quadratus

Ulna

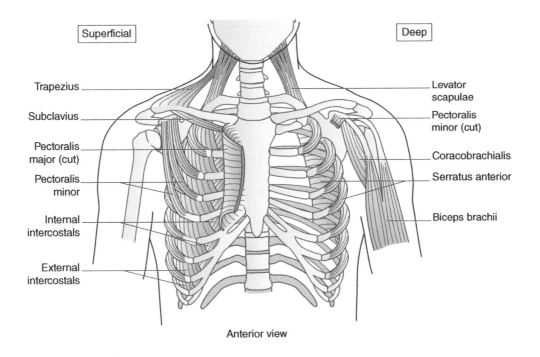

Superficial

Deep

Trapezius

Levator scapulae

Deltoid

Rhomboideus muscles

Infraspinatus

Teres minor

Teres major

Serratus anterior

Triceps brachii

Posterior view

Superficial

Deep

Trapezius

Levator scapulae

Subclavius

Pectoralis minor (cut)

Pectoralis major (cut)

Coracobrachialis

Pectoralis minor

Serratus anterior

Internal intercostals

Biceps brachii

External intercostals

Anterior view

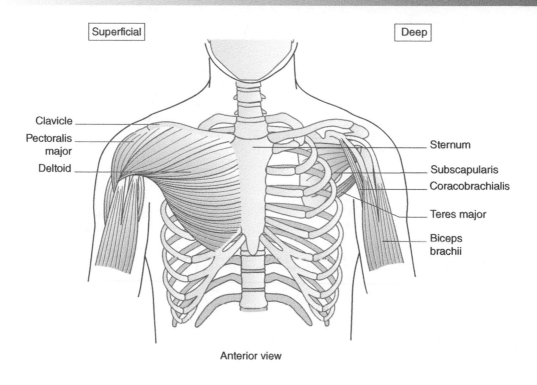

Superficial | Deep

Clavicle
Pectoralis major
Deltoid

Sternum
Subscapularis
Coracobrachialis
Teres major
Biceps brachii

Anterior view

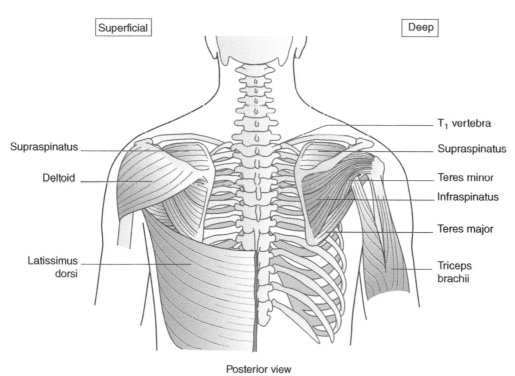

Superficial | Deep

Supraspinatus
Deltoid
Latissimus dorsi

T₁ vertebra
Supraspinatus
Teres minor
Infraspinatus
Teres major
Triceps brachii

Posterior view

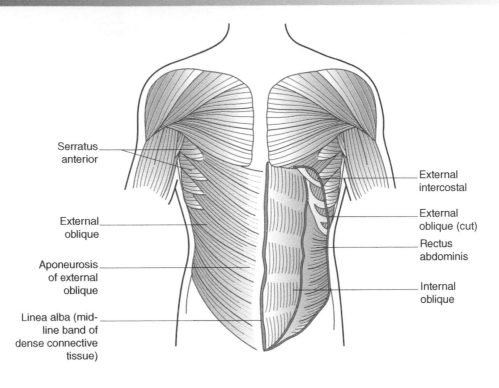

Serratus anterior

External oblique

Aponeurosis of external oblique

Linea alba (mid-line band of dense connective tissue)

External intercostal

External oblique (cut)

Rectus abdominis

Internal oblique

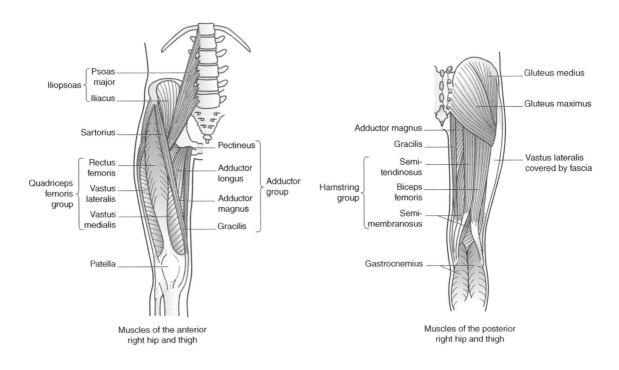

Iliopsoas {
Psoas major
Iliacus
}

Sartorius

Quadriceps femoris group {
Rectus femoris
Vastus lateralis
Vastus medialis
}

Pectineus

Adductor longus

Adductor magnus

Gracilis

Adductor group

Patella

Muscles of the anterior right hip and thigh

Adductor magnus

Gracilis

Hamstring group {
Semi-tendinosus
Biceps femoris
Semi-membranosus
}

Gastrocnemius

Gluteus medius

Gluteus maximus

Vastus lateralis covered by fascia

Muscles of the posterior right hip and thigh

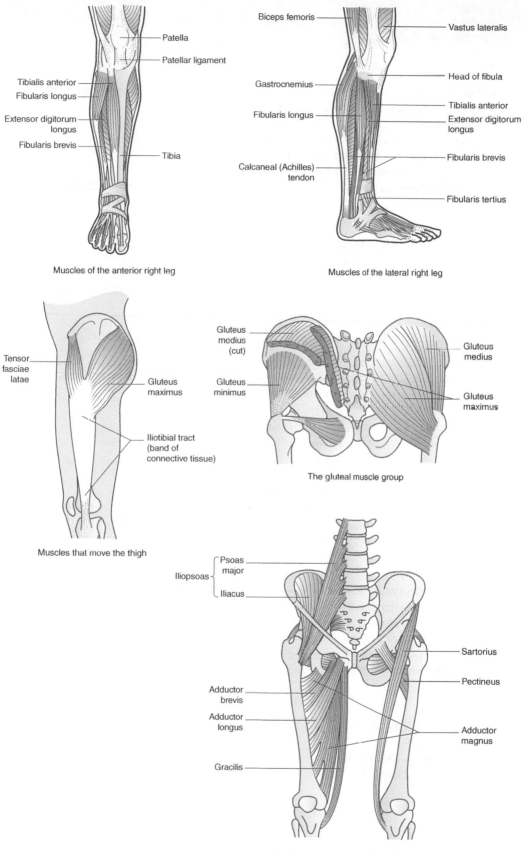

Patella

Patellar ligament

Tibialis anterior

Fibularis longus

Extensor digitorum longus

Fibularis brevis

Tibia

Muscles of the anterior right leg

Biceps femoris

Vastus lateralis

Gastrocnemius

Head of fibula

Fibularis longus

Tibialis anterior

Extensor digitorum longus

Calcaneal (Achilles) tendon

Fibularis brevis

Fibularis tertius

Muscles of the lateral right leg

Tensor fasciae latae

Gluteus maximus

Iliotibial tract (band of connective tissue)

Muscles that move the thigh

Gluteus medius (cut)

Gluteus medius

Gluteus minimus

Gluteus maximus

The gluteal muscle group

411

Iliopsoas

Psoas major

Iliacus

Sartorius

Pectineus

Adductor brevis

Adductor longus

Adductor magnus

Gracilis

The iliopsoas muscle and the adductor group

17.

- The skeletal muscles can be → named according to size, shape, location and number of origins, associated bones and the action of the muscle
- The skeletal muscles can be → divided into four areas
- The origin of a muscle → is on the stationary bone where it begins
- Muscle ends → at an insertion on the bone that moves
- The buccinator muscle → compresses cheeks
- All skeletal muscles are attached → at a minimum of two points to bone or other connective tissue

18.

CUBARINCTO → BUCCINATOR
ALANACOMIT → ANATOMICAL
LUGALTE → GLUTEAL
STRAVENSER → TRANSVERSE

LARCRUCI → CIRCULAR
PECSTRI → TRICEPS
CIBEPS → BICEPS
TRACODDU → ADDUCTOR

19.

Action	Definition
Extension	Increases the angle or distance between two bones or parts of the body
Flexion	Decreases the angle of a joint
Abduction	Moves away from the midline
Adduction	Moves closer to the midline
Circumduction	A combination of flexion, extension, abduction and adduction
Supination	Turns the palm up
Pronation	Turns the palm down
Plantar flexion	Lowers the foot (point the toes)
Dorsiflexion	Elevates the foot
Rotation	Moves a bone around its longitudinal axis

20.

- Two opposing muscles are called → agonist and antagonist
- An agonist is also called → a prime mover
- Prime movers are → mainly responsible for producing an action
- An antagonist of a prime mover → causes muscle movement in the opposite direction
- An agonist → may cause an arm to bend
- The antagonist → will cause an arm to straighten

21.

GNATOIS → AGONIST
RIPEM → PRIME
GIANTASTON → ANTAGONIST
TRAITOON → ROTATION

ELFIXON → FLEXION
STENEXION → EXTENSION
DIMNILE → MIDLINE
PARTNAL → PLANTAR

Snap shot
Intramuscular injection
This site is chosen so as to avoid unintentional damage to the sciatic nerve

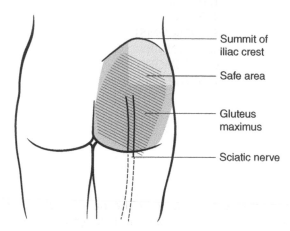

- Summit of iliac crest
- Safe area
- Gluteus maximus
- Sciatic nerve

Word search

Z	R	B	N	K	M	A	B	N	H	P	I	Q	O	X	V	Y	Z	H	S
K	R	O	T	A	N	I	C	C	U	B	E	E	D	J	Q	U	E	D	E
O	A	C	A	I	D	R	A	C	M	N	W	R	O	C	T	F	Y	G	G
T	W	C	S	R	S	M	O	O	T	H	Z	I	I	E	Y	J	Q	T	J
F	W	H	E	L	W	Z	P	R	W	P	N	M	C	M	N	G	S	X	U
H	A	E	L	T	R	V	H	L	F	T	Y	T	D	S	Y	I	P	L	N
Y	A	S	C	H	Y	I	E	L	S	O	J	M	J	G	N	S	Z	P	G
T	F	N	S	C	F	L	Q	Q	F	N	P	E	R	O	L	L	I	B	V
I	K	O	U	K	O	T	C	I	A	J	N	E	G	P	Z	O	X	U	B
L	E	D	M	W	V	N	B	H	Q	D	N	A	A	P	T	C	J	G	M
I	P	N	K	Q	J	R	D	C	O	E	D	J	S	X	K	O	M	E	I
T	I	E	H	D	I	A	J	M	M	L	W	P	I	Q	I	M	C	R	L
C	M	T	P	L	L	R	Y	E	O	H	I	J	X	S	W	O	C	E	A
A	Y	Z	S	R	W	S	K	T	B	V	C	N	J	X	Y	T	X	M	T
R	S	N	D	S	I	T	R	G	F	N	E	T	E	K	Z	I	N	O	E
T	I	C	D	U	D	U	B	O	C	M	H	M	X	G	T	O	S	C	L
N	U	E	M	P	E	P	R	K	T	L	A	A	E	A	I	N	M	R	E
O	M	A	B	L	E	Q	S	N	U	C	L	E	I	N	A	T	C	A	K
C	J	D	E	J	T	S	I	N	O	G	A	T	N	A	T	R	V	S	S
N	O	D	M	S	Y	N	A	P	T	I	C	Y	Q	E	P	J	H	U	S

Crossword

Across
2. NUCLEI
4. HEAT
7. SUPINATION
8. MUSCLES
10. CYLINDRICAL
12. EPIMYSIUM
13. CONTRACTILITY
14. BUTTOCK
15. CHEEK
16. BONE

Down
1. TENDONS
3. FOUR
5. ANTAGONIST
6. VOLUNTARY
9. LOCOMOTION
11. DORSIFLEXION

Fill in the blanks

1. It is the <u>bones</u> that provide the <u>framework</u> and leverage for the <u>body</u>. The muscles <u>pull</u> the bones; they can only pull, they cannot <u>push</u>. Bones cannot <u>move</u> body parts. Muscles <u>contract</u> and move the walls of viscera and <u>blood</u> vessels, cardiac <u>muscle</u> makes the <u>heart</u> beat. Energy is turned into <u>locomotion</u> by the muscles, helping to <u>drive</u> the body.

2. Notwithstanding the continuous <u>downward</u> pull of <u>gravity</u>, the body maintains an <u>erect</u> or seated <u>posture</u> as a result of the <u>continuous</u> small <u>adjustments</u> made by the skeletal muscles. The ability to <u>mobilise</u> occurs as a result of skeletal muscle activity and muscle <u>contraction</u>. When muscles <u>contract</u> they pull on the <u>tendons</u> and <u>bones</u> of the skeleton producing <u>movement</u>.

3. Muscle <u>tendons</u> play a role in <u>stabilising</u> and reinforcing the joints. During movement <u>skeletal</u> muscles pull on <u>bones</u> stabilising the <u>joints</u> of the skeleton. Skeletal muscle plays a key part in <u>protecting</u> the internal <u>organs</u>, as the visceral organs and internal <u>tissues</u> in the abdominal <u>cavity</u> are protected by <u>layers</u> of skeletal tissue inside the <u>abdominal</u> wall and floor of the <u>pelvic</u> cavity.

4. Heat <u>generation</u> is essential in <u>maintaining</u> normal body <u>temperature</u>. Skeletal <u>muscles</u> account for 40% of <u>body</u> mass, they are the <u>muscle</u> type primarily responsible for the <u>generation</u> of body heat. During muscle <u>contraction</u>, <u>adenosine</u> triphosphate is used to <u>release</u> the energy, with about 75% of its <u>energy</u> escaping as <u>heat</u>.

5. All <u>skeletal</u> muscles are <u>attached</u> at a minimum of two <u>points</u> to <u>bone</u> or other connective <u>tissue</u>. When one part of the skeleton is moved by muscle <u>contraction</u>, related parts are <u>steadied</u> by other muscles for <u>movement</u> to be effective. The <u>origin</u> of a muscle is on the <u>stationary</u> bone where it begins, and the muscle <u>ends</u> at an insertion on the <u>bone</u> that moves. Muscles can be named according to <u>size</u>, shape, <u>location</u> and number of origins, associated <u>bones</u> and the action of the muscle.

6. There are usually at least <u>two</u> opposing muscles, <u>agonist</u> and <u>antagonist</u>, acting on a <u>joint</u> bringing about movement in <u>opposite</u> directions. An agonist or <u>prime mover</u> is a muscle mainly responsible for producing an <u>action</u>; an <u>antagonist</u> of a prime mover causes muscle <u>movement</u> in the opposite <u>direction</u>.

Multiple choice answers

1. (a), 2. (c), 3. (b), 4. (d), 5. (b), 6. (a), 7. (b), 8. (c), 9. (a), 10. (a)

Chapter 7

1.

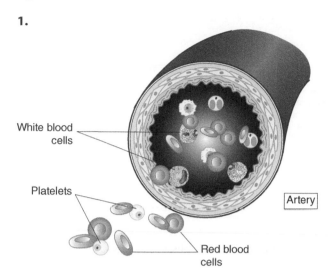

White blood cells

Platelets

Artery

Red blood cells

2.

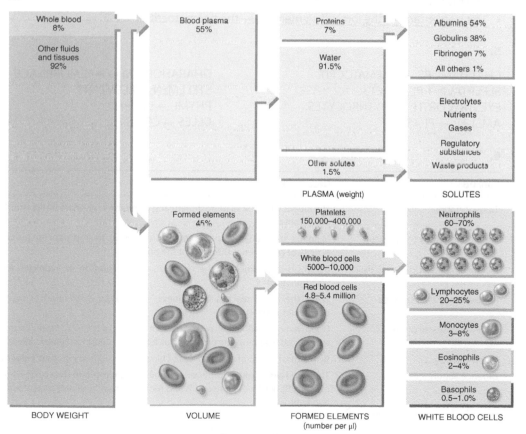

Components of blood

3.

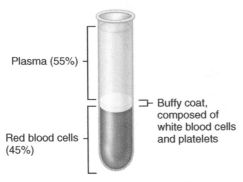

Appearance of centrifuged blood

4.

- Blood is a fluid → connective tissue
- Blood contains formed elements → such as red blood cells, white blood cells, platelets
- The fluid portion is → plasma
- Between the plasma and erythrocytes in a centrifuged sample lies → the buffy coat
- The buffy coat consists of → white blood cells and platelets
- The percentage of the formed elements is → the haematocrit

416

5.

CHATTIAMORE → HAEMATOCRIT
SLEEPTALT → PLATELETS
EYESTRYCORTH → ERYTHROCYTES
AMSLAP → PLASMA

GHARAHOREEM → HAEMORRHAGE
STEELMEN → ELEMENTS
PHYML → LYMPH
CLLES → CELLS

6.

Function	Description
Transportation	The means whereby all nourishment and respiratory gases are transported to and away from cells
Maintaining body temperature	Maintain the body temperature by distributing heat produced by chemical activity of cells evenly, throughout the body
Maintaining the acid–base balance	Blood pH maintained by the excretion or reabsorption of hydrogen ions and bicarbonate ions
Regulation of fluid balance	When the blood reaches the kidneys, excess fluid is excreted or reabsorbed maintaining fluid balance
Removal of waste products	Blood removes all waste products from tissues and cells. Waste products are transported to appropriate organs for excretion, such as lungs, kidneys, intestine, skin
Blood clotting	By the mechanism of clotting, loss of blood cells and body fluids is prevented
Defence action	The blood aids against the invasion of microorganisms and their toxins due to the phagocytic action of neutrophils and monocytes and the presence of antibodies and antitoxins

7.

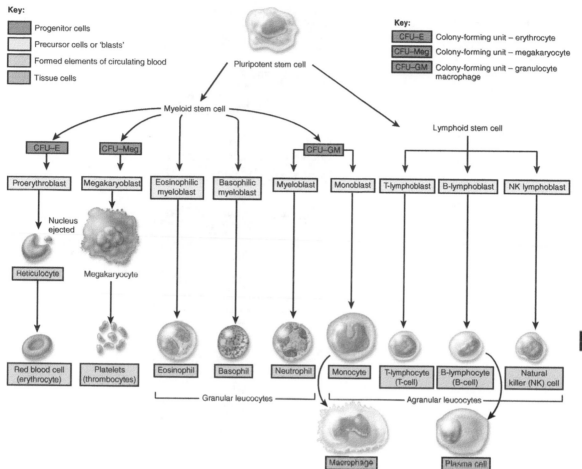

Key:
- ▮ Progenitor cells
- ▯ Precursor cells or 'blasts'
- ▮ Formed elements of circulating blood
- ▮ Tissue cells

Key:
- CFU–E Colony-forming unit – erythrocyte
- CFU–Meg Colony-forming unit – megakaryocyte
- CFU–GM Colony-forming unit – granulocyte macrophage

8.

- Blood helps to maintain the body temperature by → distributing heat produced by chemical activity of cells evenly, throughout the body
- By the mechanism of clotting → loss of blood cells and body fluids is prevented
- The process by which formed elements of blood develop is known as → haemopoiesis
- Multipotent stem cells divide into myeloid and lymphoid stem cells in the bone marrow → in order to produce blood cells
- Myeloid stem cells further subdivide in the bone marrow producing → erythrocytes
- T-lymphocytes continue their development → in the thymus and may then migrate to other lymph tissues

9.

TIPTOENUTML → MULTIPOTENT
METS → STEM
ORWARM → MARROW
DIMELOY → MYELOID

PHYMODIL → LYMPHOID
GCLINTTO → CLOTTING
NOIS → IONS

10.

8 μm

Surface view

Sectioned view

RBC shape

11.

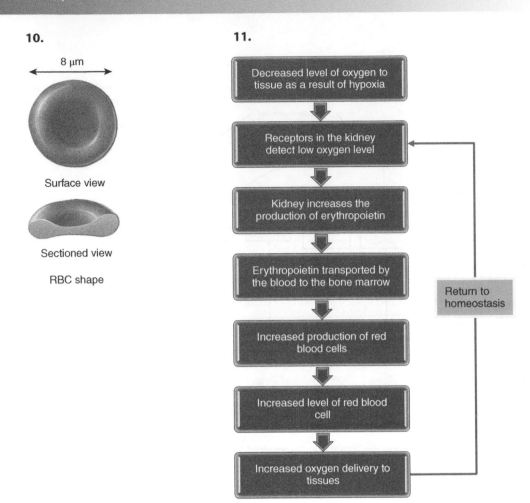

Decreased level of oxygen to tissue as a result of hypoxia

Receptors in the kidney detect low oxygen level

Kidney increases the production of erythropoietin

Erythropoietin transported by the blood to the bone marrow

Increased production of red blood cells

Increased level of red blood cell

Increased oxygen delivery to tissues

Return to homeostasis

12.

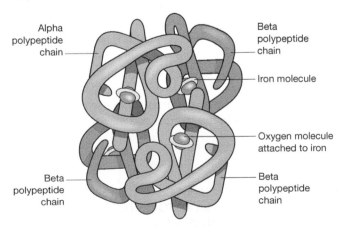

Alpha polypeptide chain

Beta polypeptide chain

Iron molecule

Oxygen molecule attached to iron

Beta polypeptide chain

Beta polypeptide chain

13.

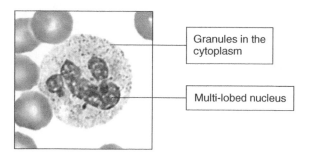

Granules in the cytoplasm

Multi-lobed nucleus

14.

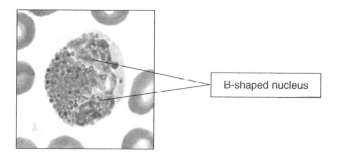

B-shaped nucleus

15.

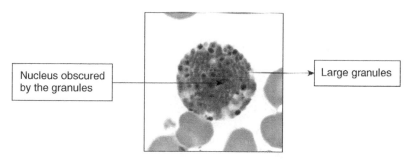

Nucleus obscured by the granules

Large granules

16.

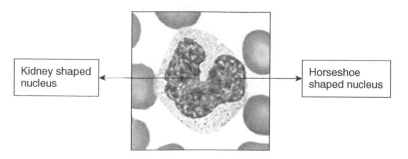

Kidney shaped nucleus

Horseshoe shaped nucleus

17.

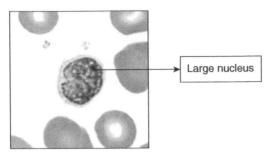

Large nucleus

18.

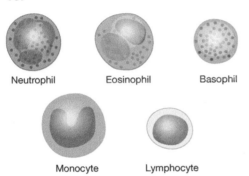

Neutrophil   Eosinophil   Basophil

Monocyte   Lymphocyte

19.

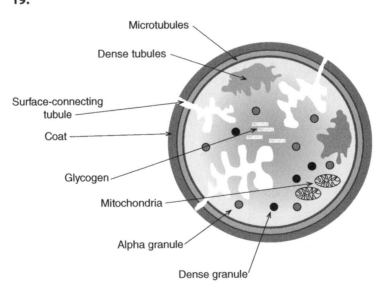

Microtubules

Dense tubules

Surface-connecting tubule

Coat

Glycogen

Mitochondria

Alpha granule

Dense granule

20.

Factor	Common name
I	Fibrinogen
II	Prothrombin
V	Proaccelerin, labile factor
VII	Proconvertin
VIII	Antihaemophilic factor A
IX	Antihaemophilic factor B
X	Thrombokinase, Stuart–Prower factor
XI	Antihaemophilic factor C
XII	Hageman factor
XIII	Fibrin stabilising factor

21.

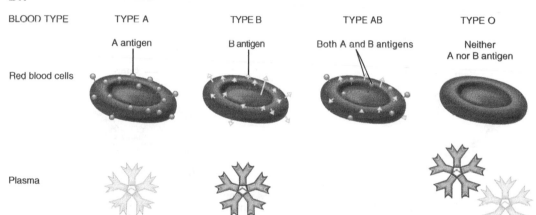

22.

Blood type	Antigens	Antibodies	Can donate blood to	Can receive blood from
A	Antigen A	Anti-B	A, AB	A, O
B	Antigen B	Anti-A	B, AB	B, O
AB	Antigen A and Antigen B	None	AB	A, B, AB, O
O	None	Anti-A and Anti-B	A, B, AB, O	O

23.

- The most abundant blood cells are the → erythrocytes
- Blood cells are produced in the → bone marrow
- Haemoglobin is composed of the protein, globin, bound to the iron-containing pigment called → haem
- All white blood cells migrate from the blood vessel by a process known as → emigration
- Platelets are produced in the bone marrow from → megakaryocytes
- On the surface of the red cells are markers called → antigens

24.

SNIGENTA → ANTIGENS   BIACEVONC → BICONCAVE
STEELLTAP → PLATELETS   RAGURANL → GRANULAR
COMSTONEY → MONOCYTES   LOGANUCOATI → COAGULATION
BOILSPHAS → BASOPHILS   RUSHES → RHESUS

25.

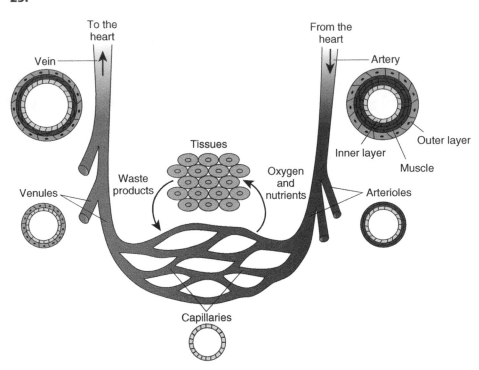

26.

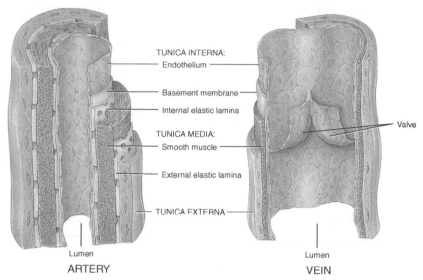

TUNICA INTERNA:
Endothelium

Basement membrane

Internal elastic lamina

TUNICA MEDIA:
Smooth muscle

External elastic lamina

TUNICA EXTERNA

Valve

Lumen
ARTERY

Lumen
VEIN

27.

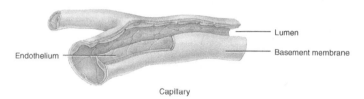

Lumen

Basement membrane

Endothelium

Capillary

28.

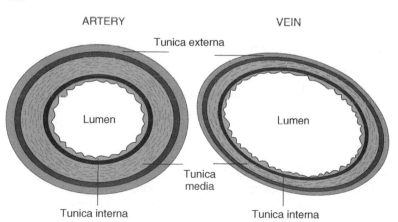

ARTERY

VEIN

Tunica externa

Lumen

Lumen

Tunica
media

Tunica interna

Tunica interna

29.

Arteries	Veins
Transport blood away from the heart	Transport blood to the heart
Carry oxygenated blood, except the umbilical and pulmonary arteries	Carry deoxygenated blood, except the umbilical and pulmonary veins
Have a narrow lumen	Have a wider lumen
Have more elastic tissue	Have less elastic tissue
Do not have valves	Have valves
Transport blood under pressure	Transport blood under low pressure

30.

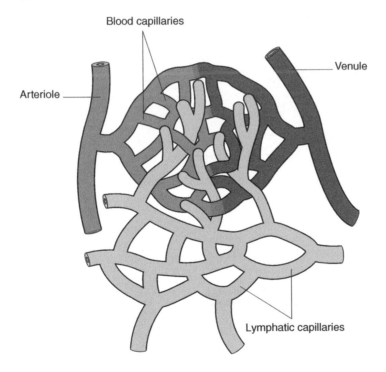

31.

- Arteries → carry the blood away from the heart
- Veins → carry blood from the capillaries back towards the heart
- Capillaries → enable the exchange of water, nutrients and chemicals between the blood and the tissues
- Capillaries are → tiny, thin-walled vessels acting as a bridge between arteries and veins
- The lymphatic system begins with very small, closed-end vessels called → lymphatic capillaries
- The lymphocytes in lymph nodes filter out → harmful substances from lymph

32.

PARCELSILIA → CAPILLARIES
RATERY → ARTERY
NEIV → VEIN
PHYLM → LYMPH
NOXGATEDEY → OXYGENATED
SALVEV → VALVES
SLAPAM → PLASMA
TRIFLATE → FILTRATE

Snap shot
Varicosities

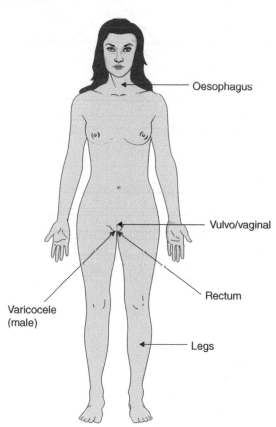

Oesophagus

Vulvo/vaginal

Rectum

Varicocele
(male)

Legs

Word search

R	N	F	J	Q	T	N	I	T	E	I	O	P	O	R	H	T	Y	R	E
Y	S	E	S	L	I	H	P	O	S	A	B	M	I	K	S	G	I	C	B
B	Z	Q	S	I	S	E	I	O	P	O	M	E	A	H	L	B	P	J	Q
X	I	H	P	M	Y	L	E	L	L	E	U	C	O	C	Y	T	E	S	B
P	L	A	S	M	A	I	S	E	T	Y	C	O	B	M	O	R	H	T	E
E	E	U	O	G	F	Q	G	N	T	I	R	C	O	T	A	M	E	A	H
O	V	A	S	O	C	O	N	S	T	R	I	C	T	I	O	N	N	S	Z
S	M	R	E	Y	H	S	L	I	H	P	O	R	T	U	E	N	E	N	L
I	H	H	T	C	W	S	F	O	O	F	G	I	E	L	U	T	N	S	M
N	A	B	Y	A	N	N	C	S	W	Y	O	O	J	P	Y	S	E	L	I
O	E	I	C	P	A	I	L	L	I	V	S	D	X	C	Z	I	X	Q	T
P	M	C	O	I	R	F	Q	Q	E	U	Q	C	O	S	D	U	S	I	E
H	O	O	R	L	T	Z	S	I	S	O	T	Y	C	O	G	A	H	P	Y
I	G	N	H	L	E	E	N	E	B	L	R	E	B	B	S	V	X	X	B
L	L	C	T	A	R	C	H	Y	X	A	I	I	H	U	Y	T	J	L	S
S	O	A	Y	R	Y	R	P	Z	K	R	T	P	O	Q	L	T	F	G	M
Y	B	V	R	I	R	C	E	A	H	N	P	L	A	T	E	L	E	T	S
T	I	E	E	E	P	X	G	Y	A	A	S	E	T	Y	C	O	N	O	M
E	N	R	C	S	X	E	N	C	O	A	G	U	L	A	T	I	O	N	I
O	I	P	B	J	M	S	N	E	G	I	T	N	A	D	K	W	M	Q	E

426

Crossword

Across
2. PLATELETS
4. THYMUS
6. ANTIGENS
10. HEART
11. THROMBOCYTES
14. VASOCONSTRICTION
16. LYMPH
17. HAEM
18. EMIGRATION

Down
1. SPLEEN
3. LEUCOCYTES
5. HAEMATOCRIT
7. HAEMOGLOBIN
8. BUFFY
9. THROMBOXANES
10. HAEMOPOIESIS
12. MEGAKARYOCYTES
13. ERYTHROCYTES
15. PLASMA

Fill in the blanks

1. The circulatory system includes the <u>heart</u>, the <u>blood</u>, the blood <u>vessels</u> and the <u>lymphatic</u> system. The blood vessels <u>transport</u> blood throughout the <u>body</u>. Blood consists of <u>formed</u> elements and a fluid <u>portion</u>, plasma. Blood has many functions, including <u>transportation</u> of <u>nutrients</u>, respiratory gases such as oxygen and carbon dioxide, <u>metabolic</u> waste such as <u>urea</u> and uric acid, <u>hormones</u>, electrolytes and antibodies. Circulation of blood occurs through a network of blood <u>vessels</u> leading away from and returning to the <u>heart</u>.

2. Blood is a <u>fluid</u> connective tissue, consisting of formed <u>elements</u> such red blood <u>cells</u>, white <u>blood</u> cells, <u>platelets</u>, and a fluid portion, <u>plasma</u>.

3. The process by which formed elements of blood develop is called <u>haemopoiesis</u>. In the last three months of gestation and throughout <u>life</u>, the red bone <u>marrow</u> is the primary centre for haemopoiesis. In order to produce blood cells, <u>multipotent</u> stem cells divide into <u>myeloid</u> and <u>lymphoid</u> stem cells in the bone marrow. Myeloid stem cells further subdivide in the bone marrow producing red blood cells, <u>platelets</u> (thrombocytes), <u>basophils</u>, eosinophils, neutrophils and <u>monocytes</u>. Lymphoid <u>stem</u> cells begin the development in the <u>bone</u> marrow as B- and T-<u>lymphocytes</u>. B-lymphocytes continue development in bone marrow, prior to migrating to <u>lymph</u> nodes, spleen or tonsils. T-lymphocytes continue their development in the <u>thymus</u> and may then <u>migrate</u> to other lymph tissues.

4. The most abundant blood cells are the <u>erythrocytes</u>; they are biconcave discs containing oxygen-carrying protein, <u>haemoglobin</u>. They live for around <u>120</u> days. Young red blood cells contain a <u>nucleus</u>; however, in a <u>mature</u> red blood cell the nucleus is <u>absent</u> and the cell has no <u>organelles</u>, this increases the <u>oxygen</u>-carrying capacity of the red blood cell.

5. White blood cells, also called <u>leucocytes</u>, only circulate for a <u>short</u> portion of their life span, spending most of their life span <u>migrating</u> through dense and loose <u>connective</u> tissues. All white blood cells migrate from the blood vessel by a process known as <u>emigration</u>. Some of the white blood cells are capable of <u>phagocytosis</u> – the neutrophils, eosinophils and <u>monocytes</u>.

6. Platelets are small blood cells, consisting of some <u>cytoplasm</u> surrounded by a plasma <u>membrane</u>, produced in the bone marrow from megakaryocytes; fragments break off to form platelets. They are around 2–4 μm in <u>diameter</u> without a <u>nucleus</u>, living for approximately 5–9 days. Platelets have a role to play in preventing blood <u>loss</u> by the formation of platelet <u>plugs</u>, sealing <u>holes</u> in blood vessels, <u>releasing</u> chemicals and aiding blood <u>clotting</u>.

7. The red blood cells define which blood <u>group</u> a person belongs to. On the <u>surface</u> of the red cells are antigens. Apart from identical twins, each person has different <u>antigens</u>, these identify blood types. The <u>ABO</u> system is the system used for defining blood groups. If an individual has blood group A, then they have <u>A</u> antigens covering their red cells. Group B has <u>B</u> antigens on their red blood <u>cell</u>; while group <u>O</u> has neither <u>antigen</u> and group <u>AB</u> has <u>both</u> antigens.

427

Multiple choice answers

1. (b), 2. (b), 3. (a), 4. (c), 5. (d), 6. (d), 7. (b), 8. (a), 9. (d), 10. (b)

Chapter 8

1.

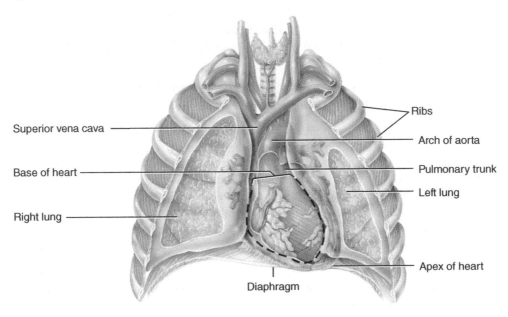

Superior vena cava

Base of heart

Right lung

Ribs

Arch of aorta

Pulmonary trunk

Left lung

Apex of heart

Diaphragm

2.

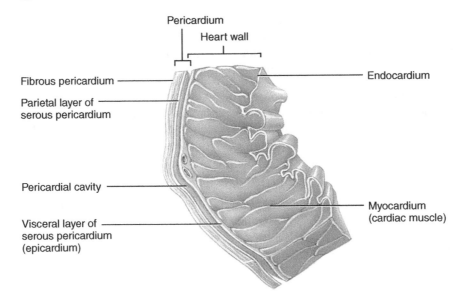

Pericardium

Heart wall

Fibrous pericardium

Parietal layer of
serous pericardium

Pericardial cavity

Visceral layer of
serous pericardium
(epicardium)

Endocardium

Myocardium
(cardiac muscle)

3.

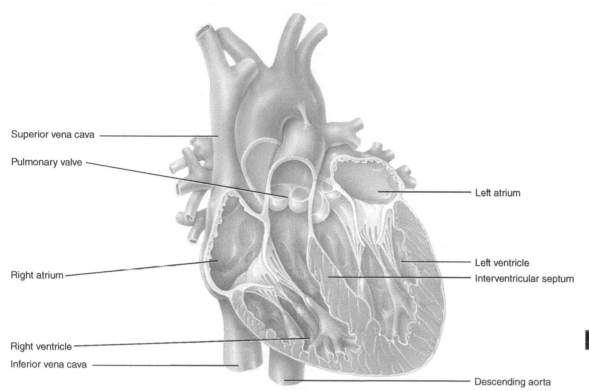

Superior vena cava

Pulmonary valve

Left atrium

Right atrium

Left ventricle

Interventricular septum

Right ventricle

Inferior vena cava

Descending aorta

4.

- The apex of the heart is below → the base of the heart, lying on the diaphragm
- Between the parietal and visceral pericardium is a thin film of pericardial fluid → this reduces friction as the heart moves during its cycle of contraction and relaxation
- The bulk of muscle in the heart is → the myocardium
- The atria are → the smaller chambers of the heart
- The atrioventricular valves → prevent the backward flow of blood from the ventricles into the atria
- The interventicular septum → divides the ventricles

5.

RATIONEXAL → RELAXATION
ARATI → ATRIA
SERVENTICL → VENTRICLES
DECARUMRIPI → PERICARDIUM

DECORUMNADI → ENDOCARDIUM
DACOMRUMIY → MYOCARDIUM
DISCUTRIP → TRICUSPID
DISCUBIP → BICUSPID

6.

Artery	Major branches	Area of the heart supplied
Left anterior descending (LAD)	Diagonals Septals	Front and side of the left ventricle, apex of the heart
Circumflex artery	Oblique marginal	Back and side of the left ventricle
Right coronary artery (RCA)	Posterior descending artery	Right ventricle, base of the heart and interventricular septum

7.

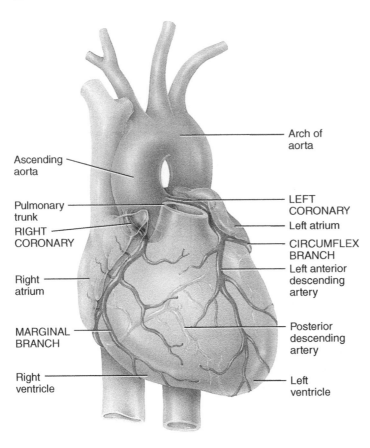

8.

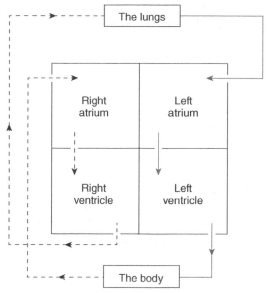

9.

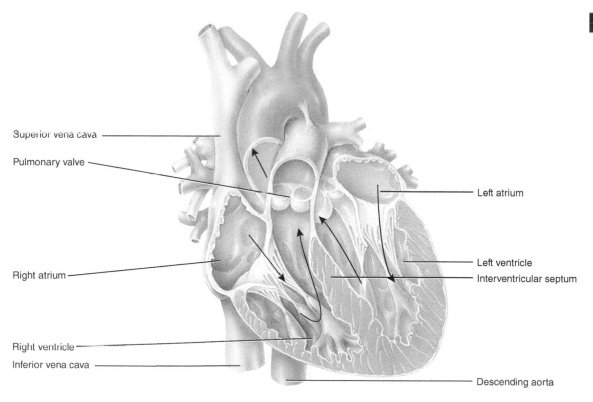

10.

CRUFMECLIX → CIRCUMFLEX
YARNCROO → CORONARY
SANCHBRE → BRANCHES
LACTIONCURI → CIRCULATION

MYSTICES → SYSTEMIC
YONEXTAGED → OXYGENATED
SEVONU → VENOUS
TRAILARE → ARTERIAL

11.

- The heart receives → approximately 5% of the body's blood supply
- The heart receives a plentiful supply of blood ensuring the constant supply of → oxygen and nutrients and the efficient removal of waste products
- The inner part of the endocardium is → supplied with blood directly from the inside of the heart chambers
- The circumflex artery supplies the → back and side of the left ventricle
- The heart is best thought of as two pumps → the right and the left pumps
- The pumps are made up of two chambers → the atrium and the ventricle, as well as their associated valves

12.

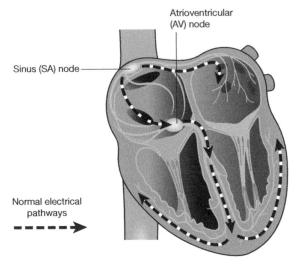

13.

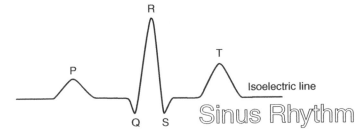

14.

ECG letter(s)	Heart electrical activity	Corresponding action
P	Atrial depolarisation	Atrial contraction
QRS	Ventricular depolarisation	Ventricular contraction (just after the peak of the R wave)
T	Ventricular repolarisation	Relaxation phase of the ventricle Atrial repolarisation cannot be seen as it is hidden by the greater electrical activity of the ventricle

15.

Hormones	Action
Epinephrine	Epinephrine is a hormone secreted by the medulla of the adrenal glands. Strong emotions such as fear or anger cause epinephrine to be released into the bloodstream, which causes an increase in heart rate, muscle strength, blood pressure and sugar metabolism. Epinephrine Is used chiefly as a stimulant In cardiac arrest
Norepinephrine	This is a hormone that is produced naturally by the body and has wide-ranging effects on many areas of the body. Often it is referred to as a 'fight or flight' chemical, as it is responsible for the body's reaction to stressful situations. It normally produces effects such as increased heart rate, increased blood pressure, widening of pupils, widening of airways in the lungs and narrowing of blood vessels in non-essential organs
Thyroid hormones	These include thyroxine (T4) and triiodothyronine (T3). Increase heart rate and contractility. These hormones affect cardiac muscle fibres in much the same way as norepinephrine by the sympathetic nervous system; they increase both heart rate and contractility

433

16.

- The cardiac cycle refers to → the mechanical activity of the heart
- Systole corresponds to → the contraction of a heart chamber (atrium or ventricle).
- Diastole corresponds to → the relaxation of a heart chamber (atrium or ventricle).
- 'Cardiac output' is a term relating to → the amount of blood the heart pumps out in one minute
- Heart rate is controlled by two main mechanisms: → the autononomic nervous system and hormone activity
- Baroreceptors are specialised mechanical receptors located → in the carotid sinus and the aortic arch, sensitive to the amount of stretch in these blood vessels

17.

REALTICCLE → ELECTRICAL
TUPTUO → OUTPUT
ROTACID → CAROTID
LAIDPOORSATINE → DEPOLARISATION

SADLIETO → DIASTOLE
YESLSTO → SYSTOLE
CAUTIONMO → AUTONOMIC

Snap shot
Taking a patient's pulse
Sites that may be used to assess a person's pulse

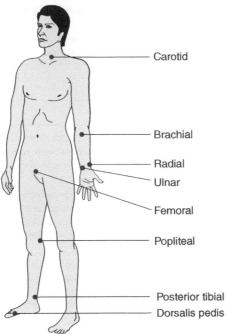

- Carotid
- Brachial
- Radial
- Ulnar
- Femoral
- Popliteal
- Posterior tibial
- Dorsalis pedis

Definitions

Term	Definition
Asystole	Complete absence of electrical and mechanical activity in the heart
Bradycardia	Heart rate less than 60 beats per minute
Tachycardia	Describes a rapid heartbeat of 100 beats per minute or more at rest
Arrhythmia	Irregular heart rhythm
Sinus rhythm	In health, the rhythm of the pulse is regular and is termed sinus rythm
Fibrillation	Rapid and irregular contractions of the heart. In fibrillation the heart fails to continue as a pump. This can be life threatening, and must always be reported

Word search

D	S	E	P	T	U	M	M	U	I	D	R	A	C	I	R	E	P	H	Q
H	I	M	R	G	N	R	M	R	J	G	C	X	K	A	P	E	F	W	D
O	W	P	G	M	X	J	Y	R	M	E	D	I	A	S	T	I	N	U	M
R	S	G	S	K	X	I	L	X	L	D	T	F	I	E	I	D	L	S	V
W	T	L	V	U	G	T	Q	L	E	X	M	R	P	T	C	I	J	T	O
C	N	W	J	A	C	R	A	T	K	T	D	I	I	O	G	Q	L	S	R
P	L	K	A	N	Z	I	A	Z	S	E	N	F	R	C	D	V	E	Y	D
S	L	H	J	O	R	N	B	E	N	E	X	O	A	H	U	N	C	E	Z
V	Z	F	K	F	F	W	I	D	P	L	N	I	O	H	O	S	K	J	N
L	Q	H	T	G	S	C	O	H	D	A	K	F	F	M	K	A	P	N	X
B	I	R	Y	G	I	C	R	H	R	Q	Q	I	R	D	A	T	R	I	A
W	A	X	C	R	A	I	O	Y	W	K	I	O	L	K	U	I	V	K	D
I	O	A	T	R	N	F	L	Z	X	W	H	H	X	A	V	X	C	R	I
G	N	N	D	E	T	A	N	E	G	Y	X	O	E	D	H	E	E	U	E
Q	E	I	B	D	V	E	N	O	U	S	G	A	Y	W	I	S	P	P	D
V	U	S	Y	B	M	M	M	Y	O	C	A	R	D	I	U	M	B	F	A
M	G	F	H	U	Q	Y	S	X	C	D	Y	I	X	V	G	T	Z	A	M
O	M	M	X	D	E	P	O	L	A	R	I	S	A	T	I	O	N	X	B
O	E	N	I	X	O	R	Y	H	T	N	T	H	F	M	A	R	I	W	M
D	S	I	H	U	E	N	Z	M	J	J	D	C	S	N	J	L	Y	B	B

435

Crossword

Across
1. AORTA
4. FIST
9. BARORECEPTORS
11. ATRIA
14. SEPTUM
16. CARDIOREGULATORY
17. PERICARDIUM
19. LEFT
21. FOUR
22. STERNUM
23. LUNG

Down
2. TRICUSPID
3. ATHEROSCLEROTIC
5. THORACIC
6. CONTRACT
7. ELECTRIC
8. HIS
10. MYOCARDIUM
12. ENDOCARDIUM
13. TWO
15. MITRAL
17. PURKINJE
18. CORONARY
20. ADRENAL

Fill in the blanks

1. The heart is made up of <u>four</u> chambers, two atria and <u>two</u> ventricles. Deoxygenated <u>blood</u> returns to the <u>right</u> side of the heart via the <u>venous</u> circulation. It is <u>pumped</u> into the right <u>ventricle</u> and then to the <u>lungs</u> where carbon <u>dioxide</u> is <u>released</u> and <u>oxygen</u> is absorbed. The oxygenated blood then travels back to the <u>left</u> side of the heart into the left <u>atrium</u>, then into the left <u>ventricle</u> from where it is pumped into the <u>aorta</u> and arterial <u>circulation</u>.

2. The heart creates its own <u>electrical</u> impulses and controls the route the <u>impulses</u> take through a specialised <u>conduction</u> pathway made up of <u>five</u> elements, the <u>sino-atrial</u> node, the <u>atrio-ventricular</u> node, the bundle of <u>His</u>, the left and right bundle branches and the <u>Purkinje</u> fibres.

3. Epinephrine is a <u>hormone</u> secreted by the <u>medulla</u> of the adrenal <u>glands</u>. Strong <u>emotions</u>, such as fear or <u>anger</u>, cause <u>epinephrine</u> to be released into the <u>bloodstream</u>, which causes an <u>increase</u> in heart rate, muscle <u>strength</u>, blood <u>pressure</u> and sugar <u>metabolism</u>. Epinephrine is used chiefly as a <u>stimulant</u> in <u>cardiac</u> arrest. <u>Thyroxine</u> released in large quantities has the effect of <u>increasing</u> the heart <u>rate</u>.

Multiple choice answers

1. (d), 2. (d), 3. (d), 4. (a), 5. (b), 6. (a), 7. (b), 8. (a), 9. (d), 10. (c)

Chapter 9

1.

Function	Description
Ingestion	Taking food into the digestive system
Propulsion	Moving the food along the length of the digestive system
Digestion	Breaking down food. This can be achieved *mechanically* as food is chewed or moved through the digestive system, or *chemically* by the action of *enzymes* mixed with the food as it moves through the digestive system
Absorption	The products of digestion exit the digestive system and enter the blood or lymph capillaries for distribution to where they are required
Elimination	The waste products of digestion are excreted from the body as faeces

2.

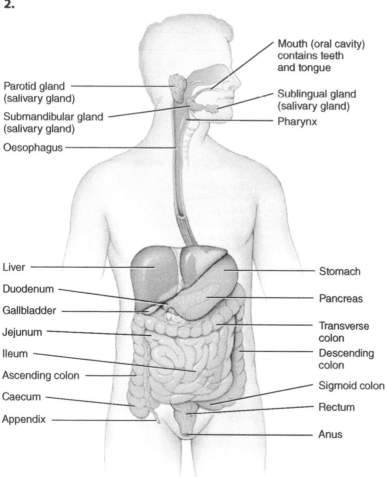

3.

Superior lip

Hard palate

Soft palate

Uvula

Cheek

Molars

Premolars

Cuspid (canine)

Incisors

Oral vestibule

Palatine tonsil

Tongue

Lingual frenulum

Opening of duct of submandibular gland

Gingivae (gums)

Inferior lip (pulled down)

Anterior view

4.

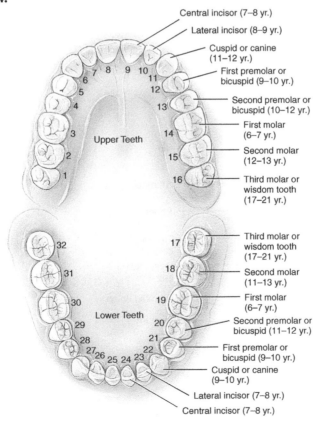

Central incisor (7–8 yr.)

Lateral incisor (8–9 yr.)

Cuspid or canine (11–12 yr.)

First premolar or bicuspid (9–10 yr.)

Second premolar or bicuspid (10–12 yr.)

First molar (6–7 yr.)

Second molar (12–13 yr.)

Third molar or wisdom tooth (17–21 yr.)

Upper Teeth

7 8 9 10
6   11
5   12
4   13
3   14
2   15
1   16

Lower Teeth

32   17
31   18
30   19
29   20
28   21
27   22
26 25 24 23

Third molar or wisdom tooth (17–21 yr.)

Second molar (11–13 yr.)

First molar (6–7 yr.)

Second premolar or bicuspid (11–12 yr.)

First premolar or bicuspid (9–10 yr.)

Cuspid or canine (9–10 yr.)

Lateral incisor (7–8 yr.)

Central incisor (7–8 yr.)

Permanent (secondary) dentition

5.

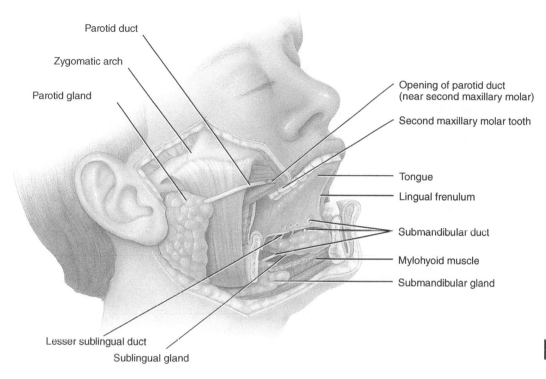

Parotid duct

Zygomatic arch

Parotid gland

Opening of parotid duct
(near second maxillary molar)

Second maxillary molar tooth

Tongue

Lingual frenulum

Submandibular duct

Mylohyoid muscle

Submandibular gland

Lesser sublingual duct

Sublingual gland

6.

1. What does saliva contain?
Saliva contains:
- water
- salivary amylase
- mucus
- mineral salts
- lysozyme
- immunoglobulins
- blood clotting factors.

2. What are the functions of saliva?
- Salivary amylase is a digestive enzyme responsible for beginning the breakdown of carbohydrate molecules from complex polysaccharides to the disaccharide maltase.
- The fluid nature of saliva helps to moisten and lubricate food making it easier to hold the food in the mouth, also assisting in forming the food into a bolus in preparation for swallowing.
- The continuous secretion of saliva is cleansing, a lack of moisture can lead to oral mucosal infections and formation of mouth ulcers.
- Lysozyme, a constituent of saliva, has an antibacterial action. Immunoglobulin and clotting factors also contribute to the prevention of infection.
- Taste is only possible when food substances are moist. Saliva is required to moisten food.

3. What is the pH of saliva?
5.8–7.4

4. In health what volume of saliva is produced daily?
1–1.5 L

7.

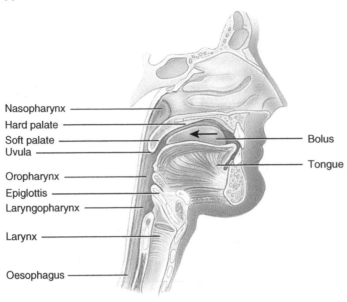

Nasopharynx

Hard palate

Soft palate

Uvula

Oropharynx

Epiglottis

Laryngopharynx

Larynx

Oesophagus

Bolus

Tongue

Position of structures before swallowing

8.

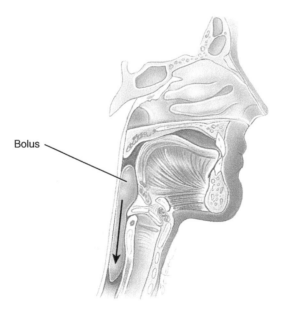

Bolus

During the pharyngeal stage of swallowing

9.

- The tongue is a large → voluntary muscular structure which occupies much of the oral cavity
- The palate → forms the roof of the mouth and consists of two parts: the hard palate and the soft palate
- The parotid glands are the largest of the salivary glands and are → located anterior to the ears
- The activity of the parasympathetic fibres → leads to an increased production of saliva in response to the sight, smell or taste of food
- The pharynx consists of → three parts
- The food bolus leaves the oropharynx → and enters the oesophagus

10.

LUPISPORON → PROPULSION

LAXIAML → MAXILLA

VASAIL → SALIVA

LAMESAY → AMYLASE

YESYMOLZ → LYSOZYME

GASHOSOUPE → OESOPHAGUS

XNYRAHP → PHARYNX

USLOB → BOLUS

11.

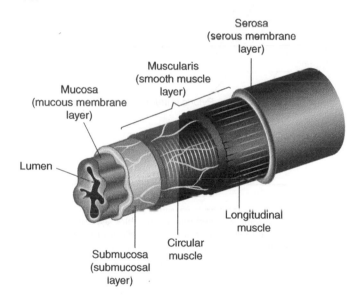

12.

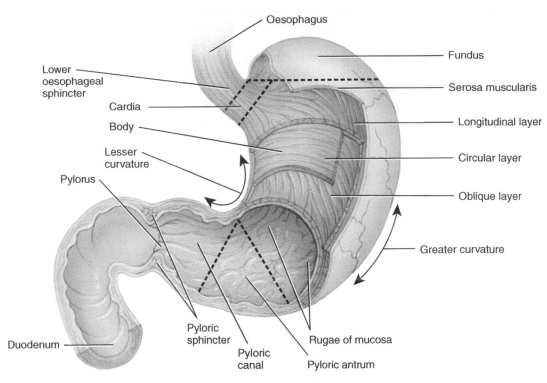

Anterior view of regions of stomach

13.

Component	Functions
Surface mucous cells	Produce thick bicarbonate-coated mucus. This thick layer of mucus protects the stomach mucosal epithelia from corrosion by acidic gastric juice. When these cells become damaged they are quickly shed and replaced
Mucous neck cells	Also secrete mucus – this mucus is different from surface neck cell mucus
Parietal cells	Produce hydrochloric acid and intrinsic factor. Intrinsic factor is necessary for the absorption of vitamin B12. This vitamin is essential for the production of mature erythrocytes. Hydrochloric acid creates the acidic environment of the stomach (pH 1–3) and begins denaturing dietary protein in preparation for the action of pepsin
Chief cells	Produce pepsinogen which is converted to *pepsin* in the presence of hydrochloric acid. Pepsin is necessary for the breakdown of protein into smaller peptide chains
Enteroendocrine cells (G cells)	Produce a variety of hormones including *gastrin*. These hormones help regulate gastric motility

14.

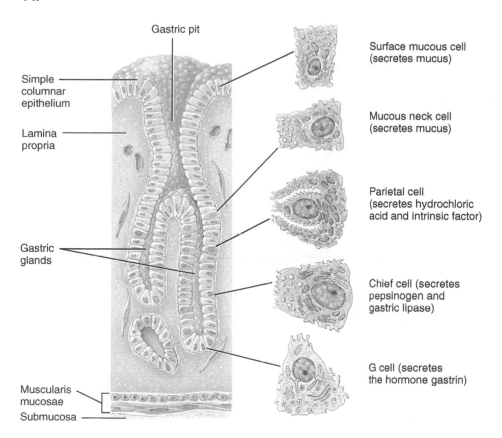

Gastric pit

Simple
columnar
epithelium

Lamina
propria

Gastric
glands

Muscularis
mucosae

Submucosa

Surface mucous cell
(secretes mucus)

Mucous neck cell
(secretes mucus)

Parietal cell
(secretes hydrochloric
acid and intrinsic factor)

Chief cell (secretes
pepsinogen and
gastric lipase)

G cell (secretes
the hormone gastrin)

15.

NOSINGPEPE → PEPSINOGEN
SHOTMAC → STOMACH
LATERPAI → PARIETAL
TIRESONCE → SECRETION

GSTARIC → GASTRIC
URAGE → RUGAE
DRCHOOYCHIRL → HYDROCHLORIC

16.

- The stomach is a muscular organ located → on the left side of the upper abdomen
- The stomach receives food from → the oesophagus
- As food reaches the end of the oesophagus, it enters the stomach through a muscular valve called → the lower oesophageal sphincter
- The stomach secretes acid → and enzymes that digest food
- Ridges of muscle tissue that line the stomach are called → rugae
- The stomach muscles contract periodically → churning food to enhance digestion

17.

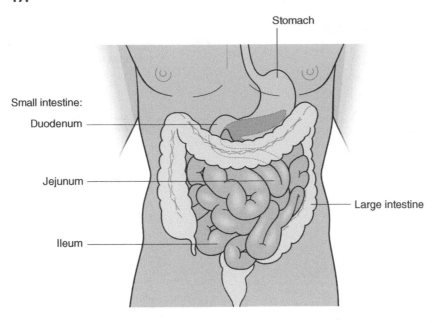

18.

Section	Function/description
The duodenum	Approximately 25 cm long. It is the entrance to the small intestine
	The duodenum is largely responsible for the breakdown of food in the small intestine, using enzymes. The duodenum wall is composed of a very thin layer of cells that form the muscularis mucosae
	The duodenum also regulates the rate of emptying of the stomach. Secretin and cholecystokinin are released from cells in the duodenal epithelium in response to acidic and fatty stimuli when the pylorus opens and releases gastric chyme into the duodenum for further digestion
The jejunum	Measures 2.5 m and is the middle part of the small intestine
	The inner surface of the jejunum, its mucous membrane, is covered in projections called villi, these increase the surface area of tissue available to absorb nutrients from the gut contents. The transport of nutrients across epithelial cells through the jejunum and ileum includes the passive transport of fructose and the active transport of amino acids, small peptides, vitamins and most glucose
The ileum	Measures 3.5 m. It meets the large intestine at the ileocaecal valve. This valve prevents the backflow of the products of digestion from the large intestine back into the small intestine
	The final and longest segment of the small intestine, specifically responsible for the absorption of vitamin B12 and the reabsorption of conjugated bile salts. The smooth muscle of the ileum is thinner than the walls of other parts of the intestine, peristaltic contractions are slower

19.

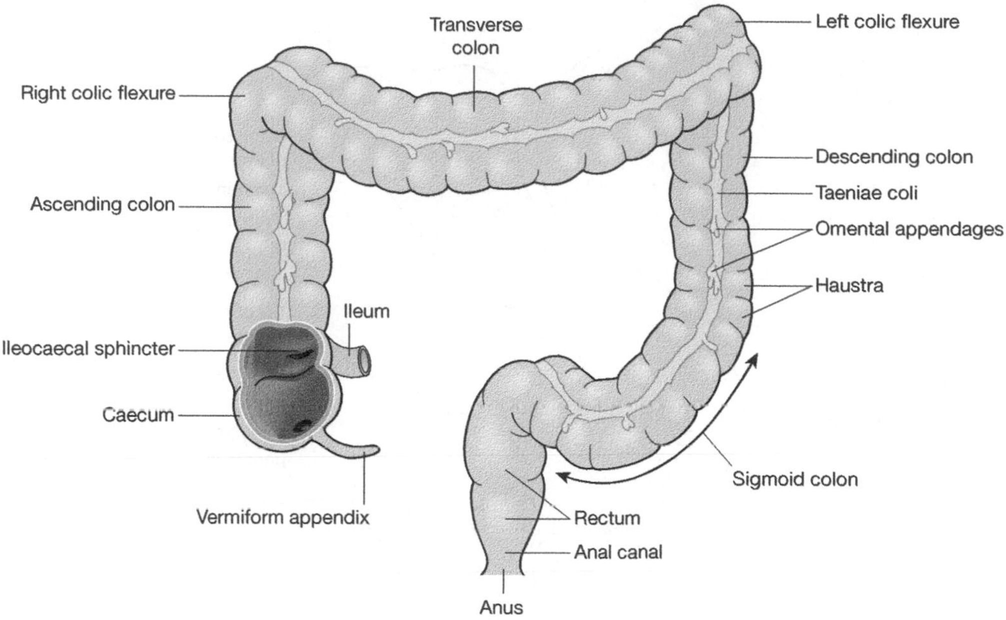

20.

- The small intestine consists of → three sections
- The first section of the small intestine is called → the duodenum
- The large intestine consists of → four sections
- The large intestine mucosa contains large numbers of goblet cells that secrete mucus to → ease the passage of faeces and protect the walls of the colon
- The simple columnar epithelium changes to stratified squamous epithelium at the → anal canal
- The large intestine absorbs → some vitamins, minerals, electrolytes and drugs

21.

MUDDUONE → DUODENUM
MILEU → ILEUM
NUMEJJU → JEJUNUM
TINESCRE → SECRETIN

LIVLI → VILLI
AMUCEC → CAECUM
SAFECE → FAECES
BLOGET → GOBLET

22.

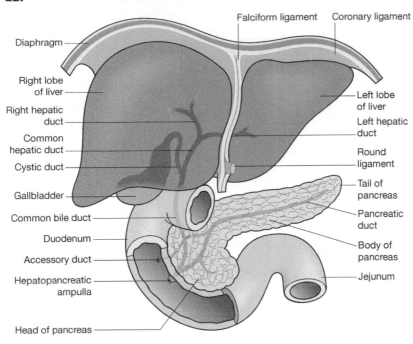

Falciform ligament

Coronary ligament

Diaphragm

Right lobe of liver

Right hepatic duct

Common hepatic duct

Cystic duct

Gallbladder

Common bile duct

Duodenum

Accessory duct

Hepatopancreatic ampulla

Head of pancreas

Left lobe of liver

Left hepatic duct

Round ligament

Tail of pancreas

Pancreatic duct

Body of pancreas

Jejunum

23.

Production and storage of bile

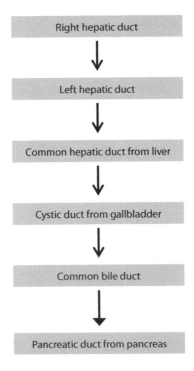

Right hepatic duct

↓

Left hepatic duct

↓

Common hepatic duct from liver

↓

Cystic duct from gallbladder

↓

Common bile duct

↓

Pancreatic duct from pancreas

24.

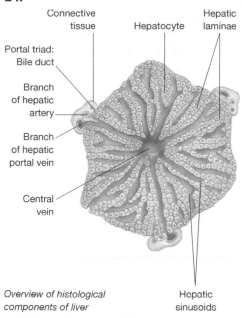

Connective tissue   Hepatocyte   Hepatic laminae

Portal triad:
Bile duct

Branch of hepatic artery

Branch of hepatic portal vein

Central vein

Overview of histological components of liver

Hepatic sinusoids

25.

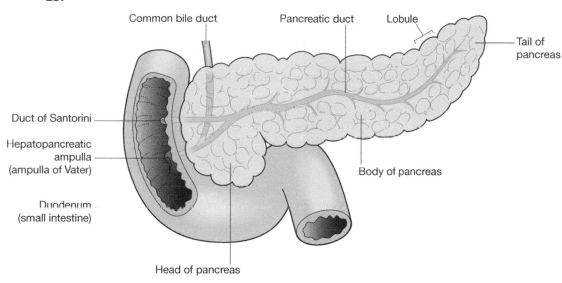

Common bile duct   Pancreatic duct   Lobule

Tail of pancreas

Duct of Santorini

Hepatopancreatic ampulla (ampulla of Vater)

Body of pancreas

Duodenum (small intestine)

Head of pancreas

26.

- The liver is located → in the right upper quadrant
- The liver is involved in lipid metabolism, lipogenesis and → the synthesis of cholesterol
- The gallbladder functions as a → reservoir for bile
- When the walls of the gallbladder contract, bile is expelled into the cystic duct and down into the common bile duct before entering the duodenum via the → hepatopancreatic ampulla
- The cells of the pancreas are responsible for making → the endocrine and exocrine products
- Parasympathetic vagus nerve stimulation promotes → the release of pancreatic juice

27.

ELIB → BILE
PONGIISLEES → LIPOGENESIS
APHOTESTYEC → HEPATOCYTES
CHEPATI → HEPATIC

SHOOTCLLEER → CHOLESTEROL
DOCREENIN → ENDOCRINE
REXONEIC → EXOCRINE
ICEJU → JUICE

Snap shot

Drug-induced gastric irritation

Diclofenac can cause gastric or intestinal bleeding, which can be fatal.

The nurse should undertake a full assessment of Ms Hernandez's needs. The medication should not be given if the person is known to have an allergy to diclofenac and misoprostol, aspirin or any other NSAID. This medication should not be given if the patient has active bleeding in the stomach or the intestines.

Arthrotec should be used as directed by the prescriber and Ms Hernandez should be advised to follow all directions on the prescription label. The dose prescribed should be adhered to and she should not take the medicine in larger or smaller amounts or for longer than recommended.

Arthrotec should be taken with food or milk in order to reduce the risk of stomach upset. The tablet should be swallowed whole; the drug should not be crushed, broken or chewed.

Ms Hernandez should be advised not to share her medicines with anyone else, even if they have the same symptoms that she has.

If Arthrotec is used long-term, Ms Hernandez may need frequent medical tests at the general practice.

She should be reminded to store the medication at room temperature away from moisture and heat.

Word search

T	H	H	Z	G	V	I	U	S	U	G	A	H	P	O	S	E	O	C	L
E	L	C	D	K	D	N	A	L	U	C	O	S	J	D	X	N	U	Q	W
L	Y	M	A	F	G	G	S	T	C	Z	E	N	I	R	C	O	X	E	Y
B	S	K	O	M	N	E	D	I	O	M	G	I	S	L	A	U	P	R	R
O	O	R	X	S	O	S	C	C	I	B	I	D	O	B	I	A	A	V	J
G	Z	E	Y	W	T	T	D	D	K	A	E	K	B	M	R	T	O	X	T
B	Y	V	S	S	X	I	S	Z	X	N	L	U	M	O	N	H	F	I	F
Y	M	I	E	X	A	O	O	P	T	J	R	G	T	E	B	W	A	Y	S
V	E	L	N	I	M	N	O	I	T	A	N	I	M	I	L	E	E	Y	V
M	I	Z	A	M	G	O	T	Q	Z	M	D	I	C	I	Y	G	C	F	O
K	O	T	K	Y	M	I	A	T	O	C	L	F	Y	P	N	H	E	S	E
E	R	U	H	M	O	Q	U	G	V	A	O	C	J	U	G	M	S	K	C
Y	A	A	T	N	I	D	I	J	E	J	E	N	I	T	S	E	T	N	I
S	V	O	D	H	Y	D	R	O	C	H	L	O	R	I	C	F	R	O	Y
U	O	D	G	C	V	P	A	N	C	R	E	A	S	Z	Y	W	M	V	Y
O	O	M	X	I	L	E	O	C	A	E	C	A	L	B	V	K	I	B	E
C	K	B	P	U	X	Q	T	A	V	I	L	A	S	E	A	R	L	G	F
U	Y	P	C	G	U	B	O	L	U	S	N	S	C	W	X	O	I	U	F
M	G	Z	G	V	U	N	B	W	B	R	U	G	A	E	O	X	T	D	K
V	J	E	J	U	N	U	M	B	U	L	N	O	I	T	S	E	G	I	D

Crossword

Across
3. RUGAE
7. LYSOZYME
10. SUBMANDIBULAR
11. PALATE
13. PARIETAL
17. DIGESTION
18. ANUS
19. HEPATOCYTES
20. DUODENUM

Down
1. FOUR
2. PANCREAS
4. RECTUM
5. AMYLASE
6. WATER
8. ELIMINATION
9. BILE
12. THREE
14. INGESTION
15. LIVER
16. QUADRANT

449

Fill in the blanks

1. The gastrointestinal <u>tract</u> is approximately 10 <u>metres</u> long. Travelling the <u>length</u> of the <u>body</u> from the <u>mouth</u>, through the thoracic, abdominal and pelvic cavities, ending at the anus. The digestive system has one major function: to <u>convert</u> food into a form that can be utilised by the <u>cells</u> of the body.

2. The lips and <u>cheeks</u> are formed of <u>muscle</u> and <u>connective</u> tissue allowing the lips and cheeks to move <u>food</u> mixed with <u>saliva</u> around the mouth and begin <u>mechanical</u> digestion. The <u>teeth</u> contribute to mechanical digestion, chewing and mixing food with <u>saliva</u> is called <u>mastication</u>.

3. There are <u>three</u> pairs of <u>salivary</u> glands. The <u>parotid</u> glands are the largest, located anterior to the <u>ears</u>; saliva from the parotid glands enters the oral <u>cavity</u>. The <u>submandibular</u> glands are located below the <u>jaw</u> on each side of the face. <u>Sublingual</u> glands are the smallest, located in the <u>floor</u> of the mouth.

4. The food <u>bolus</u> leaves the oropharynx entering the <u>oesophagus</u>; this extends from the <u>laryngopharynx</u> to the stomach, measuring about <u>25</u> cm in length. The function is to <u>transport</u> substances. Thick <u>mucus</u> is secreted by the mucosa of the <u>oesophagus</u>, aiding the passage of the bolus, protecting the oesophagus from <u>abrasion</u>.

5. The stomach can <u>expand</u> to temporarily <u>store</u> food, partially digesting food. The <u>churning</u> action of the stomach muscles mechanically breaks down the food, acids and <u>enzymes</u> are released for <u>chemical</u> breakdown. The <u>enzyme</u> pepsin is responsible for protein breakdown. The passage of food from the stomach to the small <u>intestine</u> is controlled by the <u>pyloric</u> sphincter.

6. The small <u>intestine</u> is approximately 6 <u>metres</u> long. Here food is further broken down by <u>mechanical</u> and <u>chemical</u> digestion, and <u>absorption</u> of the products of digestion takes place. The small intestine is divided into <u>three</u> parts, <u>duodenum</u>, jejunum and <u>ileum</u>. The small intestine joins the large intestine at the <u>ileocaecal</u> valve.

7. Accessory organs of <u>digestion</u> are the <u>liver</u>, <u>gallbladder</u> and pancreas.

8. Once food residue has reached the <u>large</u> intestine it cannot flow back into the <u>ileum</u>. The large intestine measures <u>1.5</u> m in length and <u>7</u> cm in diameter. It reabsorbs <u>water</u> and maintains the <u>fluid</u> balance of the body, it absorbs certain <u>vitamins</u>, processes undigested material and <u>stores</u> waste before it is <u>eliminated</u> via the <u>anus</u>.

Multiple choice answers

1. (c), 2. (d), 3. (c), 4. (d), 5. (c), 6. (c), 7. (a), 8. (b), 9. (d), 10. (b)

Chapter 10

1.

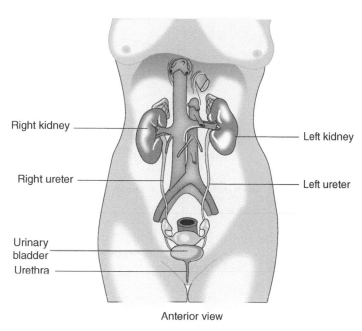

Right kidney

Left kidney

Right ureter

Left ureter

Urinary bladder

Urethra

Anterior view

2.

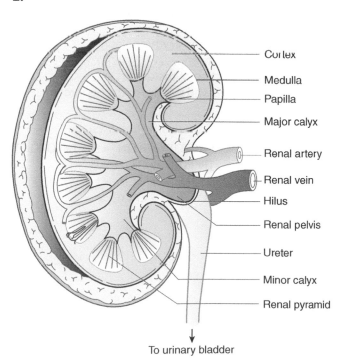

Cortex

Medulla

Papilla

Major calyx

Renal artery

Renal vein

Hilus

Renal pelvis

Ureter

Minor calyx

Renal pyramid

↓

To urinary bladder

3.

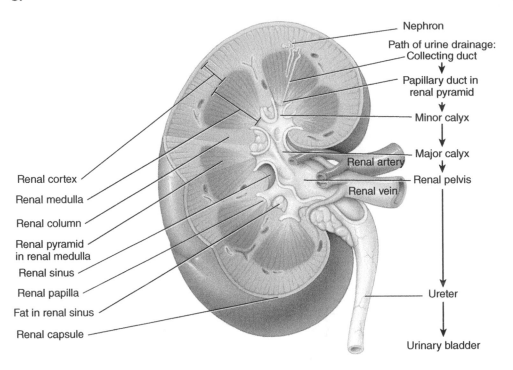

Nephron

Path of urine drainage:
Collecting duct
↓
Papillary duct in
renal pyramid
↓
Minor calyx
↓
Major calyx
↓
Renal pelvis

Renal artery

Renal vein

Renal cortex

Renal medulla

Renal column

Renal pyramid
in renal medulla

Renal sinus

Renal papilla

Fat in renal sinus

Renal capsule

Ureter
↓
Urinary bladder

4.

- The kidneys play an important role in → maintaining homeostasis
- The kidneys have → an endocrine function
- Hormones secreted by the kidneys include → renin and erythropoietin
- The renal cortex → is the outermost part of the kidney
- The renal pelvis → forms the expanded upper portion of the ureter
- The medulla has → an abundance of blood vessels and tubules of the nephrons

5.

DELLAMU → MEDULLA
SPLIVE → PELVIS
LIFTRATION → FILTRATION
BAPTISRONREO → REABSORPTION

PHOTOTYRERIEIN → ERYTHROPOIETIN
TREEUR → URETER
CASAFI → FASCIA
SLYCACE → CALYCES

6.

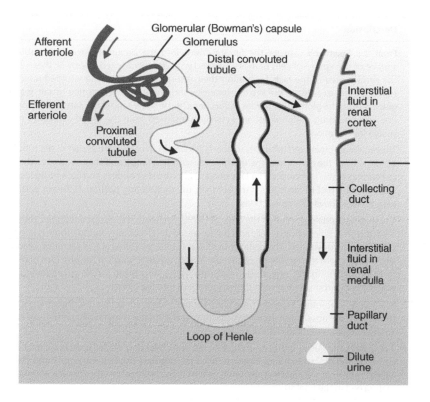

Afferent arteriole

Glomerular (Bowman's) capsule

Glomerulus

Distal convoluted tubule

Efferent arteriole

Proximal convoluted tubule

Interstitial fluid in renal cortex

Collecting duct

Interstitial fluid in renal medulla

Papillary duct

Loop of Henle

Dilute urine

7.

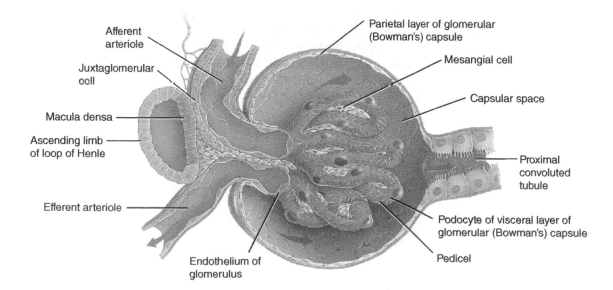

Afferent arteriole

Juxtaglomerular ooll

Macula densa

Ascending limb of loop of Henle

Efferent arteriole

Endothelium of glomerulus

Parietal layer of glomerular (Bowman's) capsule

Mesangial cell

Capsular space

Proximal convoluted tubule

Podocyte of visceral layer of glomerular (Bowman's) capsule

Pedicel

8.

Component	Description
Proximal convoluted tubule	From the Bowman's capsule, the filtrate drains into the proximal convoluted tubule. The surface of the epithelial cells here are covered with densely packed microvilli; these increase the surface area of the cells facilitating their resorptive function. The infolded membranes forming the microvilli are the site of numerous sodium pumps. Resorption of salt, water and glucose from the glomerular filtrate occurs here; at the same time some substances, including uric acid and drug metabolites, are actively transferred from the blood capillaries into the tubule for excretion
Loop of Henle	The proximal convoluted tubule then bends into the loop of Henle; this part of the tubule dips or 'loops' from the cortex into the medulla (descending limb), and then returns to the cortex (ascending limb). The loop of Henle is divided into the descending and ascending loops. The ascending loop of Henle is much thicker than the descending portion. Different parts of the loop of Henle have different actions
Distal convoluted tubule	The thick ascending portion of the loop of Henle leads into the distal convoluted tubule; this is lined with simple cuboidal cells and the lumen of the distal convoluted tubule is larger than the proximal convoluted. The distal convoluted tubule performs active secretion of ions and acids, assists with the regulation of calcium ions by excreting excess calcium ions in response to calcitonin hormone, selectively reabsorbs water and plays a role in regulating pH by absorbing bicarbonate and secreting protons (H^+) into the filtrate
	If antidiuretic hormone is present, the distal tubule and the collecting duct become permeable to water. In the absence of antidiuretic hormone the tubule is minimally permeable to water so large volumes of diluted urine are formed
Collecting duct	The distal convoluted tubule then drains into the collecting ducts; several collecting ducts converge and drain into a larger system called the papillary ducts, these empty into the minor calyx. From here the filtrate, now urine, drains into the renal pelvis. Sodium and water are reabsorbed in the final stage

9.

- These are small structures, forming the functional units of the kidney → nephrons
- There are over → one million nephrons per kidney
- When blood reaches the kidneys for filtration → it enters the Bowman's capsule
- From the Bowman's capsule, the filtrate drains into the → proximal convoluted tubule
- The loop of Henle → is divided into the descending and ascending loops
- Sodium and water → are reabsorbed in the final stage

10.

Function	Description
Regulation of electrolytes	Helps to regulate ions such as sodium, potassium, calcium, chloride and phosphate
Regulation of blood pH	Excretes hydrogen ions into the urine and conserves bicarbonate ions, thus helping to regulate pH of blood
Regulation of blood volume	By conserving or eliminating water in the urine
Secretion	Secretes renin (regulates blood pressure) and erythropoietin (production of red blood cells)
Production	Produces calcitriol for the regulation of calcium level
Gluconeogenesis	Aids in regulation of blood glucose
Detoxification	Detoxifies free radicals and drugs
Excretion	Excretes waste products such as urea, uric acid and creatinine

11.

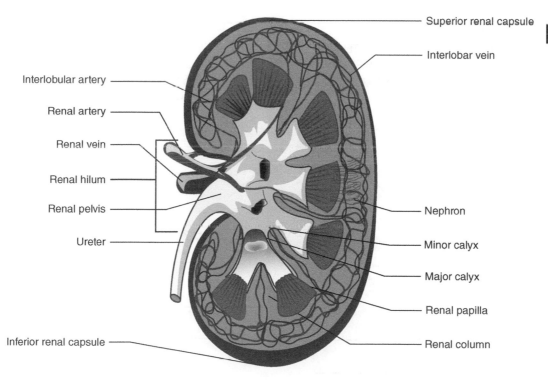

12.

Hormone	Secreted by	Function
Aldosterone	Adrenal cortex	Stimulates reabsorption of sodium and water, stimulates excretion of potassium, acts primarily on the distal tubule
Atrial natriuretic peptide	Atria of the heart	Decreases the reabsorption of sodium, causes greater excretion of sodium and water by the kidneys
Brain natriuretic peptide	Ventricles of the heart	Decreases the reabsorption of sodium, causes greater excretion of sodium and water by the kidneys
Antidiuretic hormone	Posterior pituitary gland	Stimulates the reabsorption of water, mainly by the collecting ducts
Parathyroid hormone	Parathyroid gland	Stimulates the reabsorption of calcium and the excretion of phosphate

13.

- The kidneys → maintain fluid balance, electrolyte balance and the acid–base balance of the blood
- Kidneys synthesise hormones such as → renin and angiotensin
- Kidneys produce erythropoietin, this is → a hormone that stimulates the production of red blood cells
- Healthy kidneys keep bones strong by producing → the hormone calcitriol
- The renal artery → arises from the abdominal aorta at the level of first lumbar vertebra
- Urine is 96% → water

14.

TOADSLERONE → ALDOSTERONE   SLIVEP → PELVIS
MORULESLUG → GLOMERULUS   DELLAUM → MEDULLA
HORENPN → NEPHRON   LUBETU → TUBULE
TROXEC → CORTEX   SOOTSISHAME → HOMEOSTASIS

15.

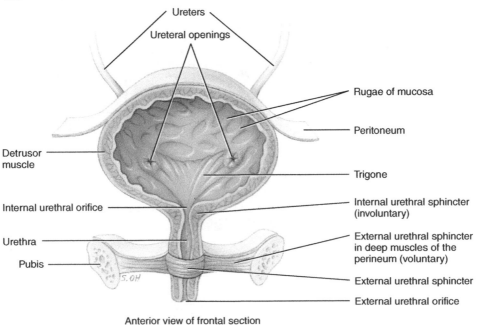

Anterior view of frontal section

16.

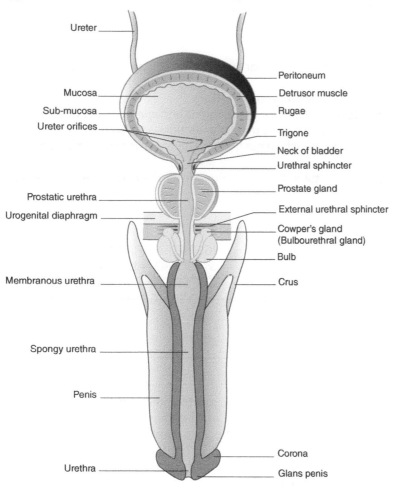

Ureter

Mucosa

Sub-mucosa

Ureter orifices

Prostatic urethra

Urogenital diaphragm

Membranous urethra

Spongy urethra

Penis

Urethra

Peritoneum

Detrusor muscle

Rugae

Trigone

Neck of bladder

Urethral sphincter

Prostate gland

External urethral sphincter

Cowper's gland
(Bulbourethral gland)

Bulb

Crus

Corona

Glans penis

17.

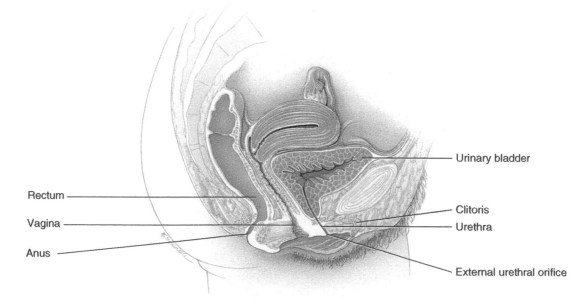

Rectum

Vagina

Anus

Urinary bladder

Clitoris

Urethra

External urethral orifice

18.

- The urinary bladder is → a hollow muscular organ and is located in the pelvic cavity posterior to the symphysis pubis
- In the male the bladder lies → anterior to the rectum
- In the female the bladder lies → anterior to the vagina and inferior to the uterus
- The inner floor of the bladder includes a triangular section → called the trigone
- The ureters are → tubular organs which run from the renal pelvis to the posterolateral base of the urinary bladder
- The urethra is → a muscular tube that drains urine from the bladder and conveys it out of the body

19.

THERAUR → URETHRA

TRUERE → URETER

SIPBU → PUBIS

UAGER → RUGAE

IGRONTE → TRIGONE

STRUDERO → DETRUSOR

CHIPSTERN → SPHINCTER

VACYTI → CAVITY

Snap shot
Urinalysis

Urinalysis is used as a screening and/or diagnostic tool to detect substances or cellular material in the urine associated with metabolic disorders, renal dysfunction or urinary tract infections. Often, substances such as protein or glucose will begin to appear in the urine before patients are aware that they may have a problem.

Urinalysis was performed in order to detect any abnormalities and was done so in the context of Andy's illness. The result of the test revealed:

pH: 4.5
protein: +++ positive
leucocytes: ++ positive
blood: ++ positive
ketones: negative
glucose: negative

Andy's urine appeared concentrated and was malodorous.

Undertaking a detailed history, examining Andy, observing his urine and the results of the urinalysis led the practice nurse to suspect a urinary tract infection.

Word search

B	L	A	D	D	E	R	B	Q	G	F	I	L	T	R	A	T	I	O	N
P	X	O	R	W	N	P	S	L	Q	R	C	S	I	E	K	O	K	M	Y
U	U	B	O	S	O	Y	O	A	T	M	E	B	K	S	I	F	J	E	R
B	S	S	J	A	R	M	E	T	E	P	E	N	M	I	D	P	Y	D	E
O	W	J	R	P	E	J	M	S	H	F	R	S	A	V	N	J	J	U	T
W	L	C	Z	R	T	D	G	I	Y	P	Y	N	H	L	E	B	X	L	E
M	V	G	U	A	S	T	T	D	A	S	T	T	M	E	Y	L	B	L	R
A	K	L	P	B	O	R	G	V	Z	E	H	L	H	P	S	O	E	A	U
N	U	J	T	K	D	G	Q	G	V	T	R	G	U	F	H	J	H	L	M
S	T	Z	P	I	L	W	K	N	C	Y	O	K	R	L	G	K	C	M	B
E	N	L	J	R	A	S	Z	S	E	L	P	U	E	U	K	X	R	C	L
C	M	O	A	Y	O	R	I	J	C	O	O	N	T	R	O	E	E	H	R
U	F	S	R	E	A	X	H	I	Q	R	I	C	H	I	S	T	N	E	T
C	L	K	K	H	M	I	H	W	T	E	K	R	N	E	R	I	N	Q
K	I	L	K	I	P	Z	K	M	J	C	T	D	A	E	E	O	N	L	L
R	V	J	N	R	V	E	L	I	A	E	I	Z	U	D	K	C	G	E	K
X	C	L	Z	E	I	E	N	S	Y	L	N	H	H	E	Y	K	Z	I	L
C	P	F	Y	B	B	V	E	O	I	E	E	N	O	G	I	R	T	Z	J
B	Z	D	E	T	U	L	O	V	N	O	C	O	A	R	M	I	V	O	E
M	P	R	O	K	C	Q	L	C	H	N	W	K	Q	P	F	Q	F	U	J

Crossword

Across
3. HENLE
4. HAEMATURIA
6. URETHRA
8. PYELONEPHRITIS
9. URETERS
12. TRIGONE
15. ANGIOTENSINOGEN
16. CALCITRIOL
18. FILTRATION

Down
1. BLADDER
2. NEPHRONS
5. ERYTHROPOIETIN
7. CORTEX
10. KIDNEYS
11. RENAL
13. MICTURITION
14. BOWMANS
17. CYSTITIS

Fill in the blanks

1. The kidneys play an important role in maintaining <u>homeostasis</u>. They remove <u>waste</u> products through the <u>production</u> and <u>excretion</u> of urine and regulate fluid <u>balance</u> in the body. The kidneys <u>filter</u> essential substances, such as <u>sodium</u> and potassium, from the <u>blood</u>, and selectively <u>reabsorb</u> substances essential to maintain <u>homeostasis</u>. Any substances not essential are <u>excreted</u> in the urine. The formation of urine is achieved through the processes of <u>filtration</u>, selective reabsorption and <u>excretion</u>. The kidneys also have an <u>endocrine</u> function, secreting hormones such as renin and <u>erythropoietin</u>.

2. Nephrons are small structures and they form the <u>functional</u> units of the <u>kidney</u>. The nephron consists of a <u>glomerulus</u> and a renal <u>tubule</u>. There are approximately one <u>million</u> nephrons per kidney and it is in these structures where <u>urine</u> is formed. The nephrons <u>filter</u> blood, perform <u>selective</u> reabsorption and <u>excrete</u> unwanted waste products from the blood.

3. The ureters are <u>tubular</u> in shape running from the renal <u>pelvis</u> to the base of the <u>urinary</u> bladder. They are approximately 25–30 cm in length and 5 mm in <u>diameter</u>. The ureters enter obliquely through the muscle <u>wall</u> of the <u>bladder</u>.

4. The <u>urinary</u> bladder is a <u>hollow</u> muscular organ and is located in the <u>pelvic</u> cavity posterior to the symphysis <u>pubis</u>; it is a smooth <u>muscular</u> sac which stores <u>urine</u>. When the bladder is empty, the <u>inner</u> wall of the bladder forms <u>folds</u>, but as the bladder fills with urine the <u>walls</u> of the <u>bladder</u> become smoother.

5. The urethra is a <u>muscular</u> tube which <u>drains</u> urine from the bladder and conveys it out of the <u>body</u>. Its wall has <u>three</u> coats: <u>muscular</u>, erectile and <u>mucous</u>. The <u>muscular</u> coat is the continuation of the bladder muscle layer. The urethra is encompassed by two separate urethral sphincter <u>muscles</u>. The <u>internal</u> urethral sphincter muscle is formed by <u>involuntary</u> smooth muscle, while <u>voluntary</u> muscles make up the external <u>sphincter</u>. The internal sphincter is created by the <u>detrusor</u> muscle. The urethra is different in <u>length</u> in males and <u>females</u>.

Multiple choice answers

1. (d), 2. (d), 3. (d), 4. (c), 5. (c), 6. (b), 7. (b), 8. (b), 9. (d), 10. (b)

Chapter 11

1.

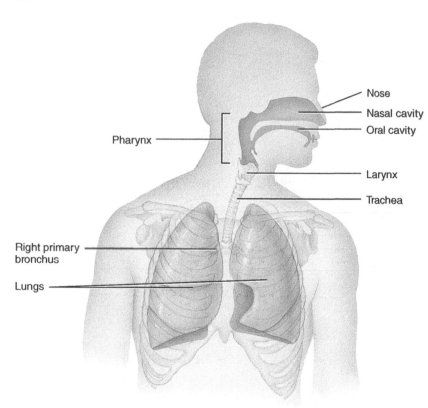

Nose

Nasal cavity

Oral cavity

Pharynx

Larynx

Trachea

Right primary
bronchus

Lungs

Anterior view showing organs of respiration

2.

Frontal bone
Frontal sinus
Olfactory epithelium
Sphenoidal sinus
Sphenoid bone
Pharyngeal tonsil
Superior ⎤
Middle ⎬ Nasal conchae
Inferior ⎦
Opening of auditory tube
External naris
Nasopharynx
Maxilla
Uvula
Oral cavity
Palatine tonsil
Palatine bone
Oropharynx
Tongue
Soft palate
Epiglottis
Mandible
Laryngopharynx
Lingual tonsil
Hyoid bone
Thyroid cartilage
Oesophagus
Larynx
Cricoid cartilage
Thyroid gland
Trachea

3.

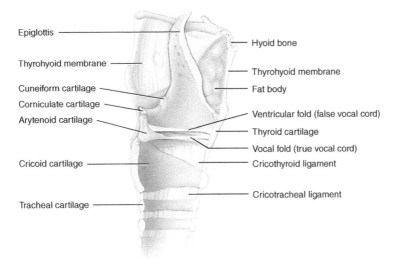

Epiglottis
Hyoid bone
Thyrohyoid membrane
Thyrohyoid membrane
Cuneiform cartilage
Fat body
Corniculate cartilage
Ventricular fold (false vocal cord)
Arytenoid cartilage
Thyroid cartilage
Vocal fold (true vocal cord)
Cricoid cartilage
Cricothyroid ligament
Cricotracheal ligament
Tracheal cartilage

Sagittal section

4.

Trachea

Primary bronchi

Secondary bronchi

Tertiary bronchi

Bronchioles

Terminal bronchioles

5.

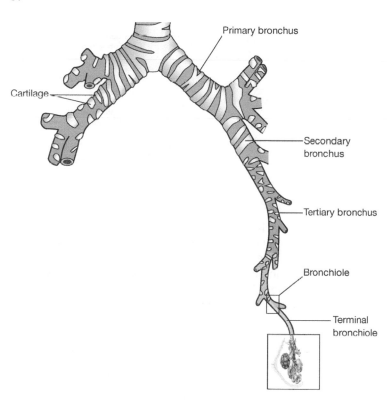

Primary bronchus

Cartilage

Secondary bronchus

Tertiary bronchus

Bronchiole

Terminal bronchiole

6.

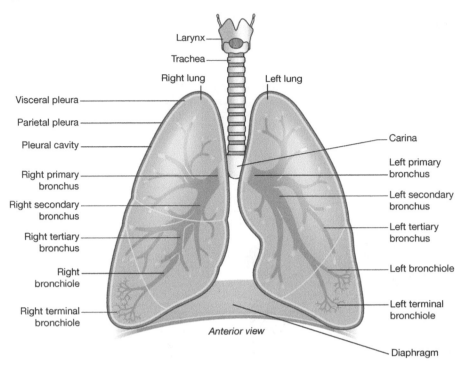

Larynx

Trachea

Right lung   Left lung

Visceral pleura

Parietal pleura

Pleural cavity   Carina

Left primary
bronchus

Right primary
bronchus   Left secondary
                                                  bronchus
Right secondary
bronchus   Left tertiary
                                                  bronchus
Right tertiary
bronchus

Right
bronchiole   Left bronchiole

Right terminal   Left terminal
bronchiole   bronchiole

Anterior view

                                                  Diaphragm

7.

- As cells use oxygen → carbon dioxide is produced as waste
- The organs of the upper respiratory tract are the → mouth, nose, nasal cavity and pharynx
- The upper respiratory tract → warms, filters and moistens the inhaled air
- Nine pieces of cartilage tissue, three single pieces and three pairs, → form the larynx
- The trachea → extends from the laryngopharynx to the carina
- The lungs are divided into lobes, → three lobes in the right lung and two in the left

8.

CHEATAR → TRACHEA   RULEAP → PLEURA
SHURCONB → BRONCHUS   CGARATILE → CARTILAGE
NARXYPH → PHARYNX   SHOENCROBIL → BRONCHIOLES
NARCIA → CARINA   VEILOLA → ALVEOLI

9.

Phase	Description
Pulmonary ventilation	How air gets in and out of the lungs
External respiration	How oxygen diffuses from the lungs to the bloodstream and how carbon dioxide diffuses from blood and to the lungs
Transport of gases	How oxygen and carbon dioxide are transported between the lungs and body tissues
Internal respiration	How oxygen is delivered to and carbon dioxide collected from body cells

10.

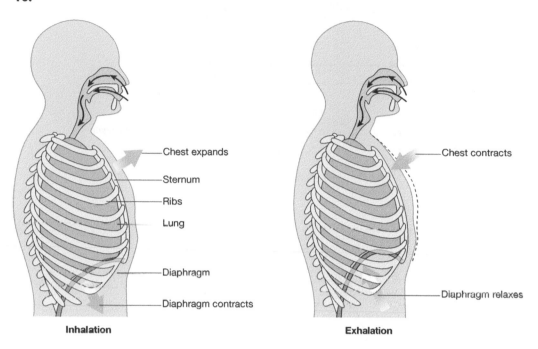

Chest expands

Sternum

Ribs

Lung

Diaphragm

Diaphragm contracts

Inhalation

Chest contracts

Diaphragm relaxes

Exhalation

11.

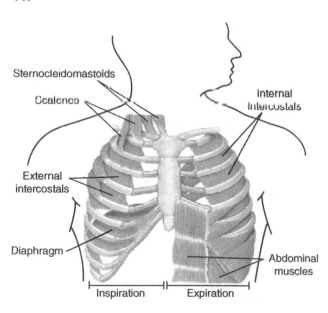

Sternocleidomastoids

Scalenes

Internal
Intercostals

External
intercostals

Diaphragm

Abdominal
muscles

Inspiration   Expiration

12.

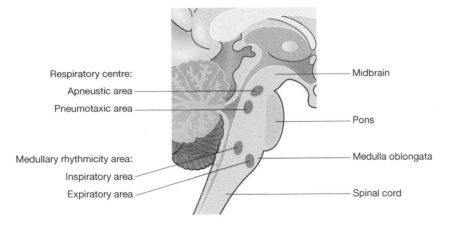

Respiratory centre:
　Apneustic area
　Pneumotaxic area

Medullary rhythmicity area:
　Inspiratory area
　Expiratory area

Midbrain

Pons

Medulla oblongata

Spinal cord

13.

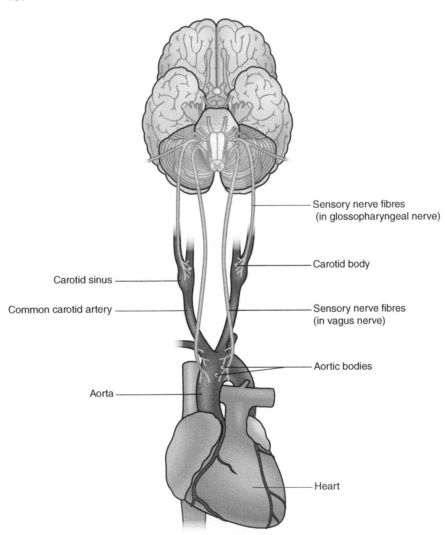

Sensory nerve fibres
(in glossopharyngeal nerve)

Carotid body

Carotid sinus

Common carotid artery

Sensory nerve fibres
(in vagus nerve)

Aortic bodies

Aorta

Heart

14.

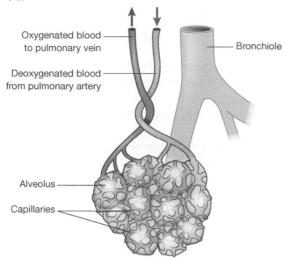

Oxygenated blood to pulmonary vein

Deoxygenated blood from pulmonary artery

Bronchiole

Alveolus

Capillaries

15.

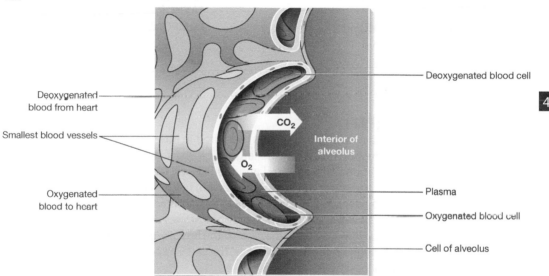

Deoxygenated blood from heart

Smallest blood vessels

Oxygenated blood to heart

Deoxygenated blood cell

CO_2

O_2

Interior of alveolus

Plasma

Oxygenated blood cell

Cell of alveolus

16.

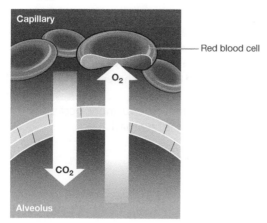

Capillary

Red blood cell

O_2

CO_2

Alveolus

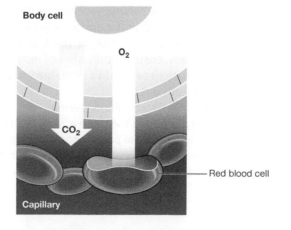

Body cell

O_2

CO_2

Red blood cell

Capillary

17.

- Pulmonary ventilation concerns → how air gets in and out of the lungs
- External respiration concerns → how oxygen diffuses from the lungs to the blood and how carbon dioxide diffuses from blood to the lungs
- During inspiration → the thorax expands and intrapulmonary pressure falls below atmospheric pressure
- When intrapulmonary pressure is less than atmospheric pressure → air will naturally enter the lungs until the pressure difference no longer exists
- The rate and depth of breathing are controlled by → the respiratory centres
- Exchange of gases in the lungs → takes place between alveolar air and the blood flowing through the lung capillaries

18.

TREPIRAISON → RESPIRATION
LAIVENTNOTI → VENTILATION
SESAG → GASES
PHISECAMORT → ATMOSPHERIC

VALORELA → ALVEOLAR
PROTECMECHORES → CHEMORECEPTORS
TAXHOR → THORAX
RAMPONYLU → PULMONARY

468 Snap shot

Peak expiratory flow (PEF)

This is usually referred to as 'peak flow'; it is measured in litres and is an objective measure that helps to detect airflow obstruction in the larger airways. If there is constriction of the airways then the rate of expiration will be limited and the PEF will be lower than the predicted normal value, which takes into account the age of the person, height and gender.

The health care provider has a responsibility to ensure that the measurement is accurate and the patient is taught how to perform the test. For best results the patient should stand or be seated in an upright position, a seal is made with the lips around the mouthpiece prior to forcefully exhaling. If the patient's condition permits, the test is repeated three times and the highest result recorded using local policy and procedure.

- Explain the procedure to the patient.
- Wash hands
- Fit a disposable mouthpiece to a peak flow meter.
- With the patient in the upright position (standing or sitting), zero the indicator on the peak flow meter (it should be at the bottom of the scale). The patient should hold the meter horizontally, ensuring they are not restricting the sliding marker on the device.
- Ask the patient to take in a deep breath, seal the lips around the mouthpiece and give a short, sharp breath out.
- If the patient's condition permits, this should be performed on two more occasions. The highest reading of the three attempts should be the one that is recorded.
- If needed, make the patient comfortable.
- Dispose of the disposable mouthpiece in line with local policy.
- Wash hands

Word search

M	Z	C	F	Z	V	A	H	B	J	Y	N	I	I	R	L	M	R	T	S
E	X	I	Q	G	L	P	Y	X	I	D	N	F	Q	A	X	Z	E	R	O
M	D	X	L	U	C	N	J	N	X	U	U	G	Y	B	H	U	O	Z	H
G	Y	A	Z	O	M	E	S	E	Y	C	P	E	R	C	B	T	B	R	I
A	A	T	X	Y	U	U	U	G	P	N	T	O	P	S	P	L	L	E	K
R	Z	O	Q	K	W	S	H	Y	S	I	N	Z	P	E	E	E	U	S	S
H	E	M	D	E	B	T	K	X	U	C	E	C	C	I	P	V	N	P	T
P	Z	U	V	V	B	I	T	O	H	L	L	E	N	R	F	C	G	I	N
A	Q	E	L	Q	R	C	Q	I	O	K	R	N	O	A	B	X	U	R	P
I	F	N	U	K	R	O	O	X	V	O	V	E	I	L	B	R	Q	A	F
D	A	P	M	Z	B	L	A	K	M	C	A	Y	S	L	B	S	L	T	I
O	J	I	U	B	E	M	Y	E	Q	M	A	B	U	I	U	F	A	I	P
D	J	D	K	S	L	P	H	A	H	R	G	U	F	P	H	R	R	O	O
A	R	U	E	I	P	C	P	V	E	Y	C	B	F	A	L	D	Y	N	E
L	S	A	N	G	A	S	E	S	Z	H	Z	J	I	C	R	D	N	X	M
V	V	T	T	O	Y	C	N	Z	B	Z	C	J	D	X	T	Z	X	I	Y
Z	P	H	A	R	Y	N	X	P	J	B	T	A	I	U	L	P	H	R	W
M	Q	E	V	B	A	I	T	Z	T	N	V	L	R	D	V	T	A	C	K
D	L	V	J	U	M	D	V	E	N	T	I	L	A	T	I	O	N	T	C
H	A	B	F	O	J	I	L	O	E	V	L	A	U	K	E	D	Y	U	D

Crossword

Across

2. PULMONARY
5. DIFFUSION
6. LITRES
7. DIAPHRAGM
9. ERYTHROCYTE
11. CHEMORECEPTORS
14. HYDROGEN
16. LARYNX
18. LUNGS

Down

1. SEPTUM
2. PLEURA
3. RESPIRATORY
4. PALATINE
8. HYPOXIA
10. THORACIC
12. TRACHEA
13. PHARYNX
15. EXPANDS
17. BLOOD

Fill in the blanks

1. The <u>respiratory</u> system is responsible for <u>gaseous</u> exchange between the <u>circulatory</u> system and the <u>atmosphere</u>. <u>Air</u> is taken in via the <u>upper</u> airways, through the lower airways and into the small <u>bronchioles</u> and <u>alveoli</u> within the lung <u>tissue</u>.

2. The lungs are divided into <u>lobes</u>. There are <u>three</u> lobes in the right lung and <u>two</u> in the left. Each is surrounded by two thin protective <u>membranes</u>: the <u>parietal</u> and <u>visceral</u> pleura. The <u>parietal</u> pleura lines the wall of the thorax, the <u>visceral</u> pleura covers the <u>lungs</u>. The space between the two <u>pleura</u>, the pleural <u>space</u>, is minute, and contains a thin film of <u>lubricating</u> fluid, which <u>reduces</u> friction between the two pleura, allowing both layers to slide over one another during <u>breathing</u>.

3. Pulmonary <u>ventilation</u> involves physical movement of <u>air</u> in and out of the <u>lungs</u>. The primary function is to maintain adequate <u>alveolar</u> ventilation. This <u>prevents</u> the build-up of carbon <u>dioxide</u> in the <u>alveoli</u> and achieves a constant supply of <u>oxygen</u> to the <u>tissues</u>. Air flows between the atmosphere and the <u>alveoli</u> of the <u>lungs</u> as a result of pressure difference created by the <u>contraction</u> and <u>relaxation</u> of the respiratory <u>muscles</u>. The rate of <u>air</u> flow and the effort needed for breathing is influenced by the alveolar surface <u>tension</u> and integrity of the lungs.

Multiple choice answers

1. (c), 2. (c), 3. (c), 4. (c), 5. (b), 6. (d), 7. (a), 8. (c), 9. (c), 10. (a)

Chapter 12

1.

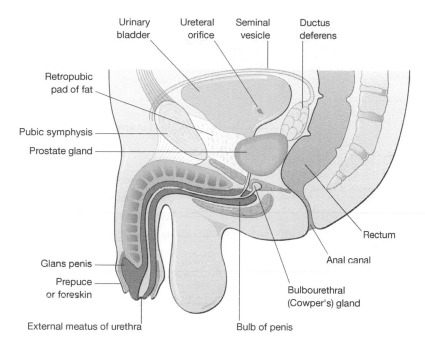

2.

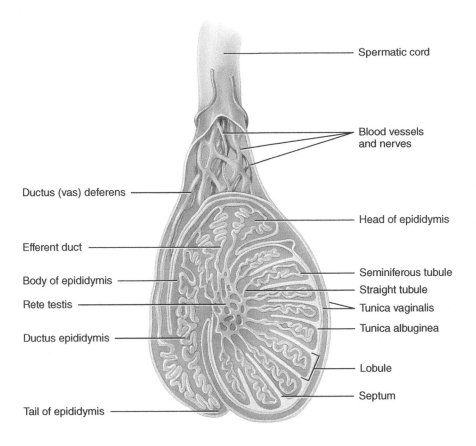

Spermatic cord

Blood vessels and nerves

Ductus (vas) deferens

Head of epididymis

Efferent duct

Body of epididymis

Seminiferous tubule

Rete testis

Straight tubule

Tunica vaginalis

Tunica albuginea

Ductus epididymis

Lobule

Septum

Tail of epididymis

3.

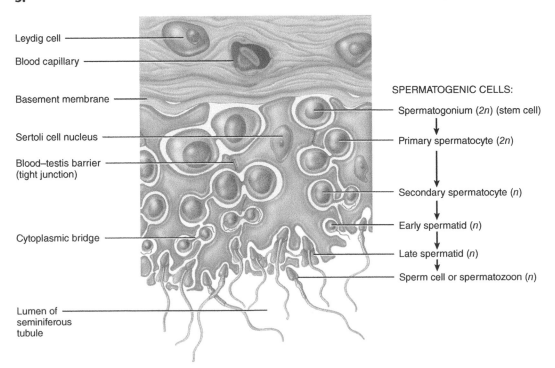

Leydig cell

Blood capillary

Basement membrane

Sertoli cell nucleus

Blood–testis barrier (tight junction)

Cytoplasmic bridge

Lumen of seminiferous tubule

SPERMATOGENIC CELLS:

Spermatogonium (2*n*) (stem cell)
↓
Primary spermatocyte (2*n*)
↓
Secondary spermatocyte (*n*)
↓
Early spermatid (*n*)
↓
Late spermatid (*n*)
↓
Sperm cell or spermatozoon (*n*)

4.

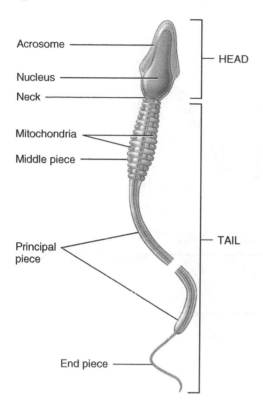

Acrosome

Nucleus

Neck

Mitochondria

Middle piece

Principal
piece

End piece

HEAD

TAIL

5.

Skin:
• Hair growth

Brain:
• Libido
• Levels of
  aggression

Bone marrow:
• Production of
  red blood cells

Male sex organs:
• Spermatogenesis
• Prostatic growth
• Erectile function

Muscle:
• Muscle mass

Bone:
• Bone density

6.

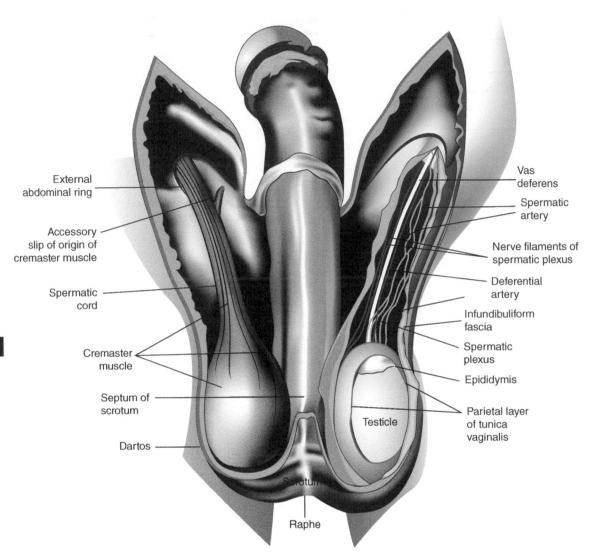

External abdominal ring

Accessory slip of origin of cremaster muscle

Spermatic cord

Cremaster muscle

Septum of scrotum

Dartos

Vas deferens

Spermatic artery

Nerve filaments of spermatic plexus

Deferential artery

Infundibuliform fascia

Spermatic plexus

Epididymis

Testicle

Parietal layer of tunica vaginalis

Scrotum

Raphe

7.

Dorsal

— Corpora cavernosa

— Tunica albuginea of
corpora cavernosum

— Deep artery of penis

— Corpus spongiosum

— Spongy urethra

— Tunica albuginea of
corpus spongiosum

Ventral

8.

- The reproductive glands of the male are the testes → these are the male equivalent of the ovaries
- Leydig cells, between the seminiferous tubules, → manufacture and secrete testosterone and other androgens
- Spermatogenesis turns each diploid spermatogonium into → four haploid sperm cells, quadrupling is accomplished through meiotic cell division
- The epididymis brings sperm to maturity → as sperm leaving the testes are immature, and are unable to fertilise the egg
- The vas deferens is a long, muscular tube → which transports sperm from the epididymis to the urethra
- The seminal vesicles are sac-like pouches attached to the vas deferens → near the base of the bladder; they provide sperm with a source of energy and assist with motility

475

9.

LANESIM → SEMINAL   PERMS → SPERM
YIDDIMSEPI → EPIDIDYMIS   PLIODID → DIPLOID
SNIPE → PENIS   PLIODAH → HAPLOID
SLANG → GLANS   PARHE → RAPHE

10.

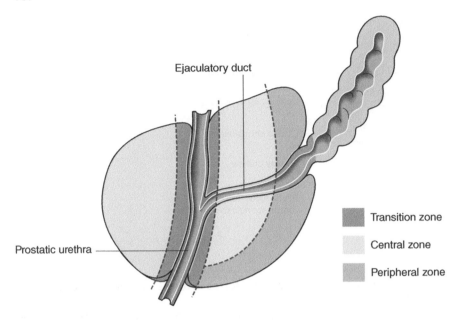

Ejaculatory duct

Prostatic urethra

Transition zone

Central zone

Peripheral zone

11.

Zone	Description
Peripheral	This is the area of the prostate that is closest to the rectum. It is the largest zone of the prostate gland and accounts for 70% of the total gland
Transition	This zone is the middle area of the prostate, located between the peripheral and central zones, surrounding the urethra as it passes through the prostate. Up until 40 years this zone makes up approximately 20% of the prostate gland. As a man ages, the transition zone begins to enlarge, until it becomes the largest area of the prostate. As the transition zone enlarges, it then pushes the peripheral zone of the prostate toward the rectum
Central	The central zone is in front of the transition zone. This zone is farthest from the rectum and contains approximately one third of the ducts that secrete fluid that helps create semen

12.

- The peripheral zone of the prostate gland → is the area of the prostate that is closest to the rectum
- As the transition zone enlarges, it then pushes → the peripheral zone of the prostate toward the rectum
- The central zone is in front of the transition zone → and is farthest from the rectum
- The gland cells within the prostate produce a → thin fluid that is rich in proteins and minerals that maintain and nourish the sperm
- Prostate-specific antigen counteracts the clotting enzyme in the seminal vesicle fluid → which principally glues the semen to the cervix, located next to the uterine entrance inside the vagina
- Digital rectal examination is usually performed to → check for growths in or enlargement of the prostate gland

13.

GIANTEN → ANTIGEN
OPTRATSE → PROSTATE
REARPHILEP → PERIPHERAL
LATERNC → CENTRAL

TRAITSINON → TRANSITION
GATDILI → DIGITAL
ONEZ → ZONE
MUTERC → RECTUM

14.

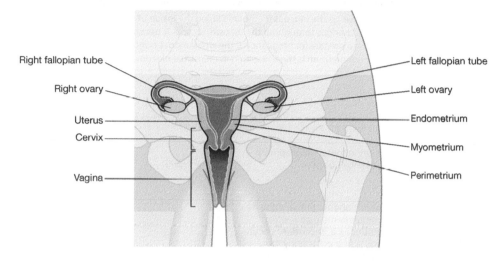

15.

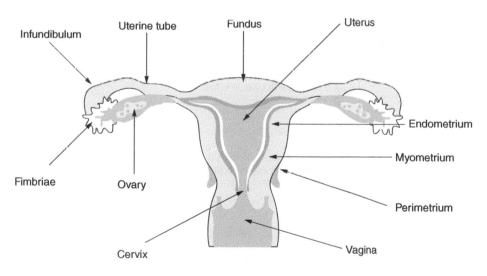

16.

Layers	Description
Perimetrium	A serous membrane that envelopes the uterus, the outer layer; provides support to the uterus located within the pelvis. Also known as the parietal peritoneum
Myometrium	The middle layer, made up of smooth muscle. Throughout pregnancy and childbirth the uterus has to stretch and the muscular layer permits this. The muscle will contract during labour, and postnatally this muscular layer contracts forcefully to eject the placenta
Endometrium	The endometrium is the mucous membrane lining the inside of the uterus. The endometrium changes throughout the menstrual cycle. It becomes thick and rich with blood vessels to prepare for pregnancy. If the woman does not become pregnant then part of the endometrium is shed, resulting in menstrual bleeding

17.

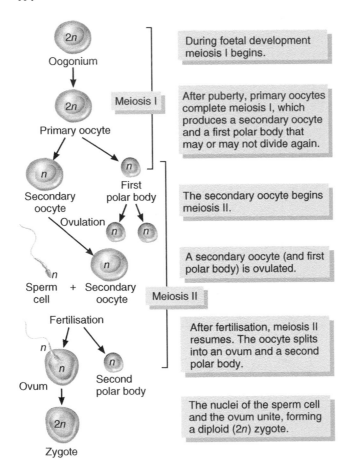

18.

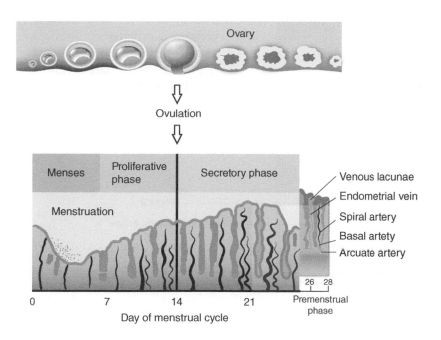

19.

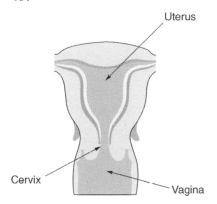

20.

- The female reproductive system produces the ova → and is designed to transport the ova to the site of fertilisation
- The vagina is a canal that joins the → cervix to the outside of the body; it is also known as the birth canal
- The uterus is a hollow, pear-shaped organ divided into two parts → the cervix, which is the lower part that opens into the vagina, and the main body of the uterus, called the corpus
- The ovaries are small, oval-shaped glands → located on either side of the uterus; they produce eggs and hormones
- Fallopian tubes are narrow tubes → attached to the upper part of the uterus and serve to transport the ova from the ovaries to the uterus
- Conception is the fertilisation of an egg by a sperm; it normally → occurs in the fallopian tubes. The fertilised egg moves to the uterus, and implants into the lining of the uterine wall

21.

REVIXC → CERVIX
IANPOLLAF → FALLOPIAN
YAROV → OVARY
USTURE → UTERUS

SPORCU → CORPUS
ANIVAG → VAGINA
TAUTSOMENRIN → MENSTRUATION
LICELLOF → FOLLICLE

22.

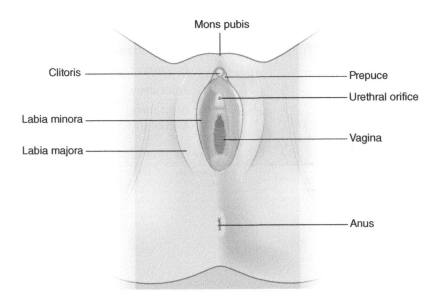

Mons pubis

Clitoris

Prepuce

Urethral orifice

Labia minora

Vagina

Labia majora

Anus

480

23.

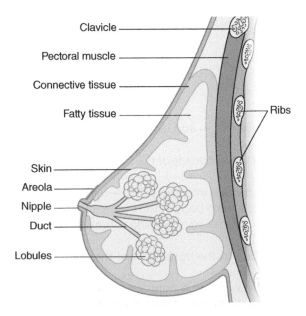

Clavicle

Pectoral muscle

Connective tissue

Fatty tissue

Ribs

Skin

Areola

Nipple

Duct

Lobules

24.

Intraclavicular (subclavicular) nodes

Supraclavicular nodes

Clavicle

Axillary nodes

Internal mammary nodes

Lymph vessels

25.

NATALOCTI → LACTATION

GRONERESTEPO → PROGESTERONE

ABIAL → LABIA

LUVVA → VULVA

SCUDT → DUCTS

SONM → MONS

RAJMAO → MAJORA

RAMION → MINORA

26.

- The labia majora are the outer lips of the vulva made of two symmetrical pads of fatty tissue → providing protection for the urethral and vaginal openings
- Labia minora are thin folds of tissue within the labia majora → functioning as protective structures that surround the clitoris, urinary orifice and vaginal orifice
- The clitoris is a small white body of oval tissue located at the top of the labia minora and the clitoral hood → it is composed of spongy tissue and is highly sexually sensitive
- The key function of the breast is to produce, store and release milk produced in lobules located → throughout the breast following stimulation by hormones produced after the woman has given birth
- There are a number of major nerves in the breast area, → including nerves in the chest and arm, branches from the 4th, 5th and 6th thoracic nerves supply the breasts
- Progesterone prepares the uterus for pregnancy and the breasts for producing milk for lactation, → each month breast tissues are exposed to cycles of oestrogen and progesterone throughout a woman's childbearing years

Snap shot
Erectile dysfunction

- Before starting to use the medication read the manufacturer's patient instructions.
- Sit upright or slightly reclined when performing the injection.
- Choose an injection site on the side of the shaft of the penis, in the first one-half area closest to the base of the penis. Avoid visible blood vessels.
- Hold the head of the penis, and stretch it lengthwise along the thigh so as to clearly see the selected injection site. Clean the site with a new alcohol swab.
- Remove the cover from the needle. Position the penis firmly against the thigh to keep it from moving during the injection.
- Hold the syringe between the thumb and index finger. Using a steady motion, push the needle straight into the selected site until the metal part of the needle is almost entirely in the penis.
- With a steady motion, push down on the plunger so that the entire volume of solution is slowly injected. Grasping the barrel of the syringe, pull the needle out of the penis. Apply pressure to the injection site with the alcohol swab for 5 minutes.
- Safely dispose of the used syringe and needle.
- Alternate the side of the penis and vary the site of injection with each use.
- If the erection last more than 4 hours, immediately contact a doctor

Penis injection sites

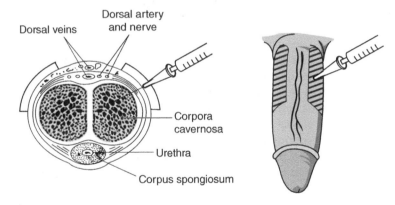

Word search

A	L	M	A	S	N	R	H	C	C	B	O	V	X	T	R	X	J	I	P
P	S	Y	K	K	G	A	T	E	A	E	M	Y	H	A	R	E	O	L	A
E	P	O	V	H	C	P	M	U	I	R	T	E	M	O	D	N	E	Z	U
N	E	M	J	S	F	H	J	E	D	K	M	P	L	Z	Z	L	O	H	M
I	R	E	D	Z	I	E	S	N	E	G	O	R	D	N	A	V	H	A	E
S	M	T	P	T	A	S	M	F	R	F	U	X	P	J	C	J	N	Z	E
M	O	R	P	Z	I	Y	E	W	P	E	A	I	R	B	M	I	F	W	O
U	K	I	M	Q	G	Q	W	N	U	P	A	W	Y	U	G	A	N	O	T
I	R	U	E	T	U	B	U	I	F	S	R	Q	L	A	H	W	T	E	Q
R	S	M	C	E	R	V	I	X	V	G	S	O	V	B	W	Z	S	S	V
T	I	E	B	N	N	O	B	H	D	E	O	E	S	W	U	T	M	T	U
E	Z	N	S	U	R	E	T	U	X	D	I	T	T	T	O	X	U	R	L
M	B	Q	A	N	O	Q	M	U	L	H	A	Q	A	S	A	X	O	O	V
I	K	J	C	V	L	D	E	P	G	O	K	P	T	M	E	T	E	G	A
R	P	B	Y	E	Y	B	Q	T	Q	L	W	E	J	U	R	T	E	E	R
E	T	I	P	R	O	G	E	S	T	E	R	O	N	E	N	E	F	N	F
P	E	N	E	S	V	W	H	X	P	O	Y	V	W	Z	O	H	P	S	H
X	P	S	E	I	R	A	V	O	N	S	T	A	W	K	P	Q	T	S	T
G	Z	N	K	R	O	V	L	E	M	T	B	A	Z	M	T	K	J	Z	W
T	V	L	I	P	L	I	M	U	T	O	R	C	S	C	V	X	J	D	I

483

Crossword

Across
2. BREASTS
5. ANDROGENS
7. PENIS
8. RUGAE
9. MYOMETRIUM
10. PROSTATE
12. UTERUS
14. CREMASTERIC
15. FIMBRIAE
18. OOGENESIS
19. OVARIES
20. VAGINA

Down
1. TESTES
3. SPERM
4. SALPINGES
6. SPERMATOGENESIS
11. CERVIX
13. OESTROGENS
16. ADNEXA
17. VASECTOMY

Fill in the blanks

1. The male <u>reproductive</u> system works with other body systems, producing <u>hormones</u> essential for biological <u>development</u>, sexual <u>behaviour</u> and <u>sexual</u> performance. Other body systems involved include the neuroendocrine system and the <u>musculoskeletal</u> system. The male reproductive system is also central to the function of the <u>urinary</u> system.

2. The <u>male</u> reproductive system includes the <u>scrotum</u>, testes, <u>spermatic</u> ducts, sex <u>glands</u> and the <u>penis</u>. Working together these organs produce <u>sperm</u>, the male <u>gamete</u>, and the other components of semen. These organs also work together to <u>deliver</u> semen out of the body and into the <u>vagina</u> where it can <u>fertilise</u> egg cells.

3. The female reproduction system produces the <u>ova</u> and the <u>female</u> sex <u>hormones</u> that maintain the <u>reproductive</u> cycle.

4. The external female <u>genitalia</u> are known collectively as the <u>vulva</u>. They include the <u>mons</u> pubis, the <u>labia</u>, the clitoris, the <u>vaginal</u> and <u>urethral</u> openings, and glands. The external genitalia enable <u>sperm</u> to enter the body, protect the <u>internal</u> genital organs from <u>infectious</u> organisms and provide <u>sexual</u> pleasure.

Multiple choice answers

1. (c), 2. (c), 3. (b), 4. (b), 5. (b), 6. (c), 7. (b), 8. (d), 9. (b), 10. (d)

Chapter 13

1.

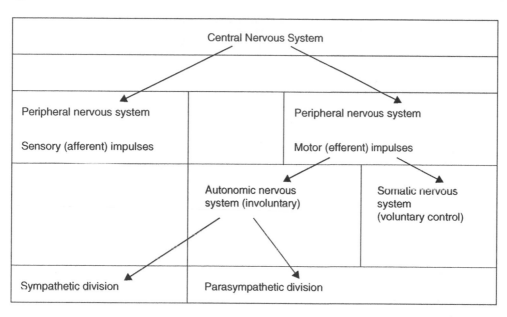

2.

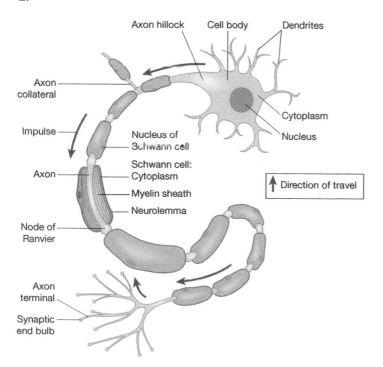

3.

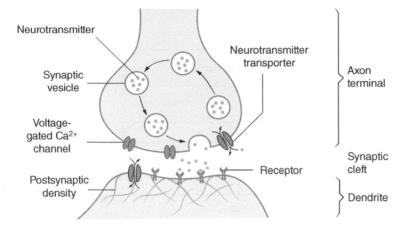

Neurotransmitter

Synaptic
vesicle

Voltage-
gated Ca²⁺
channel

Postsynaptic
density

Neurotransmitter
transporter

Axon
terminal

Synaptic
cleft

Receptor

Dendrite

4.

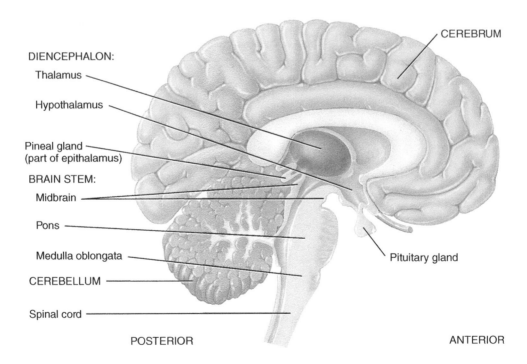

DIENCEPHALON:

Thalamus

Hypothalamus

Pineal gland
(part of epithalamus)

BRAIN STEM:

Midbrain

Pons

Medulla oblongata

CEREBELLUM

Spinal cord

CEREBRUM

Pituitary gland

POSTERIOR

ANTERIOR

5.

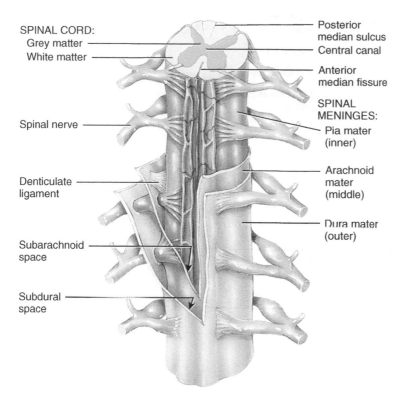

SPINAL CORD:
Grey matter
White matter

Posterior median sulcus
Central canal
Anterior median fissure

SPINAL MENINGES:
Pia mater (inner)

Spinal nerve

Arachnoid mater (middle)

Denticulate ligament

Dura mater (outer)

Subarachnoid space

Subdural space

6.

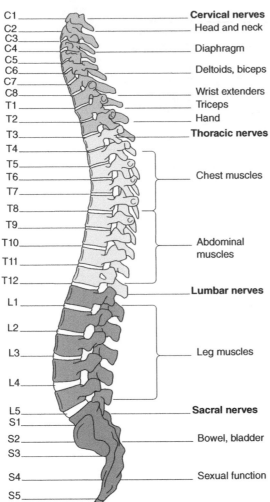

C1	**Cervical nerves**
C2	Head and neck
C3	
C4	Diaphragm
C5	
C6	Deltoids, biceps
C7	
C8	Wrist extenders
T1	Triceps
T2	Hand
T3	**Thoracic nerves**
T4	
T5	
T6	Chest muscles
T7	
T8	
T9	
T10	Abdominal
T11	muscles
T12	
L1	**Lumbar nerves**
L2	
L3	Leg muscles
L4	
L5	**Sacral nerves**
S1	
S2	Bowel, bladder
S3	
S4	Sexual function
S5	

7.

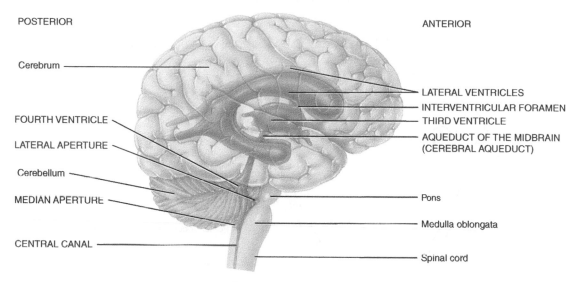

POSTERIOR

ANTERIOR

Cerebrum

LATERAL VENTRICLES

INTERVENTRICULAR FORAMEN

THIRD VENTRICLE

FOURTH VENTRICLE

AQUEDUCT OF THE MIDBRAIN
(CEREBRAL AQUEDUCT)

LATERAL APERTURE

Cerebellum

MEDIAN APERTURE

Pons

Medulla oblongata

CENTRAL CANAL

Spinal cord

8.

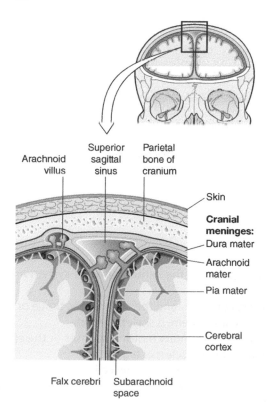

Arachnoid
villus

Superior
sagittal
sinus

Parietal
bone of
cranium

Skin

**Cranial
meninges:**
Dura mater

Arachnoid
mater

Pia mater

Cerebral
cortex

Falx cerebri

Subarachnoid
space

9.

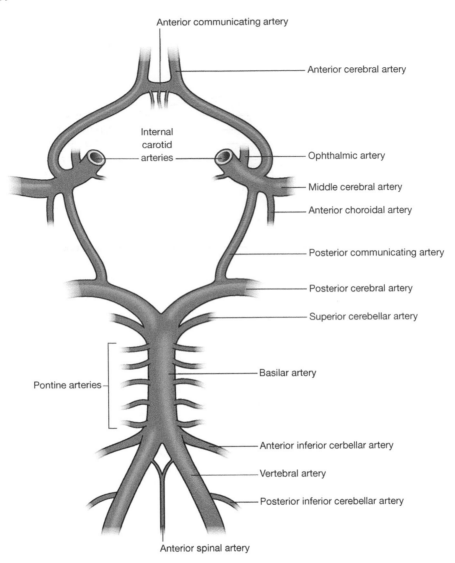

Anterior communicating artery

Anterior cerebral artery

Internal carotid arteries

Ophthalmic artery

Middle cerebral artery

Anterior choroidal artery

Posterior communicating artery

Posterior cerebral artery

Superior cerebellar artery

Pontine arteries

Basilar artery

Anterior inferior cerbellar artery

Vertebral artery

Posterior inferior cerebellar artery

Anterior spinal artery

10.

- The nervous system can be divided into two parts: → the central nervous system and the peripheral nervous system
- The somatic nervous system is under voluntary control → and the effector, the tissue or organ responding to instruction from the central nervous system, is skeletal muscle
- The autonomic nervous system is responsible for involuntary motor responses → the effector may be smooth or cardiac muscle (both involuntary muscles) or a gland
- The functional unit of the nervous system is → the neurone or nerve cell
- The meninges protect the blood vessels that serve nervous tissue → there is a layer of cerebrospinal fluid between the meninges
- The choroid plexus in the ventricles of the brain → produces cerebrospinal fluid

11.

SNIGEMEN → MENINGES
LIVETRENC → VENTRICLE
SEXPLU → PLEXUS
BEERSLAPCROIN → CEREBROSPINAL

UREOSENN → NEURONES
MISTRUTTEREROSNAN → NEUROTRANSMITTERS
COMSATI → SOMATIC
MOOTNUICA → AUTONOMIC

12.

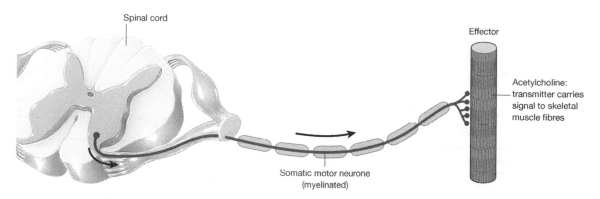

Spinal cord

Effector

Acetylcholine:
transmitter carries
signal to skeletal
muscle fibres

Somatic motor neurone
(myelinated)

13.

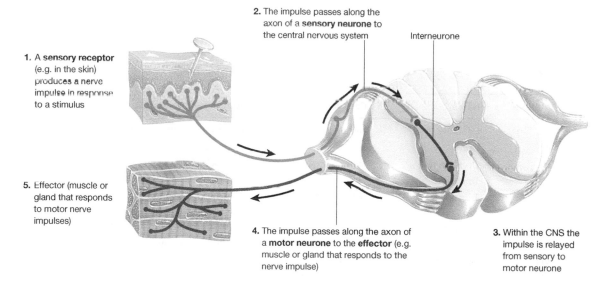

2. The impulse passes along the
axon of a **sensory neurone** to
the central nervous system

Interneurone

1. A **sensory receptor**
(e.g. in the skin)
produces a nerve
impulse in response
to a stimulus

5. Effector (muscle or
gland that responds
to motor nerve
impulses)

4. The impulse passes along the axon of
a **motor neurone** to the **effector** (e.g.
muscle or gland that responds to the
nerve impulse)

3. Within the CNS the
impulse is relayed
from sensory to
motor neurone

14.

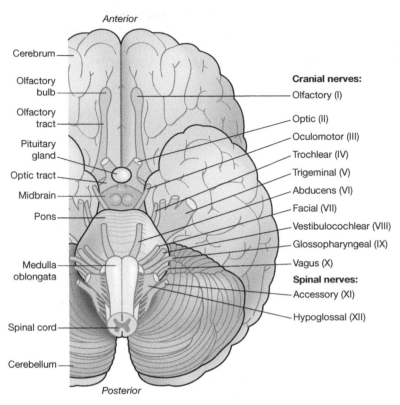

Anterior

Cerebrum

Olfactory bulb

Olfactory tract

Pituitary gland

Optic tract

Midbrain

Pons

Medulla oblongata

Spinal cord

Cerebellum

Posterior

Cranial nerves:
Olfactory (I)
Optic (II)
Oculomotor (III)
Trochlear (IV)
Trigeminal (V)
Abducens (VI)
Facial (VII)
Vestibulocochlear (VIII)
Glossopharyngeal (IX)
Vagus (X)
Spinal nerves:
Accessory (XI)
Hypoglossal (XII)

15.

Number	Name	Components	Location/function
I	Olfactory	Sensory	Olfactory receptors for sense of smell
II	Optic	Sensory	Retina (sight)
III	Occulomotor	Motor	Eye muscles (including eye lids and lens, pupil)
IV	Trochlear	Motor	Eye muscles
V	Trigeminal	Sensory and motor	Teeth, eyes, skin, tongue for sensation of touch, pain and temperature
VI	Abducens	Motor	Jaw muscles (chewing), eye muscles
VII	Facial	Sensory and motor	Taste buds, facial muscles, tear and salivary glands
VIII	Vestibulocochlear	Sensory	Inner ear (hearing and balance)
IX	Glossopharyngeal	Sensory and motor	Pharyngeal muscles (swallowing)
X	Vagus	Sensory and motor	Internal organs
XI	Spinal accessory	Motor	Neck and back muscles
XII	Hypoglossal	Motor	Tongue muscles

16.

Organ/system	Sympathetic effects	Parasympathetic effects
Cell metabolism	Increases metabolic rate and stimulates fat breakdown and increases blood sugar levels	No effect
Blood vessels	Constricts blood vessels in the viscera/skin Dilates blood vessels in the heart and skeletal muscle	No effect
Eye	Dilates pupils	Constricts pupils
Heart	Increases rate and force of contraction	Decreases rate
Lungs	Dilates bronchioles	Constricts bronchioles
Kidneys	Decreases urine output	No effect
Liver	Causes the release of glucose	No effect
Digestive system	Decreases peristalsis and constricts digestive sphincters	Increases peristalsis and dilates digestive sphincters
Adrenal medulla	Stimulates cells to secrete epinephrine and norepinephrine	No effect
Lacrimal glands	Inhibits the production of tears	Increases the production of tears
Salivary glands	Inhibits the production of saliva	Increases the production of saliva
Sweat glands	Stimulates to produce perspiration	No effect

17.

- The 12 pairs of cranial nerves differ in their functions → some are sensory nerves, some are motor nerves and some are mixed nerves
- The brain can be divided into → four anatomical regions
- The cerebrum is → the largest brain structure, divided into the left and right hemispheres
- The diencephalon is the part of the brain surrounded by → the cerebrum, containing three paired structures
- The cerebellum coordinates → voluntary muscle movement, balance and posture
- The spinal cord is → enclosed within the vertebral canal, which forms a protective ring of bone around the cord

18.

PHILDEACONNE → DIENCEPHALON
CRUMBEER → CEREBRUM
EREBELLCUM → CEREBELLUM
SWILIL → WILLIS
PSYCHETMATI → SYMPATHETIC
CHYMEPAPARATTSI → PARASYMPATHETIC
AILNARC → CRANIAL
TOXERC → CORTEX

Snap shot
Ageing and the nervous system

Structural changes
- Weight of the brain decreases
- Thickening and fibrotic changes associated with the meninges
- Ventricles expand in size

Cellular changes
- There is a decrease in the number of neurones
- Decreased myelin sheath
- Decreases are evident in dendritic processes and synaptic connections
- Intracellular neurofibrillary tangles with significant accumulation in the cortex; this is associated with Alzheimer dementia
- There is an imbalance of neurotransmitter activity

Cerebrovascular changes
- Arterial atherosclerosis can lead to cerebral infarct
- Permeability of the blood–brain barrier is increased
- Decreased vascular density

Functional changes
- Cognitive alterations related to chronic disease
- Memory impairments
- Sleep disruption
- Reduction in tendon reflexes
- Deficit in taste and smell (progressive)
- Visual disturbance related to accommodation and colour vision
- Alteration in gait due to decrease in neuromuscular control

Word search

I	D	S	Z	J	N	E	U	R	O	M	U	S	C	U	L	A	R	X	M
E	N	E	L	N	A	H	S	C	S	H	Z	G	N	I	A	R	B	U	E
E	S	N	E	T	V	U	U	I	O	G	R	Z	W	H	M	A	A	W	P
U	Y	S	O	M	T	L	K	M	M	U	Y	Y	C	J	R	F	T	Z	A
M	M	O	A	U	I	A	E	O	A	T	Q	N	W	N	E	C	G	E	R
S	P	R	W	L	T	N	N	N	T	T	H	S	E	R	I	Z	V	S	A
H	A	Y	X	L	Z	I	I	O	I	E	T	M	P	E	V	N	Y	V	S
G	T	V	Y	E	N	P	P	T	C	E	X	J	J	C	N	N	O	T	Y
J	H	U	P	B	L	S	S	U	P	J	B	L	B	E	A	M	C	U	M
S	E	T	S	E	X	O	T	A	Y	D	R	N	S	P	R	P	E	R	P
X	T	Z	L	R	H	R	Z	S	N	E	O	S	S	T	Y	L	E	E	A
Y	I	E	Q	E	O	B	M	N	G	N	T	E	E	O	H	F	A	N	T
X	C	G	T	C	E	E	N	O	A	D	O	Z	K	R	L	E	I	O	H
N	O	X	A	R	C	R	A	P	T	R	M	J	O	E	X	D	L	R	E
N	G	A	G	U	B	E	O	K	I	I	N	T	X	K	C	S	G	U	T
R	F	K	P	P	G	C	S	F	Z	T	C	I	X	X	R	Q	O	E	I
L	A	R	E	H	P	I	R	E	P	E	E	Q	L	O	A	K	R	N	C
F	C	R	A	N	I	A	L	Y	F	S	O	R	R	E	O	P	U	J	A
J	B	Z	S	O	G	E	F	I	C	K	G	U	M	M	Y	M	E	I	F
J	P	O	L	C	K	W	E	N	C	X	Y	Z	K	Z	F	M	N	V	W

Crossword

Across

2. TASTE
4. EFFECTOR
6. OLFACTORY
7. HOMEOSTASIS
11. ACETYLCHOLINE
12. ASTROCYTES
14. VENTRICLES
16. DURA
18. RECEPTORS
19. MYELIN
20. NUCLEI

Down

1. CEREBRUM
3. NEUROTRANSMITTER
5. PONS
8. NEURILEMMA
9. WILLIS
10. MENINGITIS
13. MENINGES
15. NERVES
17. CRANIAL

Fill in the blanks

1. The <u>brain</u> and <u>spinal</u> cord comprise the central nervous <u>system</u>. The network of <u>nerves</u> connecting at different levels of the <u>spinal</u> cord controls <u>conscious</u> and unconscious activities. It is through the spinal cord that <u>information</u> flows from these <u>nerves</u> to the <u>brain</u> and back again.

2. Neurones communicate with each other through their <u>axons</u> and <u>dendrites</u>. When a <u>neurone</u> receives a message from another neurone, it sends an <u>electrical</u> signal down the <u>length</u> of its <u>axon</u>. At the end of the axon, the electrical <u>signal</u> is converted into a <u>chemical</u> signal, and the axon releases chemical <u>messengers</u> called <u>neurotransmitters</u>.

3. The brain sends messages via the <u>spinal</u> cord to peripheral <u>nerves</u> throughout the body that serve to control the <u>muscles</u> and internal <u>organs</u>. The <u>somatic</u> nervous system is made up of <u>neurones</u> connecting the central <u>nervous</u> system with the parts of the body that interact with the <u>outside</u> world. <u>Somatic</u> nerves in the cervical region are related to the <u>neck</u> and <u>arms</u>; those in the thoracic region serve the <u>chest</u>; and those in the <u>lumbar</u> and <u>sacral</u> regions interact with the legs.

Multiple choice answers

1. (b), 2. (c), 3. (a), 4. (b), 5. (c), 6. (b), 7. (d), 8. (d), 9. (c), 10. (a)

Chapter 14

1.

Receptor	Stimulus	Example
Chemoreceptors	Alterations in concentrations of chemical substances	Taste and smell
Nociceptors (pain receptors)	Damage to tissues	Pain
Thermoreceptors	Heat changes	Heat and cold
Sensory receptor (mechanoreceptors)	Changes in pressures (can also include change in the movement of fluids)	Hearing and balance
Photoreceptors	Light energy	Sight and vision

2.

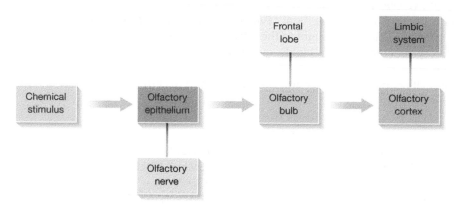

3.

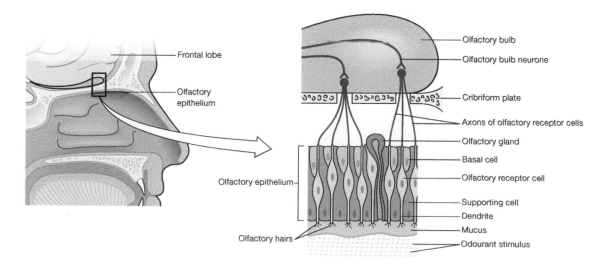

4.

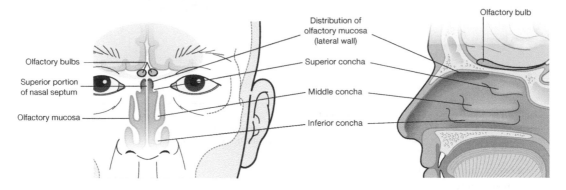

5.

- The sense of smell is useful for → the identification of food that is safe to eat and that which has gone rotten
- Olfaction is dependent on → receptors that respond to airborne particles
- On either side of the nasal septum → in the nasal cavity there are paired olfactory organs made up of two layers.
- When air is inhaled through the nasal cavity → it is subject to turbulent flow ensuring that airborne smell particles are brought to the olfactory organs
- The olfactory receptors are → highly modified neurones contained within the olfactory epithelium
- The nasal cavity contains pain receptors → that respond to certain irritants such as ammonia, chillies and menthol

6.

TAYFORCLO → OLFACTORY
CREEPROST → RECEPTORS
LUBB → BULB
BLICIM → LIMBIC

IMCHELAC → CHEMICAL
LLEMS → SMELL
IRCIMBFOR → CRIBIFORM
DRATOON → ODORANT

7.

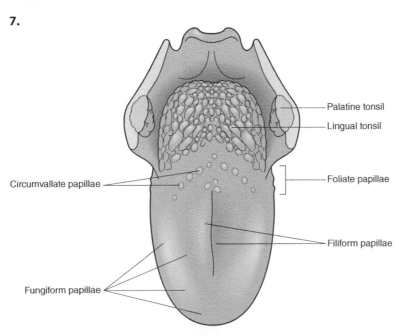

8.

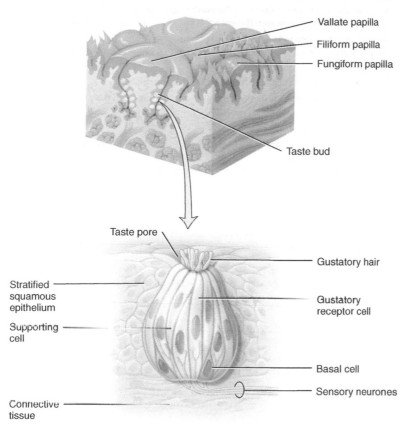

Vallate papilla

Filiform papilla

Fungiform papilla

Taste bud

Taste pore

Gustatory hair

Stratified
squamous
epithelium

Gustatory
receptor cell

Supporting
cell

Basal cell

Sensory neurones

Connective
tissue

499

9.

- Mostly when we taste bitter or sour this causes dislike because most → poisons are bitter, while foods that have gone off taste acidic
- The tongue is a muscular structure → papillae give the tongue its rough texture with thousands of taste buds covering the surfaces of the papillae
- The papillae are projections of a connective tissue core covered → with squamous epithelium
- The taste cells within a bud are arranged so that their tips form a small taste pore → through this pore extend microvilli from the taste cells
- When the taste signals are transmitted to the brain, → a number of efferent neural pathways are activated; these are important to digestive function
- Taste preferences often change → in conjunction with the needs of the body

10.

DUBS → BUDS
TOSINGUTA → GUSTATION
ORCHERTECEMPO → CHEMORECEPTOR
IMAMU → UMAMI

ALPEALIP → PAPILLAE
UNGOTE → TONGUE
SIPONO → POISON

11.

Structure	Function
Eyelids (palpebrae)	A continuation of the skin. Continual blinking keeps the surface of the eye lubricated and removes dirt. The gap between the eyelids is known as the palpebral fissure
Eyelashes	Robust hairs that help to keep foreign matter out of the eyes. They are associated with the tarsal glands which produce a lipid-rich secretion that helps to prevent the eyelids from sticking together
Lacrimal caruncle	A small collection of soft tissue that contains accessory glands
Commissure	The point where the eyelids meet; there are two, the lateral and the medial
Conjunctiva	The epithelial cell layer that lines the inside of the eyelids and the outer surface of the eye. Protects the delicate cornea
Eyebrows	Arched ridges of the supraorbital margins of the frontal bone. Protect the eyeball from foreign bodies, dust and sweat

12.

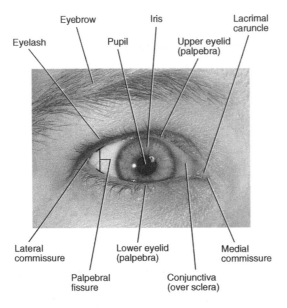

13.

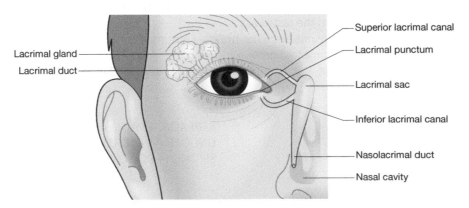

14.

Flow of tears:	Lacrimal gland		Lacrimal ducts		Superior or inferior lacrimal canal		Lacrimal sac		Nasolacrimal duct		Nasal cavity

15.

- Continual blinking keeps the surface of the eye → lubricated and removes dirt. The gap between the eyelids is known as the palpebral fissure
- Eyelashes are robust hairs that help to keep foreign matter out of the eyes associated with → the tarsal glands which produce a lipid-rich secretion that helps to prevent the eyelids from sticking together
- Conjunctiva is → the epithelial cell layer that lines the inside of the eyelids and the outer surface of the eye
- The eyebrows are → arched protecting the eyeball from foreign bodies, dust and sweat
- The organ of sight is the eye which is supplied by → the optic nerve (cranial nerve II)
- The space between the eye and the orbital cavity is → occupied by adipose tissue

16.

TAILORB → ORBITAL
POISEDA → ADIPOSE
PREPABALL → PALPEBRAL
IFSURES → FISSURE

RATSAL → TARSAL
VACUNJONTIC → CONJUNCTIVA
BREWSYEO → EYEBROWS
SPHEROPROTECTO → PHOTORECEPTORS

17.

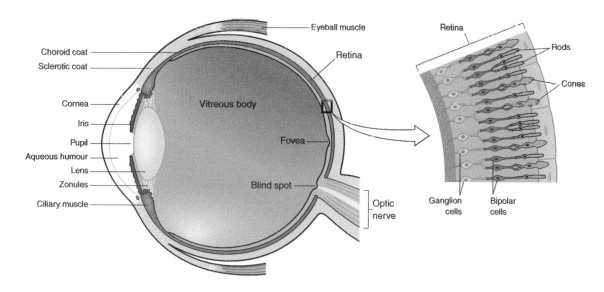

18.

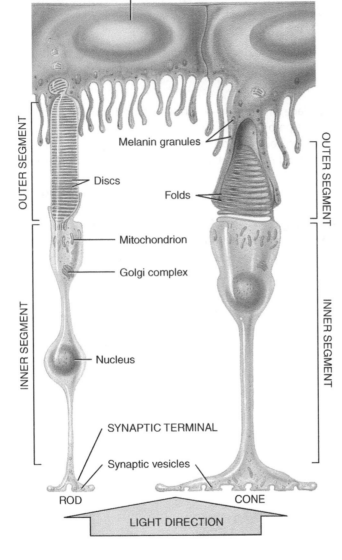

Pigment epithelial cell

Melanin granules

OUTER SEGMENT

Discs

Folds

OUTER SEGMENT

Mitochondrion

Golgi complex

INNER SEGMENT

Nucleus

INNER SEGMENT

SYNAPTIC TERMINAL

Synaptic vesicles

ROD

CONE

LIGHT DIRECTION

19.

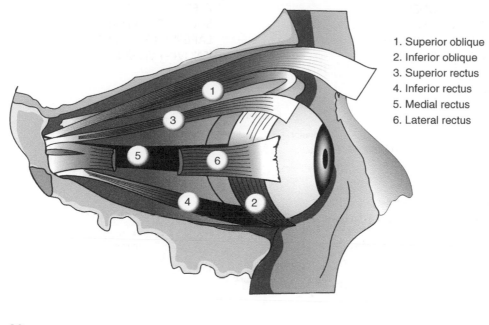

1. Superior oblique
2. Inferior oblique
3. Superior rectus
4. Inferior rectus
5. Medial rectus
6. Lateral rectus

20.

Visual pathways

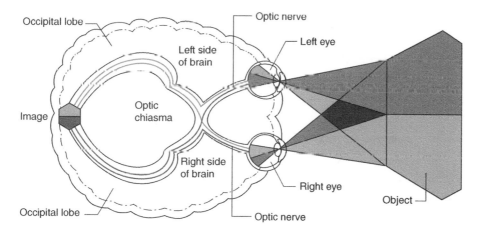

21.

- The retina is a transparent thin tissue → designed to capture photons of light and initiate processing of the image by the brain
- In the retina there are two types of receptors → rods and cones
- Cones provide the ability → to discern colour and the ability to see fine detail
- Rods are mainly responsible → for peripheral vision and vision under low light conditions
- The extrinsic eye muscles move → the eyeball in the bony orbit
- The intrinsic muscles move → those structures within the eyeball

22.

SCONE → CONES
RIPERSUO → SUPERIOR
QUILBEO → OBLIQUE
TRIBO → ORBIT

ATERIN → RETINA
SHOOTNP → PHOTONS
LAPERHIREP → PERIPHERAL
ISNOVI → VISION

23.

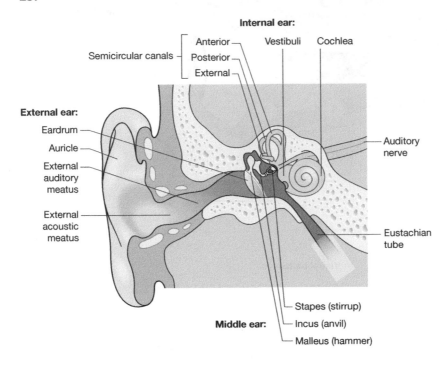

Internal ear:

Semicircular canals — Anterior — Posterior — External

Vestibuli   Cochlea

External ear:

Eardrum
Auricle
External auditory meatus
External acoustic meatus

Auditory nerve

Eustachian tube

Stapes (stirrup)
Middle ear: Incus (anvil)
Malleus (hammer)

24.

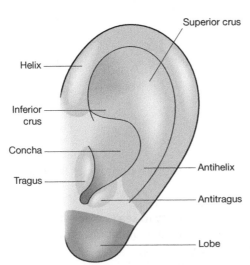

Superior crus

Helix

Inferior crus

Concha

Tragus

Antihelix

Antitragus

Lobe

25.

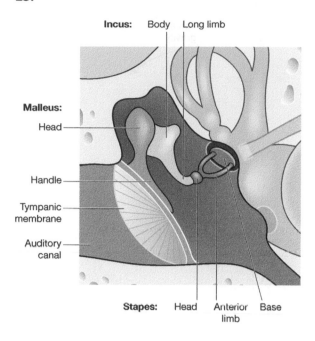

Incus: Body   Long limb

Malleus:
Head

Handle

Tympanic
membrane

Auditory
canal

Stapes: Head   Anterior   Base
limb

26.

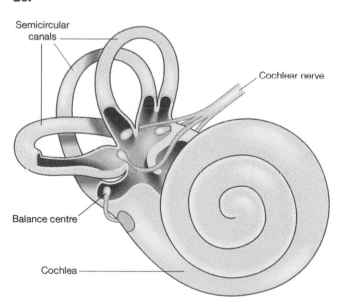

Semicircular
canals

Cochlear nerve

Balance centre

Cochlea

27.

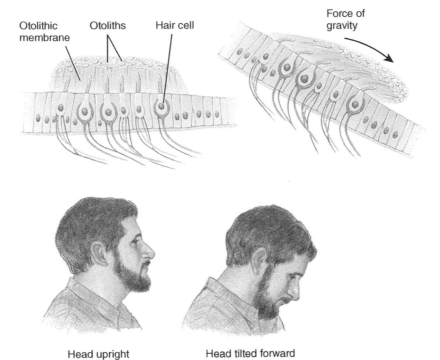

Otolithic membrane   Otoliths   Hair cell

Force of gravity

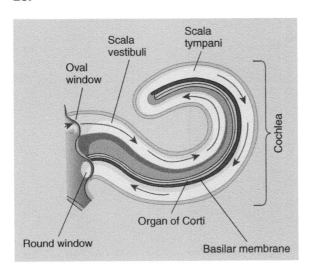

Head upright   Head tilted forward

Position of macula with head upright (left) and tilted forward (right)

28.

Scala vestibuli   Scala tympani

Oval window

Cochlea

Organ of Corti

Round window   Basilar membrane

29.

- The cochlea is a bony, spiral-shaped chamber → containing the cochlear duct of the membranous labyrinth
- The purpose of the oils and the cerumen is to lubricate the ear canal → kill bacteria and, in conjunction with the hairs, keep the canal free of debris
- The tympanic cavity is a small, air-filled cavity → lined with mucosa and contained within the temporal bone
- The inner ear is also known as the labyrinth due to the complicated series of canals it contains → it is composed of two main fluid-filled parts
- The sense of equilibrium is part of the sense of balance → and is controlled by receptors in the semicircular ducts, the utricle and the saccule of the inner ear
- The sense of hearing is provided by receptors in the cochlear duct, → they are hair cells similar to those of the semicircular canals and vestibule

30.

LEACHOC → COCHLEA
IRUBIQMILEU → EQUILIBRIUM
TOTHLIO → OTOLITH
SMALLUE → MALLEUS

SUCIN → INCUS
PASTES → STAPES
THYINLABR → LABYRINTH
CAMPYTIN → TYMPANIC

Snap shot
Visual acuity

An eye chart is used to measure visual acuity.

The classic example of an eye chart is the Snellen eye chart, this was developed in the 1860s by Dutch eye doctor Hermann Snellen. There are a number of types of the Snellen eye chart in use, but in general they show 11 rows of capital letters. The top row contains one letter (this is usually the 'big E' but other letters can be used). The other rows contain letters that become progressively smaller.

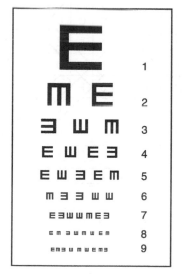

The Snellen fraction (numerator/denominator) describes the smallest size of letter that the person can identify correctly. The fraction compares the person's result (denominator) with the result expected from the 'normal' visual system (numerator).

- 6/6 means that at 6 m test distance the person is able to correctly identify a letter that a 'normal' sighted person should see at 6 m, i.e. 'normal' vision
- 6/60 means that the person is only able to see at 6 m what a 'normal' sighted person should see at 60 m. In this case the person's sight is approximately ten times poorer than 'normal' or requires detail to be brought ten times closer before it can be seen
- 6/15 means that the person could only see at 6 m what a 'normal' sighted person should see at 15 m

Word search

Crossword

Across

3. IRIS
4. AGEUSIA
6. CERUMEN
8. PARKINSON'S
9. OLFACTION
15. INCUS
16. GUSTATION
20. COCHLEA
21. CILIA

Down

1. RETINA
2. MACULA
5. EUSTACHIAN
6. CHEMORECEPTORS
7. IRRITANTS
10. LABYRINTH
11. PAPILLA
12. ANOSMIA
13. BALANCE
14. SCLERA
17. UMAMI
18. THREE
19. CHOROID

Fill in the blanks

1. The sense of <u>smell</u> is one of the oldest senses. The sense of smell is useful to us for the <u>identification</u> of food that is <u>safe</u> to eat and that which has gone <u>rotten</u>; it helps us to identify <u>dangers</u>, such as dangerous <u>chemicals</u>, and gives us pleasure through the smell of <u>flowers</u> and <u>perfume</u>. Olfaction is dependent on <u>receptors</u> that respond to <u>airborne</u> particles. In the nasal <u>cavity</u>, either side of the nasal septum, there are <u>paired</u> olfactory <u>organs</u> made up of two <u>layers</u>.

509

2. <u>Gustation</u> is the formal term for the sense of taste. In order to create the sensation of <u>taste</u>, a substance has to be in <u>solution</u> of <u>saliva</u> so that it can enter the taste pores. Taste drives the <u>appetite</u> and also protects us from <u>poison</u>. Mostly when we taste <u>bitter</u> or sour this causes <u>dislike</u>, most poisons are <u>bitter</u>, while foods that have gone off taste <u>acidic</u>.

3. The eye permits us to <u>see</u> and understand <u>shapes</u>, colours and <u>dimensions</u> of objects by processing the <u>light</u> reflected or <u>emitted</u>. The eye consists of the <u>cornea</u>, iris, <u>pupil</u>, lens and retina. The lens focuses <u>light</u> on the <u>retina</u>. The retina is covered with <u>two</u> basic types of light-sensitive <u>cells</u> – <u>rods</u> and cones. The <u>eye</u> is connected to the brain through the <u>optic</u> nerve. The point of this connection is called the "<u>blind</u> spot" because it is <u>insensitive</u> to light.

4. Sound represents a combination of <u>waves</u> generated by a <u>vibrating</u> sound <u>source(s)</u>, prop-agated through the air until they reach the <u>ear</u>. Wave <u>frequency</u> corresponds to what is perceived as pitch, amplitude corresponds to the <u>loudness</u> or intensity of <u>sound</u>. The ear has two key functions: to assist <u>equilibrium</u> and to allow us to <u>hear</u> the sounds around us. The ear is composed of <u>three</u> sections: the <u>external</u>, middle and <u>inner</u> ear.

Multiple choice answers

1. (b), 2. (c), 3. (b), 4. (c), 5. (a), 6. (b), 7. (c), 8. (b), 9. (d), 10. (a)

Chapter 15

1.

	Nervous system	Endocrine system
Speed of action	Seconds	Minutes to hours (even days)
Duration of action	Seconds to minutes	Minutes to days
Method of transmitting messages	Electrical	Chemical
Transport method	Neurones	Hormones

2.

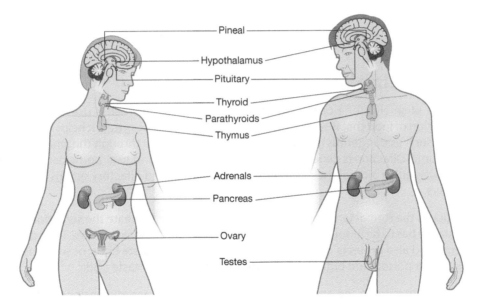

Pineal
Hypothalamus
Pituitary
Thyroid
Parathyroids
Thymus
Adrenals
Pancreas
Ovary
Testes

3.

	Definition
Endocrine	Usually means hormones that are secreted into the blood and have an effect on cells distant from those that release the hormone. However, many endocrine hormones are known to act locally and even on the cells that secrete them
Paracrine	Hormones that act locally and diffuse to the cells in the immediate neighbourhood to produce their action
Autocrine	Hormones that act on the cells that produce them
Exocrine	Glands/organs that secrete substances into ducts that eventually lead to the outside of the body (for instance, the sweat glands, the part of the pancreas that secretes digestive juices, the gallbladder)

4.

```
┌─────────────────────────────────┐ ┌─┐
│ Initial stimulus leads to release of │ │─│
│ hormone (e.g. insulin)          │ └─┘
└─────────────────────────────────┘
              │                    ┌─────────────┐
              │                    │ Negative    │
              ▼                    │ feedback    │
┌─────────────────────────────────┐│ inhibiting  │
│ Hormone exerts its effect on target ││ further     │
│ organ (e.g. liver)              ││ hormone     │
└─────────────────────────────────┘│ release     │
              │                    └─────────────┘
              ▼
┌─────────────────────────────────┐
│ Some aspect of the organ function │
│ (e.g. reduced blood sugar) feeds  │
│ back to the endocrine organ       │
└─────────────────────────────────┘
```

5.

- Homeostasis refers to → the maintenance of normal physiological balance and functioning within the body
- The endocrine system is made up of → a collection of small organs scattered throughout the body, each of which releases hormones into the blood supply
- Paracrine refers to → hormones that act locally and diffuse to the cells in the immediate neighbourhood to produce their action
- Hormones are chemical → messengers that are secreted into the blood or the extracellular fluid by one cell and have an effect on the functioning of other cells
- Changes in the number of receptors are known → as up-regulation and down-regulation
- Most hormones are inactivated by enzyme systems in the liver and kidneys → and excreted mostly in the urine, some are excreted in the faeces

6.

SHOREMON → HORMONES
CREEDINON → ENDOCRINE
CROXEINE → EXOCRINE
RATGET → TARGET

BEEFCAKD → FEEDBACK
USMUTLIS → STIMULUS
PORCESTER → RECEPTORS
RINCETOAU → AUTOCRINE

7.

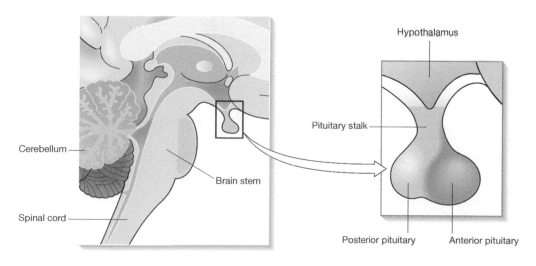

Hypothalamus
Pituitary stalk
Cerebellum
Brain stem
Spinal cord
Posterior pituitary
Anterior pituitary

8.

Hypothalamus	Anterior pituitary gland	Target organ or tissues	Action
Growth hormone releasing factor	Growth hormone	Many (especially bones)	Stimulates growth of body cells
Growth hormone release inhibiting factor	Growth hormone (inhibits release)	Many	–
Thyroid releasing hormone (TRH)	Thyroid stimulating hormone (TSH)	Thyroid gland	Stimulates thyroid hormone release
Corticotropin releasing hormone (CRH)	Adrenocorticotropic hormone (ACTH)	Adrenal cortex	Stimulates corticosteroid release
Prolactin releasing hormone	Prolactin	Breasts	Stimulates milk production
Prolactin inhibiting hormone	Prolactin (inhibits release)	Breasts	–
Gonadotropin releasing hormone	Follicle stimulating hormone Luteinising hormone	Gonads	Various reproductive functions

9.

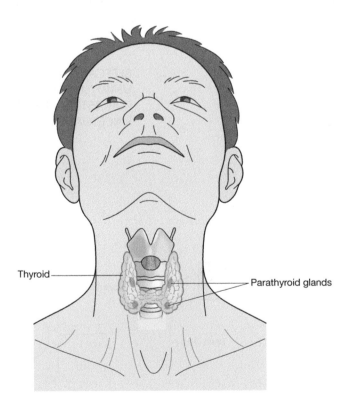

Thyroid — Parathyroid glands

10.

Increased secretion of T$_3$ and T$_4$ (hyperthyroidism)	Decreased secretion of T$_3$ and T$_4$ (hypothyroidism)
Increased basal metabolic rate	Decreased basal metabolic rate
Weight loss (despite good/increased appetite)	Weight gain (despite anorexia)
Tachycardia, palpitations, arrhythmia	Bradycardia
Excitability, nervousness, irritability	Tiredness, depression
Tremor	Numbness in the hands
Hair loss	Lifeless hair
Changes in menstruation patterns	Irregular menstrual periods
Goitre	Deep voice
Diarrhoea	Constipation
Exophthalmos	Feeling cold

11.

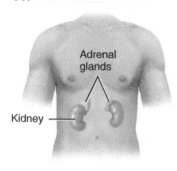

12.

Transverse section

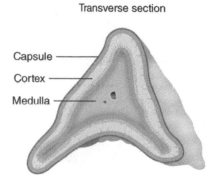

13.

Microscopic section

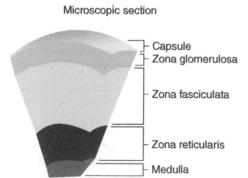

14.

- The thyroid is made up of two lobes → joined by an isthmus
- One unique factor of the thyroid gland is → its ability to create and store large amounts of hormone
- The parathyroid glands are small glands located on → the posterior of the thyroid gland
- The two adrenal glands are found on → the top of each of the two kidneys
- The outer part of each adrenal gland is → made up of three distinct functional layers
- Mineralocorticoids are the group of hormones whose main function is → the regulation of the concentration of electrolytes in the blood

15.

IDRYTHO → THYROID
RECXOT → CORTEX
ANDRIOILOCOMETCRI → MINERALOCORTICOID
SMUTHSI → ISTHMUS

SUGERMOLAOL → GLOMERULOSA
NOIDEI → IODINE
DALELUM → MEDULLA
ASLUPEC → CAPSULE

16.

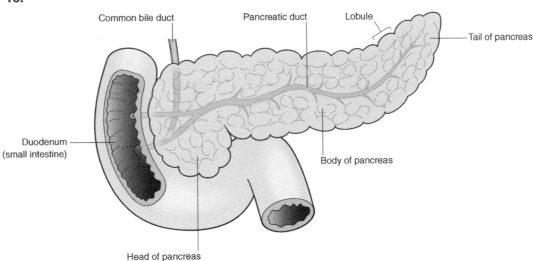

17.

Organ	Description
Thymus gland	Thymosin, a hormone produced by the thymus gland, has an important role in the development of the immune system
Stomach	The lining of the stomach, the gastric mucosa, produces gastrin when food is present in the stomach. This stimulates the production of hydrochloric acid and the enzyme pepsin, used in the digestion of food
Small intestine	The mucosa of the small intestine secretes secretin and cholecystokinin. Secretin stimulates the pancreas to produce a fluid that neutralises the stomach acid. Cholecystokinin stimulates contraction of the gallbladder, releasing bile, and stimulates the pancreas to secrete digestive enzymes
Heart	The heart also acts as an endocrine organ as well as pumping blood. Special cells in the wall of the atria produce atrial natriuretic hormone, or atriopeptin
Placenta	The placenta develops as a source of nourishment and gas exchange for the developing foetus. It also serves as a temporary endocrine gland. One hormone it secretes is human chorionic gonadotropin which signals the woman's ovaries to secrete hormones to maintain the uterine lining so that it des not degenerate and slough off in menstruation

18.

- The gonads are the primary reproductive organs: → the testes in the male and the ovaries in the female
- The pancreas is an elongated organ and → is found next to the first part of the small intestine
- The pancreas is innervated → by the parasympathetic and sympathetic nervous systems
- Special cells in the wall of the atria produce → atrial natriuretic hormone
- The majority of the pancreas is made up of → exocrine tissue and the associated ducts
- When food is present in the stomach → the gastric mucosa produces gastrin

19.

REANCAPS → PANCREAS
STEETS → TESTES
VARSIEO → OVARIES
MOYSTHIN → THYMOSIN
TAPACELN → PLACENTA
ANALSHERGN → LANGERHANS
PALAH → ALPHA
TEDAL → DELTA

Snap shot
Polydipsia and polyuria

Based on the two symptoms and John's past history of polydipsia and polyuria it likely that the condition is diabetes insipidus. However polydipsia polyuria can be caused by other conditions; a number of tests will need to be performed to make a definitive diagnosis.

If diabetes insipidus is suspected there is a need to determine which type of diabetes insipidus John has, as the treatment is different for each form of the condition. There are two types of diabetes insipidus:

1. Cranial diabetes insipidus is usually due to disease of the hypothalamus or surrounding tissues.
2. Nephrogenic diabetes insipidus occurs when there is a defect in the kidney tubules making the kidneys unable to properly respond to ADH. The defect may be due to a genetic disorder or a chronic kidney disorder. Certain drugs, such as lithium, can cause nephrogenic diabetes insipidus.

Treatment of cranial diabetes insipidus
As the key issue is hormone deficiency, then physiological replacement with desmopressin is usually effective. This can be administered orally, intranasally or parenterally.

Treatment of nephrogenic diabetes insipidus
Correct any metabolic abnormality caused by polydipsia. Ensure that any medication that may be causing the problem (for example, lithium) are changed.

High-dose desmopressin may be used for mild to moderate cases of nephrogenic diabetes insipidus in reducing the volume of urine produced. A combination of treatment with a thiazide diuretic and a non-steroidal anti-inflammatory drug may be effective. Dehydration should be prevented.

Word search

J	M	L	H	J	H	Y	P	O	T	H	A	L	A	M	U	S	O	G	S
D	I	Q	A	D	R	E	N	A	L	I	N	E	V	P	W	K	R	Y	T
J	K	B	L	I	N	F	U	N	D	I	B	U	L	U	M	Q	S	F	I
G	W	N	P	I	T	U	I	T	A	R	Y	Y	H	L	L	A	Q	S	S
U	H	U	H	O	J	C	D	T	S	A	E	R	C	N	A	P	Y	T	T
L	A	R	O	T	H	Y	R	O	X	I	N	E	E	K	V	D	Y	E	H
N	M	D	M	Z	T	T	F	B	Y	L	Q	T	Q	I	W	H	T	R	M
O	H	S	E	N	I	M	A	L	O	H	C	E	T	A	C	E	D	O	U
R	Y	D	O	N	N	E	U	R	O	H	Y	P	O	P	H	Y	S	I	S
A	T	N	S	F	O	T	D	I	O	R	Y	H	T	A	R	A	P	D	U
D	E	A	T	P	S	H	E	N	I	R	C	O	D	N	E	R	J	Y	A
R	N	L	A	P	G	H	Y	P	O	T	H	Y	R	O	I	D	I	S	M
E	I	G	S	K	P	B	P	M	V	B	E	T	T	B	S	Q	G	M
N	R	D	I	H	H	O	R	M	O	N	E	S	E	V	P	N	E	I	H
A	C	P	S	Q	G	Y	D	Y	F	P	B	U	L	S	I	J	N	K	N
L	O	C	M	U	K	R	T	B	P	B	H	I	T	M	O	S	N	X	W
I	T	N	C	L	A	N	E	R	D	A	Y	Y	E	R	U	C	Z	S	O
N	U	X	D	H	C	R	J	L	I	W	D	A	S	L	I	F	U	A	O
E	A	J	B	L	T	H	Y	R	O	I	D	Q	I	I	S	S	A	L	A
M	G	L	T	B	A	R	E	E	L	T	M	N	N	F	S	T	D	C	G

Crossword

Across
5. THYROXINE
7. ISTHMUS
9. PITUITARY
10. THYROID
11. LANGERHANS
15. ADRENALINE
16. NEURAL
17. MINERALOCORTICOIDS
19. ADENOHYPOPHYSIS
20. EUVOLAEMIA
22. PARACRINE
23. CORTEX
24. PANCREAS
25. INSULIN
26. EXOCRINE

Down
1. MEDULLA
2. STEROID
3. PROLACTIN
4. OXYTOCIN
6. HYPERTHYROIDISM
8. HYPOTHALAMUS
12. NEUROHYPOPHYSIS
13. ENDOCRINE
14. CATECHOLAMINES
18. HOMEOSTASIS
21. ADRENAL

Fill in the blanks

1. The <u>endocrine</u> system is the collection of glands producing <u>hormones</u> that regulate <u>metabolism</u>, growth and <u>development</u>, tissue <u>function</u>, sexual function, <u>reproduction</u>, sleep and mood, and other things. The endocrine system is made up of the <u>pituitary</u> gland, thyroid gland, parathyroid glands, <u>adrenal</u> glands, pancreas, <u>ovaries</u> and testes.

2. The pituitary gland is connected to the <u>hypothalamus</u> by the <u>infundibulum</u>. The pituitary gland and the hypothalamus act as a unit, controlling most of the other <u>endocrine</u> glands. Within the pituitary there are two distinct areas: the <u>adenohypophysis</u>, composed of <u>glandular</u> epithelium, and the <u>neurohypophysis</u> made of a down-growth of <u>nervous</u> tissue from the brain.

3. The thyroid gland is located in the <u>neck</u>, anterior to the <u>larynx</u> and the trachea. This is a <u>butterfly</u>-shaped gland with two <u>lobes</u> on either side of the <u>thyroid</u> cartilage and the upper incomplete cartilaginous <u>rings</u> of the <u>trachea</u>. Lying in front of the trachea is the narrow <u>isthmus</u> joining the left and right lobes. The thyroid gland secretes several hormones, collectively called thyroid <u>hormones</u>. The main hormone is <u>thyroxine</u>, also called <u>T4</u>.

4. The <u>pancreas</u> has both <u>endocrine</u> and exocrine <u>functions</u>. The bulk of the pancreas is composed of <u>exocrine</u> cells producing enzymes to help with the <u>digestion</u> of food. These release their enzymes into a series of progressively larger <u>ducts</u> that eventually join together to form the <u>main</u> pancreatic duct, this runs the length of the pancreas and drains into the <u>duodenum</u>. The second functional component of the pancreas is the endocrine pancreas, composed of small <u>islands</u> of cells, the islets of <u>Langerhans</u>. Hormones, such as <u>insulin</u> and <u>glucagon</u>, are <u>released</u> into the bloodstream. These <u>hormones</u> help control glucose <u>levels</u>.

Multiple choice answers

1. (b), 2. (a), 3. (c), 4. (d), 5. (d), 6. (a), 7. (a), 8. (b), 9. (b), 10. (c)

Chapter 16

1.

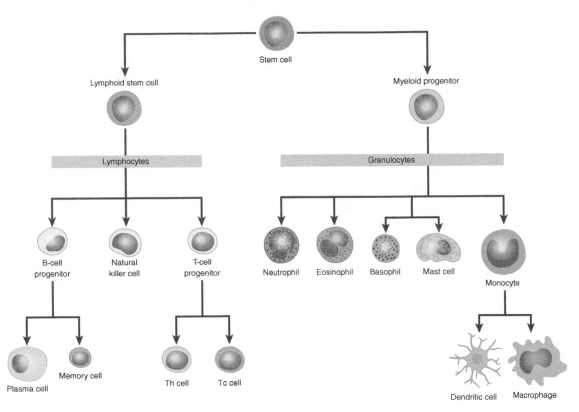

2.

Component of the immune system	Description
B-lymphocytes	Arise in the bone marrow and differentiate into plasma cells, which in turn produce immunoglobulins (antibodies)
Bone marrow	The site in the body where most of the cells of the immune system are produced as immature (stem) cells
Immunoglobulins	Also known as antibodies. Highly specialised protein molecules, they connect with and hold on to foreign antigens, so that they cannot escape destruction by cells of the immune system
Monocytes	White blood cells are also phagocytes. They have the ability to migrate into tissues, where they are known as macrophages
Plasma cells	These cells develop from B-lymphocytes, and produce the immunoglobulins
Polymorphonuclear leucocytes	White blood cells also known as phagocytes
Stem cells	Have the potential to differentiate and mature into the different cells of the immune system
Thymus	An organ instructing immature T-lymphocytes to become mature T-lymphocytes, which are then able to help fight infections
T-effector lymphocytes	Also called T-cytotoxic lymphocytes, have the ability to produce chemicals that can kill foreign cells and microorganisms, as well as helping in the process of inflammation
T helper lymphocytes	Whilst in the thymus they develop the ability to help other lymphocytes to mount an immune response
T-lymphocytes	T-lymphocytes arise in the bone marrow, migrate to the thymus where they mature, and learn to differentiate between 'self' and 'non-self' matter

3.

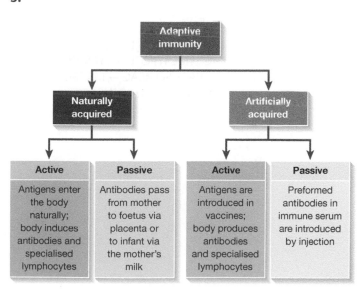

4.

Type of antibody	Functions
IgA	Found in breast milk, mucus, saliva and tears. Prevents antigens from crossing epithelial membranes and invading the deeper tissues
IgD	Produced by B cells and is displayed on their surface. Antigens bind to active B cells here
IgE	The least common antibody. Found bound to tissue cell membranes, particularly eosinophils
IgG	The most common and largest antibody. Attacks various pathogens, and crosses the placenta to protect the foetus
IgM	Produced in large quantities, is the primary response and a powerful activator of complement

5.

- Innate immunity is acquired at birth → the foetus acquires some immunity via the placenta, this is called passive immunity
- A central role of the innate immune responses is to prevent or restrict → the entrance of microorganisms into the body, so that tissue damage is limited
- Acquired immunity has the ability to remember when a particular immunological threat has → been met and overcome, known as immunological memory
- The primary response generates a slow and delayed rise in antibody levels → associated with activation of the T-lymphocyte system that stimulates B-lymphocyte separation
- The secondary response occurs on subsequent exposure to the same antigen → the response is much faster as the memory B-lymphocytes generated after the first infection divide and separate at a faster rate
- Passive immunity occurs when the person has been given antibodies → this is relatively short acting as the antibodies eventually break down

6.

VESPASI → PASSIVE

TABIESDINO → ANTIBODIES

TENAGIN → ANTIGEN

QUACREDI → ACQUIRED

TUMMYINI → IMMUNITY

CHYMESYPOTL → LYMPHOCYTES

GRAPHSOMEAC → MACROPHAGES

SYMHUT → THYMUS

7.

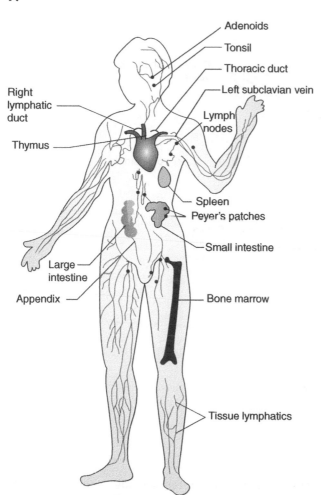

Adenoids

Tonsil

Thoracic duct

Left subclavian vein

Right lymphatic duct

Lymph nodes

Thymus

Spleen

Peyer's patches

Small intestine

Large intestine

Appendix

Bone marrow

Tissue lymphatics

8.

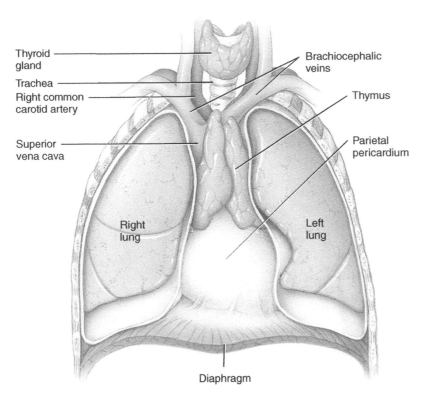

Thyroid gland

Trachea

Right common carotid artery

Superior vena cava

Brachiocephalic veins

Thymus

Parietal pericardium

Right lung

Left lung

Diaphragm

Thymus of adolescent

9.

- The key primary lymphoid organs of the immune system include → the thymus and bone marrow, they are involved in the production and early selection of lymphocytes
- The secondary lymphatic tissues include → spleen, tonsils, lymph vessels, lymph nodes, adenoids, skin and liver
- The thymus is largest and most active during the neonatal and pre-adolescent periods of development → by the early teens, the thymus begins to atrophy
- Bone marrow is the flexible tissue found in the interior of bones, the red bone marrow → is a key element of the lymphatic system, being one of the primary lymphoid organs that generates lymphocytes
- The lymphatic system is a part of the circulatory system, comprising a network of → conduits called lymphatic vessels that carry a clear fluid, called lymph, towards the heart

10.

SLEEPN → SPLEEN
RAWMOR → MARROW
PLYMH → LYMPH
REYSEP → PEYERS

HLYOPMID → LYMPHOID
ORAPHYT → ATROPHY
DIEDANSO → ADENOIDS
NOSLITS → TONSILS

11.

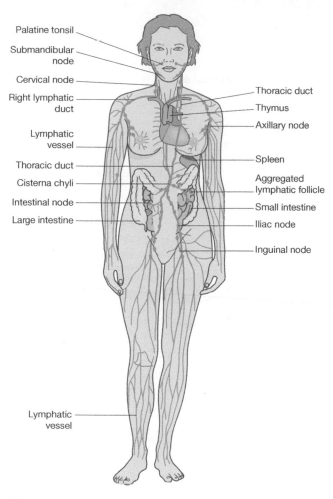

Palatine tonsil
Submandibular node
Cervical node
Right lymphatic duct
Lymphatic vessel
Thoracic duct
Cisterna chyli
Intestinal node
Large intestine
Lymphatic vessel

Thoracic duct
Thymus
Axillary node
Spleen
Aggregated lymphatic follicle
Small intestine
Iliac node
Inguinal node

12.

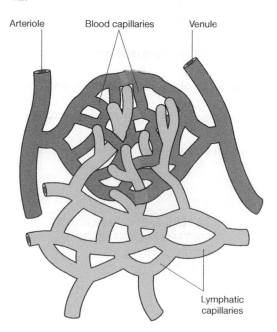

Arteriole
Blood capillaries
Venule
Lymphatic capillaries

13.

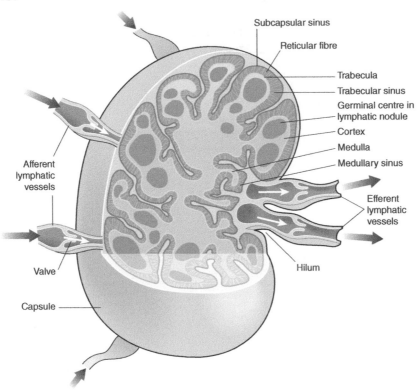

Subcapsular sinus
Reticular fibre
Trabecula
Trabecular sinus
Germinal centre in lymphatic nodule
Cortex
Medulla
Medullary sinus
Afferent lymphatic vessels
Efferent lymphatic vessels
Valve
Hilum
Capsule

14.

- The lymphatic system is a specialised system → of lymph vessels and lymph nodes
- The lymphatic vessels are drainage vessels that → collect the excess interstitial fluid and return it to the bloodstream
- The lymphatic system can be thought of as a parallel system to the blood circulatory system → but it does not have a pump like the heart
- The lymph vessels and capillaries form a network throughout the body → and connect the tissues of the body to the lymphoid organs
- Lymphatic capillaries have some anatomical similarities to blood capillaries → in that their walls consist of a layer of endothelial cells
- The lymph eventually flows into two large lymph ducts, → the right lymphatic duct and the thoracic duct

15.

TUCD → DUCT
LILIESCRAPA → CAPILLARIES
BALACUTREE → TRABECULAE
SOFILLECL → FOLLICLES

TICYCOGAHP → PHAGOCYTIC
FRETEEFN → EFFERENT
RIFTEL → FILTER
SLANGD → GLANDS

16.

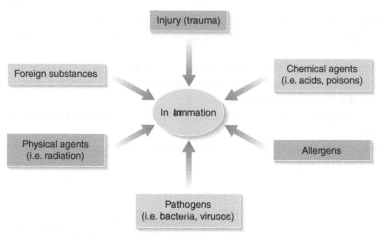

17.

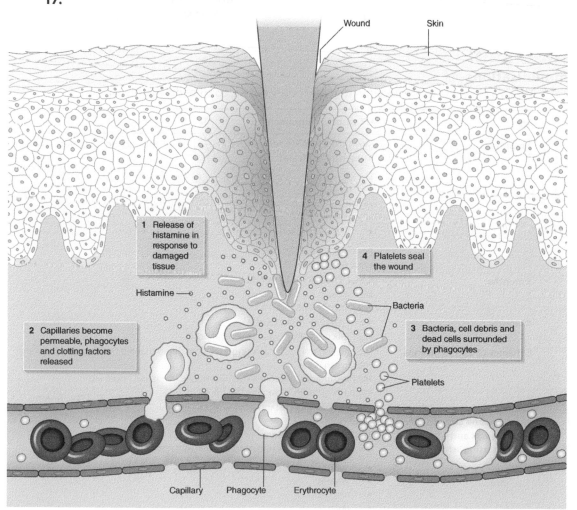

18.

- Inflammation is → the body's immediate reaction to tissue injury or damage
- The inflammatory process involves the movement of → white cells, complement and other plasma proteins
- Following injury or other damage to the body → three processes occur at the same time
- The complement system activates and assists the inflammatory and immune processes → playing a major role in the destruction of bacteria
- The kinin system helps to control vascular permeability → and immunoglobulins help in the destruction of bacteria
- Other factors involved in vascular permeability → are cytokines which promote inflammation, attracting white blood cells to the affected area

19.

SINKIN → KININS

SINKTOECY → CYTOKINES

LACRO → CALOR

PELEMMCONT → COMPLEMENT

THINEISAM → HISTAMINE

LARGENATIONDU → DEGRANULATION

STAM → MAST

POETSHANG → PATHOGENS

Snap shot
Immunisations

This is a checklist of the vaccines that are routinely offered to people in the UK.

Age	UK vaccine programme
2 months	5-in-1 (DTaP/IPV/Hib) vaccine this single jab contains vaccines to protect against five separate diseases:
	• diphtheria
	• tetanus
	• pertussis
	• polio
	• *Haemophilus influenzae* type b
	Pneumococcal (PCV) vaccine
	Rotavirus vaccine
3 months	5-in-1 (DTaP/IPV/Hib) second dose
	Meningitis C
	Rotavirus vaccine second dose
4 months	5-in-1 (DTaP/IPV/Hib) third dose
	Pneumococcal (PCV) vaccine second dose
Between 12 and 13 months	Hib/meningitis C given as a single jab containing meningitis C (second dose) and Hib (fourth dose)
	Measles, mumps and rubella (MMR) vaccine given as a single jab
	Pneumococcal (PCV) vaccine third dose
2, 3 and 4 years plus school years one and two	Children's flu vaccine (annually)
From 3 years and 4 months (up to starting school)	MMR vaccine second dose
	4-in-1 (DTaP/IPV) pre-school booster, given as a single jab containing vaccines against:
	• diphtheria
	• tetanus
	• pertussis
	• polio

Age	UK vaccine programme
Around 12–13 years (girls only)	Human papillomavirus which protects against cervical cancer – two injections given between 6 months and 2 years apart
Around 13–18 years	3-in-1 (Td/IPV) teenage booster given as a single jab and contains vaccines against: • diphtheria • tetanus • polio
Around 13–15 years	Meningitis C booster
18–25 years	Meningitis C vaccine for students
65 and over	Flu (every year) Pneumococcal (PPV) vaccine
70 years (and 78 and 79 year-olds as a catch-up)	Shingles vaccine

Vaccines for special groups

There are some vaccines that are not available routinely to everyone on the NHS, but they are available for those who fall into certain risk groups, for example, pregnant women, people with long-term health conditions and healthcare workers. These include:
• hepatitis B vaccination
• TB vaccination
• chickenpox vaccination

Travel vaccines

There are some travel vaccines that are available free on the NHS. These include:
• hepatitis A vaccine
• typhoid vaccine
• cholera vaccine

Other travel vaccines, such as yellow fever vaccination are only available privately.

527

Word search

O	W	S	Q	U	K	L	U	F	M	A	R	T	L	A	I	O	X	N	J
N	I	G	E	D	L	M	P	A	S	S	I	V	E	V	I	T	C	A	E
L	M	E	V	T	R	H	W	V	H	B	L	A	P	S	F	A	G	B	L
W	M	G	Z	U	Y	G	Y	T	I	N	U	M	M	I	B	E	G	M	G
Z	U	A	C	J	Y	C	O	Z	H	X	Z	U	S	O	S	H	R	Q	I
O	N	H	Y	Z	A	U	O	Z	O	T	U	F	H	N	Z	J	T	V	S
Z	O	P	T	F	N	Y	P	G	K	S	C	T	I	K	S	A	H	I	P
W	L	O	O	B	T	U	R	I	A	A	P	L	U	C	E	M	Y	I	L
R	O	R	T	G	I	R	O	J	S	H	U	K	S	E	T	E	M	J	E
S	G	C	O	J	G	M	S	U	C	B	P	R	A	S	Y	D	U	H	E
E	Y	A	X	E	E	Y	T	S	O	D	W	J	G	D	C	E	S	G	N
I	X	M	I	A	N	B	A	L	F	P	G	A	T	V	O	O	I	V	X
D	L	T	C	Q	S	E	G	O	J	A	Y	C	J	W	N	L	V	F	J
O	L	J	P	Z	V	O	L	N	K	Q	R	C	P	I	O	Y	K	O	K
B	R	Z	O	F	N	C	A	I	S	B	E	D	P	U	M	G	N	M	R
I	J	Z	H	U	S	D	N	X	N	S	E	N	I	K	O	T	Y	C	O
T	N	C	M	Y	L	I	D	P	C	E	Z	H	P	M	Y	L	Z	E	N
N	U	M	Z	X	N	Q	I	P	C	F	T	Y	E	N	J	T	G	U	O
A	I	H	Y	S	S	A	N	M	V	A	L	C	Q	L	P	B	L	S	D
O	N	Z	W	B	D	M	S	L	T	I	W	S	S	N	X	G	S	I	E

Crossword

Across

3. ANTIGEN
6. MULTIPOTENT
7. LYMPH
9. GRANULOCYTES
10. LYMPHOCYTE
11. THYMUS
12. CYTOTOXIC
14. NEUTROPHILS
15. PROSTAGLANDINS
16. FIVE
18. EOSINOPHILS
19. ACQUIRED
20. PASSIVE

Down

1. MONOCYTES
2. TEARS
4. IMMUNOLOGY
5. IMMUNOGLOBULINS
8. PHAGOCYTOSIS
13. PLATELETS
17. SPLEEN

Fill in the blanks

1. The immune <u>system</u> is a network of <u>cells</u>, tissues and organs working together to <u>protect</u> the body from <u>infection</u>. The body provides an ideal <u>environment</u> for many microbes, such as <u>viruses</u>, bacteria, <u>fungi</u> and <u>parasites</u>, and the <u>immune</u> system prevents and <u>limits</u> their <u>entry</u> and growth to maintain optimal <u>health</u>.

2. Lymph <u>nodes</u> are small bean-shaped structures that <u>produce</u> and store cells that <u>fight</u> infection and <u>disease</u>, and are part of the <u>lymphatic</u> system. <u>Lymph</u> is a clear fluid that carries those cells of the immune system to different parts of the <u>body</u>. When the body is fighting <u>infection</u>, lymph nodes can become <u>enlarged</u>.

3. The <u>thymus</u> is a small organ and is where <u>T-cells</u> mature. It is situated in the <u>chest</u> beneath the <u>breastbone</u>. It can <u>trigger</u> or maintain the production of <u>antibodies</u>. The <u>thymus</u> is somewhat large in <u>infants</u>, grows until <u>puberty</u>, then starts to slowly <u>shrink</u> and become replaced by <u>fat</u> with age.

Multiple choice answers

1. (b), 2. (d), 3. (a), 4. (d), 5. (b), 6. (c), 7. (c), 8. (b), 9. (c), 10. (b)

Chapter 17

1.

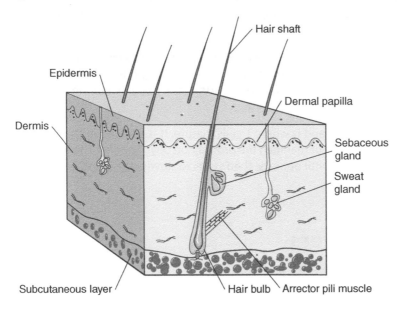

Hair shaft

Epidermis

Dermal papilla

Dermis

Sebaceous gland

Sweat gland

Subcutaneous layer

Hair bulb

Arrector pili muscle

2.

- The skin is sometimes referred to as this → the integummary system
- The thinnest part of the skin is → the epidermis
- The skin is composed of two distinct regions → the dermis and epidermis
- The skin is twice as heavy as → the brain
- The appendages are → manifestations of the skin
- The skin receives → nearly one third of all blood that flows through the body

3.

DRMIES → DERMIS
ENCOUTASSUBU → SUBCUTANEOUS
SNLAGD → GLANDS
OSCUMU → MUCOUS

SPIDEREMI → EPIDERMIS
PAILLEAP → PAPILLAE
SIREGD → RIDGES
ROPE → PORE

4.

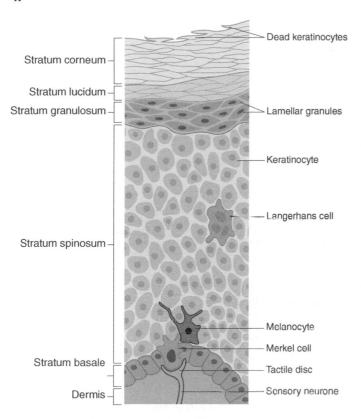

Stratum corneum — Dead keratinocytes

Stratum lucidum —

Stratum granulosum — Lamellar granules

Keratinocyte

Langerhans cell

Stratum spinosum —

Melanocyte

Merkel cell

Stratum basale — Tactile disc

Dermis — Sensory neurone

5.

- Also known as a tactile cell → Merkel cell
- The most numerous cell in the skin → keratinocytes
- Associated with immunity → Langerhans cells
- Located in the stratum basale → melanocyte

6.

YALEMCOTEN → MELANOCYTE
MUSTTAR → STRATUM
LITECAT → TACTILE
TUMMYINI → IMMUNITY

SHALENRANG → LANGERHANS
SLLEC → CELLS
NIPSMUSO → SPINOSUM
RAYELS → LAYERS

7.

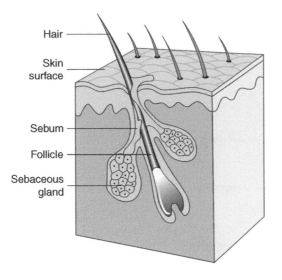

Hair

Skin surface

Sebum

Follicle

Sebaceous gland

8.

- Found on most surfaces of the body → hair
- Accompanies hair follicles → sebaceous gland
- Hair follicles are found here → skin surface
- A liquid substance exuded by the sebaceous glands → sebum
- Most of the skin has these → follicles

9.

BEMUS → SEBUM
CLIFSOLLE → FOLLICLES
CABSESEOU → SEBACEOUS
RAIH → HAIR

LAIN → NAIL
CRETORRA → ARRECTOR
BLUB → BULB
TWEAS → SWEAT

10.

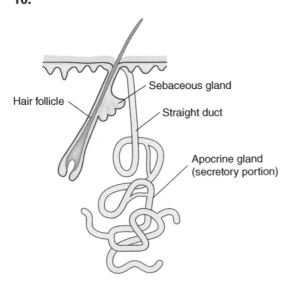

Sebaceous gland

Straight duct

Hair follicle

Apocrine gland (secretory portion)

11.

- Supplies lubrication to the skin → sebaceous gland
- Coiled glands, more prominent in localised sites such as pubic axillae → apocrine gland (secretory portion)
- Every pore is an opening for one of these → hair follicle

12.

CUBIP → PUBIC

EXALLIA → AXILLAE

OTRO → ROOT

SEXUPL → PLEXUS

SULVEL → VELLUS

TARKEIN → KERATIN

GAMPTENTINOI → PIGMENTATION

FATSH → SHAFT

13.

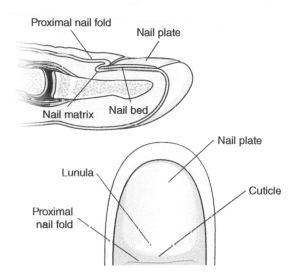

14.

- White crescent located at the proximal end of the nail → lunula
- Mainly composed of keratin → nail plate
- The formative layer of cells at the base of the fingernail or toenail → nail matrix
- Also called the eponychium → cuticle
- Tightly packed, dead, hard, keratinised epidermal cells that form a clean, solid covering over the digits → nails

15.

NULALU → LUNULA

ELICTUC → CUTICLE

TAXMIR → MATRIX

LAHAPXN → PHALANX

TASSNONEI → SENSATION

COMYPHUNHIY → HYPONYCHIUM

LAIDST → DISTAL

MIXORLAP → PROXIMAL

16.

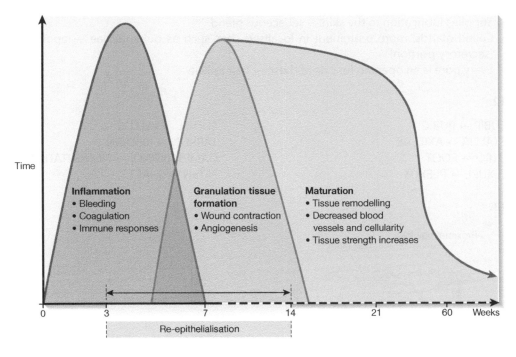

Time

Inflammation
• Bleeding
• Coagulation
• Immune responses

Granulation tissue formation
• Wound contraction
• Angiogenesis

Maturation
• Tissue remodelling
• Decreased blood vessels and cellularity
• Tissue strength increases

0   3   7   14   21   60   Weeks

Re-epithelialisation

17.

Natural skin colour		UV sensitivity and tendency to burn
1	Very fair, pale white, often freckled	**Highly sensitive** Always burns, never tans
2	Fair, white skin	**Very sensitive** Burns easily, tans minimally
3	Light brown	**Sensitive** Burns moderately, usually tans
4	Moderate brown	**Less sensitive** Burns minimally tans well
5	Dark brown	**Minimally sensitive** Rarely burns
6	Deeply pigmented, dark brown to black	**Minimal sensitivity** Never burns

Snap shot
Capillary nail bed refill (also called the nail blanch test)

1. To help determine tissue perfusion.
2. Gentle pressure is applied to the nail bed until it turns white, indicating that the blood has been forced from the tissue (blanching). Once the tissue has blanched, pressure is removed. While the patient holds their hand above their heart, the nurse measures the time it takes for blood to return to the tissue. The nail turning back to a pink colour indicates return of blood.
3. If there is a good blood flow to the nail bed, a pink colour should return in less than 2 seconds after pressure is removed.
4. Nail polish and acrylic nails should be removed prior to performing the test.
5. Any abnormalities must be reported to the person in charge.
6. The outcome of the test should be documented in the patient's notes.

Word search

G	L	Q	E	Z	T	O	X	M	E	P	I	D	E	R	M	I	S	E	N
K	U	G	K	N	V	A	C	F	T	M	U	B	E	S	K	E	W	W	A
F	N	Y	S	M	A	Q	S	U	O	E	C	A	B	E	S	N	J	S	T
Q	U	D	P	B	U	R	Q	A	P	M	Y	G	I	X	I	R	T	A	M
J	L	O	M	O	Y	I	B	D	J	B	C	L	N	Y	O	D	O	D	B
V	A	V	U	B	S	X	H	M	W	Z	A	B	R	P	J	F	J	L	U
T	C	E	B	L	M	H	I	C	E	X	R	A	G	R	L	S	A	R	U
N	M	N	E	S	V	X	P	Q	Y	M	T	K	R	U	B	N	L	E	M
R	Z	I	S	R	N	R	I	S	P	N	H	Y	U	W	G	I	V	F	G
I	B	R	O	M	D	S	G	K	E	N	O	A	T	E	Y	X	K	V	P
A	L	C	O	X	F	E	I	M	E	H	G	P	R	I	Q	F	P	M	E
H	J	O	G	A	G	L	U	L	Y	D	O	H	E	X	N	L	F	M	R
W	E	P	M	A	A	G	E	P	S	V	A	U	G	F	V	U	S	L	F
F	Q	A	C	W	E	K	O	K	M	N	E	N	R	J	V	Y	M	Z	U
K	J	N	C	T	R	D	I	Q	S	F	M	U	T	A	R	T	S	M	S
F	Y	A	N	E	E	N	R	H	M	A	G	P	E	I	C	J	T	C	I
I	Y	I	M	R	Y	U	I	W	S	O	A	C	V	W	F	L	E	U	O
B	I	L	M	S	E	T	Y	C	O	N	I	T	A	R	E	K	W	R	N
D	I	I	D	N	S	M	P	B	A	R	R	E	C	T	O	R	Y	V	I
L	S	E	T	Y	C	O	N	A	L	E	M	M	W	V	W	T	O	V	K

Crossword

Across
3. KERATIN
7. PUBERTY
11. MELANOCYTES
13. LANUGO
14. SEBUM
16. PHEROMONE
18. DERMIS

Down
1. COILED
2. LANGERHANS
4. KERATINOCYTES
5. APPENDAGES
6. HYPODERMIS
8. TACTILE
9. TWO
10. LAYER
12. EPIDERMIS
15. LUNULA
17. SEX

Fill in the blanks

1. The skin carries out a number of <u>vital</u> functions, including <u>protecting</u> the person against <u>external</u> physical, <u>chemical</u> and biological attack. It also prevents the <u>loss</u> of excess <u>water</u> from the body and plays a central role in <u>thermoregulation</u>.

2. The skin is one of the more versatile <u>organs</u> of the body. The skin is composed of distinct <u>regions</u> – the <u>dermis</u> and the epidermis. The <u>subcutaneous</u> fascia (sometimes referred to as the <u>hypodermis</u>) lies <u>under</u> the dermis. This layer of loose <u>connective</u> and <u>adipose</u> tissue has an important <u>insulating</u> role.

Multiple choice answers

1. (b), 2. (b), 3. (c), 4. (c), 5. (b), 6. (c), 7. (a), 8. (d), 9. (a), 10. (c)

The values given below are representative of the average reference range for adults in:

- blood
- cerebrospinal fluid
- urine.

The ranges shown should only be used as a guide. Reference ranges between laboratories will vary; there are many reasons for this, such as the type of analytical equipment used and the temperature, and you should always consult the ranges given by your own laboratory.

Fundamentals of Anatomy and Physiology Workbook: A Study Guide for Nursing and Healthcare Students, First Edition. Ian Peate.
© 2017 John Wiley & Sons Ltd. Published 2017 by John Wiley & Sons Ltd.

Blood (haematology)

Test	Reference range
Activated partial thromboplastin (APTT)	30–40 s
Erythrocyte sedimentation rate (ESR)	
Women	3–15 mm/h
Men	1–10 mm/h
Fibrinogen	1.5–4.0 g/L
Folate (serum)	4–18 μg/L
Haemoglobin (Hb)	
Women	11.5–16.5 g/dL
Men	13–18 g/dL
Hepatoglobins	0.3–2.0 g/L
Mean cell haemoglobin (MCH)	27–32 pg
Mean cell haemoglobin concentrate (MCHC)	30–35 g/dL
Mean cell volume (MCV)	78–95 fL
Packed cell volume (PCV or haematocrit)	
Women	0.35–0.47 (35–47%)
Men	0.4–0.54 (40–54%)
Plateletes (thrombocytes)	$150–400 \times 10^9$/L
Prothrombin time	12–16 s
Red cells (erythrocytes)	
Women	$3.8–5.3 \times 10^{12}$/L
Men	$4.5–6.5 \times 10^{12}$/L
Reticulocytes	$25–85 \times 10^9$/L
White cells total (leucocytes)	$4.0–11.0 \times 10^9$/L

Blood venous (unless stated) plasma (biochemistry)

Test	Reference range
Alanine aminotransferase (ALT)	10–40 U/L
Albumin	36–47 g/L
Alkaline phosphate	40–125 U/L
Amylase	90–300 U/L
Aspartate aminotranferase (AST)	10–35 U/L
Bicarbonate (arterial)	22–28 mmol/L
Bilirubin (total)	2–17 µmol/L
Calcium	2.1–2.6 mmol/L
Chloride	95–105 mmol/L
Cholesterol (total)	<5.2 mmol/L
HDL Cholesterol	
Women	0.6–1.9 mmol/L
Men	0.5–1.6 mmol/L
$PaCO_2$ (arterial)	4.1–6.1 kPa
Copper	13–24 µmol/L
Cortisol (at 0800 hours)	160–565 nmol/L
Creatine kinase (total)	
Women	30–150 U/L
Men	30–200 U/L
Creatinine	50 150 µmol/L
Gamma-Glutamyl-transferase (GY)	
Women	5–35 U/L
Men	10–55 U/L
Globulins	24–37 g/L
Glucose (venous blood fasting)	3.6–5.8 mmol/L
Glycosylated haemoglobin (HbA_1)	4–6%
Hydrogen ion concentration (arterial)	35–44 nmol/L

Test	Reference range
Iron	
Men	10–28 µmol/L
Women	14–32 µmol/L
Iron binding capacity, total (TIBC)	45–70 µmol/L
Lactate (arterial)	0.3–1.4 mmol/L
Lactate dehydrogenase (total)	230–460 U/L
Lead (whole blood)	<1.7 µmol/L
Magnesium	0.7–1.0 mmol/L
Osmolality	275–290 mmol/kg
PaO_2 (arterial)	12–15 kPa
Oxygen saturation (arterial)	>97%
pH	7.36–7.42
Phosphate (fasting)	0.8–1.4 mmol/L
Potassium (serum)	3.6–5.0 mmol/L
Protein (total)	60–80 g/L
Sodium	136–145 mmol/L
Transferrin	2–4 g/L
Triglycerides (fasting)	0.6–1.8 mmol/L
Urate	
Women	0.12–0.36 mmol/L
Men	0.12–0.42 mmol/L
Urea	2.5–6.5 mmol/L
Uric acid	
Women	0.09–0.36 mmol/L
Men	0.1–0.45 mmol/L
Vitamin A	0.7–3.5 µmol/L
Vitamin C	23–57 µmol/L
Zinc	11–22 µmol/L

Cerebrospinal fluid

Test	Reference range
Cells	0–5 mm^3
Chloride	120–170 mmol/L
Glucose	2.5–4.0 mmol/L
Pressure	50–180 mmH$_2$O
Protein	100–400 mg/L

Urine

Test	Reference range
Albumin/creatinine ration	<3.5 mg albumin/mmol creatinine
Calcium (diet dependent)	<12 mmol/24 h (normal diet)
Copper	0.26–0.6 µmol/24 h
Cortisol	9–50 µmol/24 h
Creatinine	9–17 mmol/24 h
5-Hydroxyindole-3-acetic acid (5H1AA)	10–45 µmol/24 h
Magnesium	3.3–5.0 mmol/24 h
Oxalate	
Women	40–320 mmol/24 h
Men	80–490 mmol/24 h
pH	4–8
Phosphate	15–50 mmol/24 h
Porphyrins (total)	90–370 mmol/24 h
Potassium*	25–100 mmol/24 h
Protein (total)	no more than 0.3 g/L
Sodium*	100–200 mmol/24 h
Urea	170–500 mmol/24 h
(*depends on intake)	

This workbook is a companion to

Fundamentals of Anatomy and Physiology

For Nursing and Healthcare Students, Second Edition

Edited by Ian Peate and Muralitharan Nair
9781119055525 | May 2016 | 656 pages

Fundamentals of Anatomy and Physiology: For Nursing and Healthcare Students is a succinct but complete overview of the structure and function of the human body, with clinical applications throughout. Designed specifically for nursing and healthcare students, the new edition of this best-selling textbook provides a user-friendly, straightforward, jargon-free introduction to the subject.

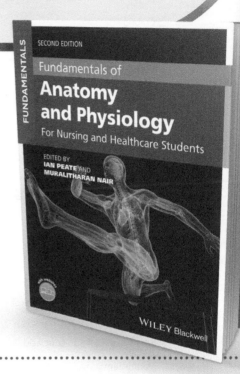

Key features:

- Clinical considerations and scenarios throughout showing how the material can be applied to daily practice

- Featuring over 300 superb full colour illustrations

- Now includes a boxed feature throughout on medicines management organized by body system, which provides information on a variety of medicines used in the care and management of patients

- The 'Conditions' feature within each chapter provides you with a list of disorders that are associated with the topics discussed, helping relate theory to practice

- Each chapter includes learning outcomes, test your knowledge, activities and summaries

- Includes a list of prefixes and suffixes, as well as normal values, and a glossary of terms

- Supported by enhanced online resources with fantastic extras for both lecturers and students, including an image bank, online glossary, flashcards, interactive multiple choice questions, interactive true or false questions, and more

Printed and bound by CPI Group (UK) Ltd, Croydon, CR0 4YY

16/09/2024

14557225-0001